Recent Advances in Psychopathology in Neurodevelopmental Disorders: From Bench to Bedside

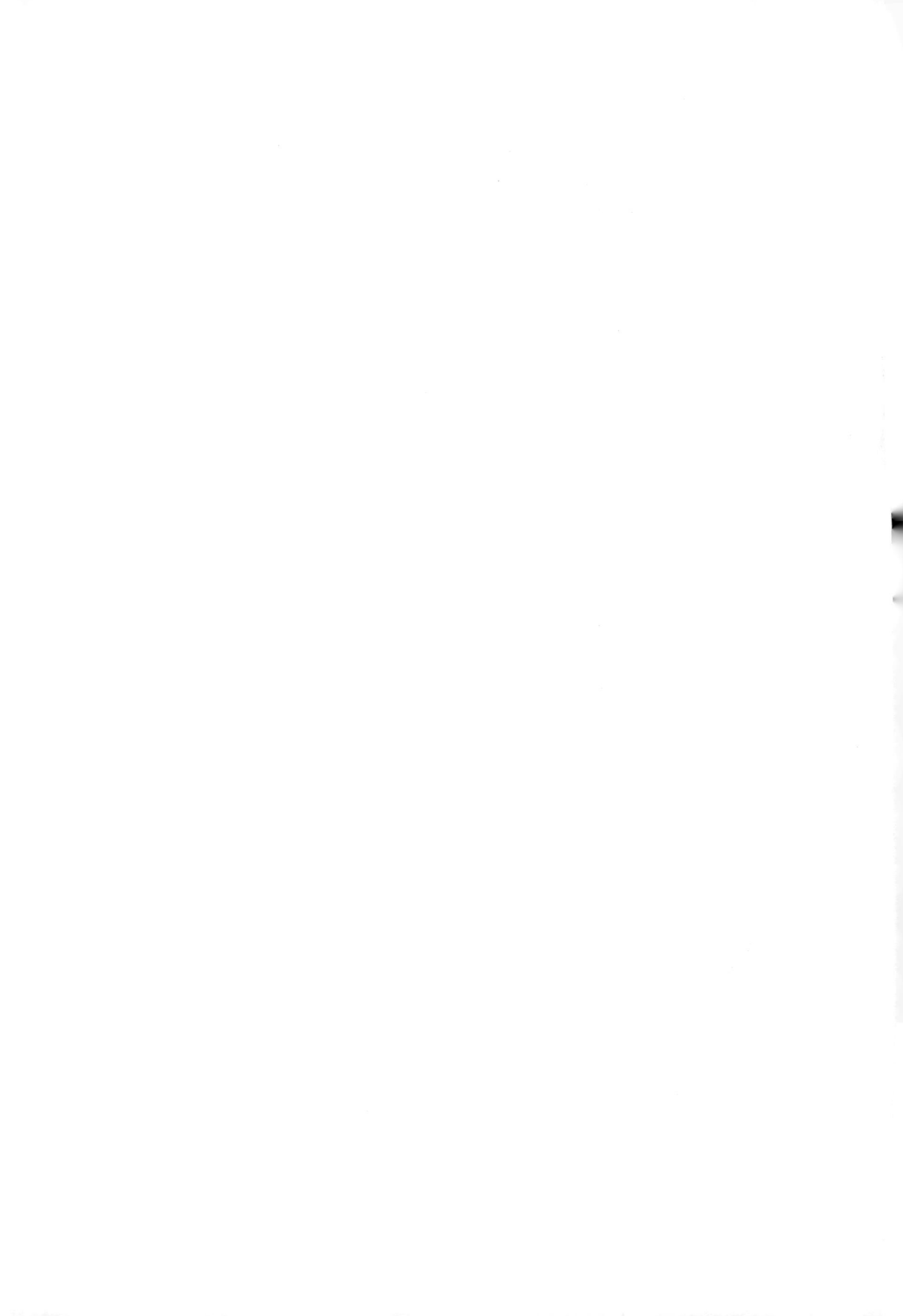

Recent Advances in Psychopathology in Neurodevelopmental Disorders: From Bench to Bedside

Editor

Shoumitro Deb

MDPI • Basel • Beijing • Wuhan • Barcelona • Belgrade • Manchester • Tokyo • Cluj • Tianjin

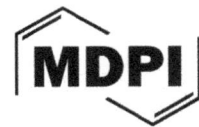

Editor
Shoumitro Deb
Imperial College London
UK

Editorial Office
MDPI
St. Alban-Anlage 66
4052 Basel, Switzerland

This is a reprint of articles from the Special Issue published online in the open access journal *International Journal of Environmental Research and Public Health* (ISSN 1660-4601) (available at: https://www.mdpi.com/journal/ijerph/special_issues/RAiPiNDFBtB).

For citation purposes, cite each article independently as indicated on the article page online and as indicated below:

LastName, A.A.; LastName, B.B.; LastName, C.C. Article Title. *Journal Name* **Year**, *Volume Number*, Page Range.

ISBN 978-3-0365-7414-1 (Hbk)
ISBN 978-3-0365-7415-8 (PDF)

© 2023 by the authors. Articles in this book are Open Access and distributed under the Creative Commons Attribution (CC BY) license, which allows users to download, copy and build upon published articles, as long as the author and publisher are properly credited, which ensures maximum dissemination and a wider impact of our publications.
The book as a whole is distributed by MDPI under the terms and conditions of the Creative Commons license CC BY-NC-ND.

Contents

About the Editor vii

Freya Tyrer, Richard Morriss, Reza Kiani, Satheesh K. Gangadharan, Harish Kundaje and Mark J. Rutherford
Health Needs and Their Relationship with Life Expectancy in People with and without Intellectual Disabilities in England
Reprinted from: *Int. J. Environ. Res. Public Health* **2022**, 19, 6602, doi:10.3390/ijerph19116602 . . . 1

Alister Baird, Bridget Candy, Eirini Flouri, Nick Tyler and Angela Hassiotis
The Association between Physical Environment and Externalising Problems in Typically Developing and Neurodiverse Children and Young People: A Narrative Review
Reprinted from: *Int. J. Environ. Res. Public Health* **2023**, 20, 2549, doi:10.3390/ijerph20032549 . . . 13

Tanja Sappok, Angela Hassiotis, Marco Bertelli, Isabel Dziobek and Paula Sterkenburg
Developmental Delays in Socio-Emotional Brain Functions in Persons with an Intellectual Disability: Impact on Treatment and Support
Reprinted from: *Int. J. Environ. Res. Public Health* **2022**, 19, 13109, doi:10.3390/ijerph192013109 . 49

Paula S. Sterkenburg, Marie Ilic, Miriam Flachsmeyer and Tanja Sappok
More than a Physical Problem: The Effects of Physical and Sensory Impairments on the Emotional Development of Adults with Intellectual Disabilities
Reprinted from: *Int. J. Environ. Res. Public Health* **2022**, 19, 17080, doi:10.3390/ijerph192417080 . 63

Johanna Eisinger, Magdalena Dall, Jason Fogler, Daniel Holzinger and Johannes Fellinger
Intellectual Disability Profiles, Quality of Life and Maladaptive Behavior in Deaf Adults: An Exploratory Study
Reprinted from: *Int. J. Environ. Res. Public Health* **2022**, 19, 9919, doi:10.3390/ijerph19169919 . . . 73

Gerda de Kuijper, Joke de Haan, Shoumitro Deb and Rohit Shankar
Withdrawing Antipsychotics for Challenging Behaviours in Adults with Intellectual Disabilities: Experiences and Views of Prescribers
Reprinted from: *Int. J. Environ. Res. Public Health* **2022**, 19, 17095, doi:10.3390/ijerph192417095 . 85

Gerda de Kuijper, Joke de Haan, Shoumitro Deb and Rohit Shankar
Withdrawing Antipsychotics for Challenging Behaviours in Adults with Intellectual Disabilities: Experiences and Views of Experts by Experience
Reprinted from: *Int. J. Environ. Res. Public Health* **2022**, 19, 15637, doi:10.3390/ijerph192315637 . 97

Shoumitro (Shoumi) Deb, Bharati Limbu, Gemma L. Unwin and Tim Weaver
Causes of and Alternatives to Medication for Behaviours That Challenge in People with Intellectual Disabilities: Direct Care Providers' Perspectives
Reprinted from: *Int. J. Environ. Res. Public Health* **2022**, 19, 9988, doi:10.3390/ijerph19169988 . . . 107

Matthew Sanders, Nam-Phuong T. Hoang, Julie Hodges, Kate Sofronoff, Stewart Einfeld, Bruce Tonge, Kylie Gray, et al.
Predictors of Change in Stepping Stones Triple Interventions: The Relationship between Parental Adjustment, Parenting Behaviors and Child Outcomes
Reprinted from: *Int. J. Environ. Res. Public Health* **2022**, 19, 13200, doi:10.3390/ijerph192013200 . 121

Emili Rodríguez-Hidalgo, Javier García-Alba, Ramon Novell and Susanna Esteba-Castillo
The Global Deterioration Scale for Down Syndrome Population (GDS-DS): A Rating Scale to Assess the Progression of Alzheimer's Disease
Reprinted from: *Int. J. Environ. Res. Public Health* **2023**, 20, 5096, doi:10.3390/ijerph20065096 . . . 133

Emili Rodríguez-Hidalgo, Javier García-Alba, Maria Buxó, Ramon Novell and Susana Esteba-Castillo
The Pictorial Screening Memory Test (P-MIS) for Adults with Moderate Intellectual Disability and Alzheimer's Disease
Reprinted from: *Int. J. Environ. Res. Public Health* **2022**, *19*, 10780, doi:10.3390/ijerph191710780 . **153**

About the Editor

Shoumitro Deb

Professor Shoumitro (Shoumi) Deb, MBBS, FRCPsych, MD, is a Visiting Professor of Neuropsychiatry at the Imperial College London, UK. Previously he was a full-time substantive Clinical Professor at the University of Birmingham and a Senior Lecturer in Psychiatry at Cardiff University. His seminal works include (a) being a member of the group that developed the first-ever evidence-based practice guidelines for intellectual disabilities (ID) in the UK NHS; (b) the first-ever comprehensive assessment of psychopathology in adults with ID and epilepsy; (c) a dementia screening questionnaire for adults with ID (DSQIID), which has been translated into more than 24 languages and validated; (d) the first-ever freely available online-accessible (easy-read) psychotropic medication information leaflets (http://www.ld-medication.bham.ac.uk); (e) the first-ever European Guideline (and recently updated in the *European Journal of Psychiatry*, 2022, 36, 11–25) on the assessment and diagnosis of psychiatric disorders in adults with ID; (f) national and international guidelines on the use of psychotropic medication in adults with ID (*World Psychiatry*, 2009, 8(3), 181–186); (g) the first-ever online training SPECTROM for caregivers to help reduce the overmedication of people with ID (https://spectrom.wixsite.com/project); (h) the first-ever comprehensive neuropsychiatric outcome study in adults with traumatic brain injury (TBI); (i) patient- and carer-determined outcome measures for patients with TBI; and (j) the only published RCT (feasibility) on risperidone versus placebo to treat aggression in adults with TBI. He has over 330 publications and has made over 250 presentations at national and international conferences (including many keynote speeches). He has also ran several MSc programmes in three UK Universities. Additionally, he was (a) a member of the first UK NICE GDG on epilepsy and other NICE guidelines, (b) a Fellow of the UK NIHR, (c) vice-chair of the World Psychiatric Association SPID, and (d) a member of the WHO Working Group on ICD-11.

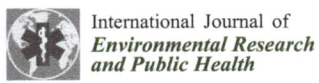

Article

Health Needs and Their Relationship with Life Expectancy in People with and without Intellectual Disabilities in England

Freya Tyrer [1,*], Richard Morriss [2], Reza Kiani [3,4], Satheesh K. Gangadharan [3,4], Harish Kundaje [5] and Mark J. Rutherford [1]

1. Biostatistics Research Group, Department of Health Sciences, University of Leicester, Leicester LE1 7RH, UK; mjr40@le.ac.uk
2. Institute of Mental Health, University of Nottingham, Nottingham NG7 2TU, UK; richard.morriss@nottingham.ac.uk
3. Leicestershire Learning Disability Services (Psychiatry), Leicestershire Partnership NHS Trust, Leicester LE4 8PQ, UK; reza.kiani@nhs.net (R.K.); s.gangadharan1@nhs.net (S.K.G.)
4. Mental Health, Ageing, Public Health and Primary Care Research Group, Department of Health Sciences, University of Leicester, Leicester LE1 7RH, UK
5. Lakeside Healthcare, Cottingham Road, Corby NN17 2UR, UK; harish.kundaje@nhs.net
* Correspondence: fct2@le.ac.uk

Abstract: Health needs are common in people living with intellectual disabilities, but we do not know how they contribute to life expectancy. We used the Clinical Practice Research Datalink (CPRD) linked with hospital/mortality data in England (2017–2019) to explore life expectancy among people with or without intellectual disabilities, indicated by the presence or absence, respectively, of: epilepsy; incontinence; severe visual loss; severe visual impairment; severe mobility difficulties; cerebral palsy and PEG feeding. Life expectancy and 95% confidence intervals were compared using flexible parametric methods. At baseline, 46.4% (total n = 7794) of individuals with intellectual disabilities compared with 9.7% (total n = 176,807) in the comparison group had ≥1 health need. Epilepsy was the most common health need (18.7% vs. 1.1%). All health needs except hearing impairment were associated with shorter life expectancy: PEG feeding and mobility difficulties were associated with the greatest loss in life years (65–68% and 41–44%, respectively). Differential life expectancy attenuated but remained (≈12% life years lost) even after restricting the population to those without health needs (additional years expected to live at 10 years: 65.5 [60.3, 71.1] vs. 74.3 [73.8, 74.7]). We conclude that health needs play a significant role but do not explain all of the differential life expectancy experienced by people with intellectual disabilities.

Keywords: intellectual disability; life expectancy; health needs; epilepsy; incontinence; visual; hearing; mobility; cerebral palsy; PEG feeding

1. Introduction

Addressing the burden of health inequalities is now a global priority [1–3]. Strategies to reduce these inequalities tend to focus on the most vulnerable, such as people living with disabilities or in areas of social deprivation [4–8]. Particularly at risk are those with intellectual disabilities (also known as learning disabilities in the UK) owing to a combination of genetic, social and behavioural factors [9,10]. Whilst there are measures in place to reduce health inequalities in this population, such as annual health checks [11], mortality data suggest that the situation has not improved, despite some deaths being potentially avoidable [12–14].

One of the challenges to reducing inequalities among people living with intellectual disabilities is that they are more likely than the general population to have severe health needs, including epilepsy, cerebral palsy and eating/feeding difficulties, which are known to shorten life expectancy [15]. Although not always life-limiting if managed well, they are relatively rare in the general population and so tend not to feature in population-level policy initiatives. Thus far, their individual contribution to life expectancy has not been formally investigated, but it is important to do so because this contribution may be over-inflated or seen as an inevitable consequence of having intellectual disabilities without seeking to improve health outcomes and/or quality of life for the individuals affected.

The aim of the current study was to investigate specific health needs and quantify their contribution to life expectancy in people with intellectual disabilities and to compare these findings with a cohort of individuals without intellectual disabilities. A further aim was to investigate people without any of the specified health needs to determine if loss in life years for people with intellectual disabilities remained.

2. Materials and Methods

2.1. Data Sources

This study followed the Reporting of studies Conducted using Observational Routinely-collected health Data (RECORD) checklist [16] (see Supplementary Table S1). We used the Clinical Practice Research Datalink (CPRD GOLD), linked (person-level) with hospital episode statistics (HES) and death registrations from the Office for National Statistics (approved study protocol number 19_267). Details of the study population have been described in a previous work [12], with the exception of 23 additional individuals identified, after an amendment to the original protocol, with Cockayne and Angelman syndrome; details of these 23 individuals were received in August 2021 (due to COVID-19 delays; please see the data flow diagram in Supplementary Figure S1 for the initial extract and the study population used for the current study). Briefly, the CPRD is an electronic health record primary care research database which is broadly representative of the national population in terms of age, gender and ethnicity [17]. Only GP surgeries in England that consented to their data being linked with hospital episode statistics (HES) and death data (approximately 75% of CPRD surgeries in England) were included in this study.

2.2. Sample Population

Initial inclusion criteria for the broader programme of work on which this study was based were: registered at the GP surgery at any point between 1 January 2000 and 29 September 2019 and 10 years old or older to account for delays in reporting of diagnoses of intellectual disability in children [18]. A random sample of 980,586 people without intellectual disabilities (initially 1 million prior to exclusions; see Supplementary Figure S1) was used for the comparison group with the same eligibility criteria (but without a diagnosis of intellectual disability). For this study, data were further restricted to the 2017–2019 observation period such that people entered the study on 1 January 2017 if this was after the original date of cohort entry or were excluded if they were last seen or died before this date. The final population comprised 7794 individuals with intellectual disabilities and 176,807 individuals without intellectual disabilities (n = 440 of whom changed status within the observation window at their first intellectual disability diagnosis).

2.3. Definition of Intellectual Disabilities and Health Needs

Diagnostic codes (Read codes and International Classification of Diseases (ICD)-10 codes) for intellectual disabilities and health needs are reported in the Supplementary Material (Table S2). These were based on a combination of previous literature [12], free text searching of diagnostic code descriptions and clinical opinion (RK, SKG, RM). The initial choice of health needs was based on the literature in this area [19] and discussions with carers and people living with intellectual disabilities as being sufficiently severe to affect life expectancy. These were: epilepsy; incontinence (urinary or faecal); severe visual loss; severe hearing impairment; severe mobility difficulties; cerebral palsy and feeding via a percutaneous endoscopic gastrostomy (PEG) tube (i.e., as a measure of severe eating/feeding difficulties). To avoid inclusion of shorter-term health needs that had resolved over time and/or been misdiagnosed in childhood, such as epilepsy [20,21], health needs were defined as being present only if their most recent diagnosis was within 10 years of cohort entry. The exception to this was cerebral palsy, which was defined by a diagnosis ever being present given that it is a life-long condition from birth/early infancy [22].

2.4. Statistical Methods

The date of entry into the cohort was defined as the latest date according to the person and practice's characteristics: the beginning (i.e., 1 January 2017) of the observation window; the date of registration with the GP practice; the date the practice was defined as being up to standard (using the CPRD's own quality indicators); or the date the individual turned 10 years old (to align with the eligibility criteria). Because there are known delays in reporting intellectual disability diagnoses [23] and to avoid conditioning on the future, an intellectual disability status was treated as an age-dependent covariate such that people with intellectual disabilities contributed to the comparison cohort prior to their first diagnosis. Health needs were also treated as age dependent, and individuals contributed to both the presence and absence of health need at different ages if they were diagnosed with a new health need during the observation period. The date of exit was defined as: the date of the last CPRD update (29 September 2019); the date of death; the date of the end of the calendar period; the date of the last practice update or the date of transfer out of practice, whichever was first. The cohort was also sub-divided into individuals without any health needs at baseline or follow-up to assess whether life expectancy was similar between people with and without intellectual disabilities (i.e., excess mortality could be explained by the health needs).

The methodology for the life expectancy work used in this study has been described in detail elsewhere [24]. Life expectancy and 95% confidence intervals (CIs) were compared for people with and without intellectual disabilities and by the presence/absence of each health need using flexible parametric models with intellectual disability and health need status treated as age-varying covariates (and an interaction term fitted). Knots were placed according to the event distribution in the intellectual disability group for greater statistical precision. All models used 5 knots (including the boundary knots; 4 degrees of freedom (df); 3df for age-varying effects) with the exception of PEG feeding, which used 4 knots (3df; 2df for age-varying effects) owing to the small sample size.

3. Results

3.1. Baseline Characteristics

Table 1 shows the characteristics of the study population over the observation period. The characteristics of the population with each individual health need are shown in Supplementary Table S3. In comparison to the rest of the population, people with intellectual disabilities were generally younger (median age 33 vs. 43 years) and more were male (57.1% vs. 49.0%). There were also more white individuals (77.0% vs. 67.5%), although this partly reflects more complete recording of ethnicity in hospital settings (only 14.0% vs. 19.6% had missing data because more people with LD were hospitalised and had their ethnicity recorded). Most individuals (73.4%) with intellectual disabilities had no cause identified: the most common genetic/chromosomal condition reported was Down syndrome (10.9% of the individuals). People with intellectual disabilities had a substantially higher proportion of all of the health needs under investigation compared to those without intellectual disabilities, as is reflected in the greater proportion without any health needs at baseline and follow-up (53.6% vs. 90.3%; intellectual disability vs. no intellectual disability).

The largest differences between people with and without intellectual disabilities were observed for cerebral palsy, which was ≈58 times more prevalent during the 2.7-year observation window (i.e., at baseline or follow-up). Epilepsy, severe visual loss, severe mobility difficulties and PEG feeding were ≈12–22 times more prevalent; and incontinence and severe health impairment were ≈2–4 times more prevalent. The most common severe health need in people with intellectual disabilities was epilepsy, which was present in 18.7% of the individuals at baseline. For people without intellectual disabilities, incontinence was the most common health need, present in 3.8% of the individuals at baseline.

Table 1. Baseline and follow-up characteristics of the study population by intellectual disability and health need status.

Characteristic			Intellectual Disability		No Intellectual Disability [1]	
			Number/ Median	Percent/ Range	Number/ Median	Percent/ Range
Total			7794	100.0	176,807	100.0
Demographic characteristics						
Age (years)			33.0	10–101	43.0	10–108
Gender		Male	4448	57.1	86,669	49.0
		Female	3346	42.9	90,138	51.0
Ethnicity		White	6002	77.0	119,403	67.5
		South Asian	211	2.7	7662	4.3
		Black	207	2.7	6236	3.5
		Other	280	3.6	8907	5.0
		Not known	1094	14.0	34,599	19.6
Observation period						
Length in cohort (years)			1.5	>0.0–2.7	1.9	>0.0–2.7
Most common genetic/chromosomal syndromes [2]						
Down syndrome			848	10.9	-	
Fragile X syndrome			151	1.9	-	
Tuberous sclerosis			60	0.8	-	
Edward syndrome			29	0.4	-	
Prader–Willi syndrome			27	0.3	-	
Severe health needs						
None (at baseline or follow-up)			4174	53.6	159,716	90.3
Epilepsy		Baseline	1456	18.7	2004	1.1
		during follow-up	55	0.7	201	0.1
Incontinence		Baseline	1039	13.3	6649	3.8
		during follow-up	214	2.7	1177	0.7
Severe visual loss		Baseline	1015	13.0	1075	0.6
		during follow-up	227	2.9	204	0.1
Severe hearing impairment		Baseline	551	7.1	5253	3.0
		during follow-up	67	0.9	592	0.3
Severe mobility difficulties		Baseline	818	10.5	1280	0.7
		during follow-up	174	2.2	570	0.3
Cerebral palsy		Baseline	658	8.4	261	0.1
		during follow-up	20	0.3	6	<0.1
PEG [3] feeding		Baseline	132	1.7	180	0.1
		during follow-up	20	0.3	54	<0.1

[1] n = 440 individuals moved from no intellectual disability to intellectual disability sample at first diagnosis during observation window. [2] n = 831 (10.7%) with phenylketonuria (not defined as a specific syndrome for this study). [3] PEG: percutaneous endoscopic gastrostomy.

3.2. Life Expectancy

Figure 1a–g shows the life expectancy estimates and percentage of life years lost (compared with the general population without health needs), for the severe health needs under investigation, by presence/absence of the health need and intellectual disability status. The final figure (Figure 1h) shows the life expectancy estimates for people without any of the health needs under investigation. Table 2 also presents the exact life expectancy estimates (with 95% CI) at 10, 20 and 40 years old.

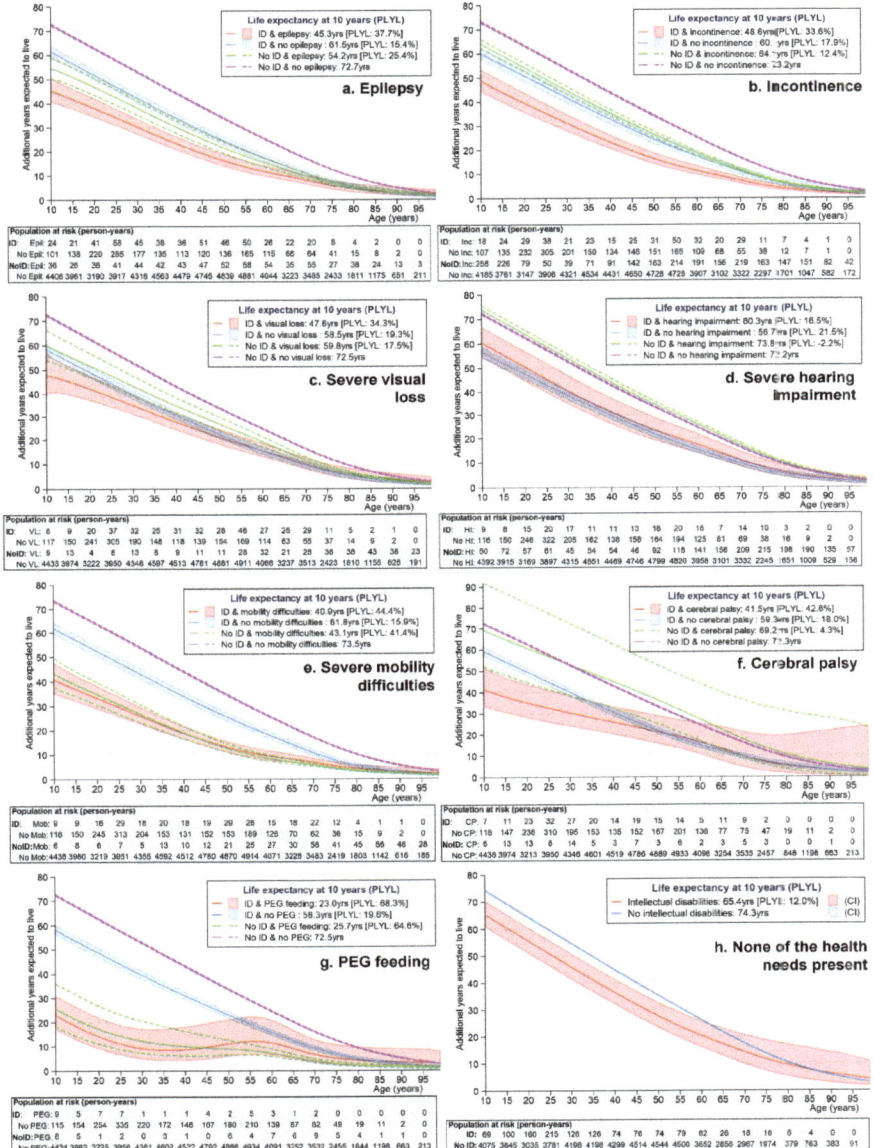

Figure 1. (a–h) Life expectancy from 10 years of age by presence/absence of intellectual disability and health needs.

Perhaps the most striking finding from the figures is that life expectancy was substantially higher across the board in people with neither intellectual disabilities nor specified health need. At 10 years of age, these individuals could expect to live between 72.2 (absence of severe health impairment) and 74.3 additional years (all of the health needs absent). At the same age, children with intellectual disabilities but without each specified health need lost ≈15–22% of life years compared to this first group, living, on average, an additional 57–62 years. Those with intellectual disabilities but without any of the health needs under investigation needs lost ≈12% of life years, living on average 8.9 years shorter than those with neither intellectual disabilities nor health needs.

We can see that the most severe of the health needs, regardless of intellectual disability status, were PEG feeding and severe mobility difficulties. Ten-year-old children with a PEG feeding tube could expect to live only an additional 23.0 years (95% CI 17.1–31.0) if they had intellectual disabilities and 25.7 years (95% CI 18.3–36.0) if they did not have intellectual disabilities, representing a loss in life years of ≈65–68% compared to those with neither condition. Similarly, children with severe mobility difficulties lost ≈41–44% of life years, living an additional 41–43 years only compared to the almost 73 years in those with neither condition. The disadvantages for individuals with PEG feeding tubes and severe mobility difficulties continued to be observed in adulthood (Table 2).

Of the remaining health needs, people with epilepsy had shorter life expectancy overall. Confidence overlapped at 10 years but, subsequently, having intellectual disability in addition to epilepsy incurred additional life expectancy disadvantages (see Table 2), with a loss in life years of ≈38%. Severe visual loss or incontinence was about equivalent to having intellectual disabilities without the health need in terms of life expectancy, but people with both intellectual disabilities and incontinence were again further disadvantaged, with a loss in life years of ≈34%. Conversely, we did not find an effect of severe hearing impairment on life expectancy. The effect of cerebral palsy on life expectancy was harder to determine, owing to small numbers, but those with cerebral palsy and intellectual disabilities had the shortest life expectancy compared with the those without cerebral palsy or with cerebral palsy but without intellectual disabilities, with a loss in life years of ≈43%. All of these findings were relatively consistent across the age range (Table 2).

Table 2. Additional years expected to live at age 10, 20 and 40 years by individual health need status and absence of health needs.

	Intellectual Disability (11,631 Person-Years)				No Intellectual Disability (296,324 Person-Years)			
	Health Need Present		Health Need Absent		Health Need Present		Health Need Absent	
Epilepsy: Additional years expected to live (95% CI): % life years lost [1]								
At 10 years:	45.3 (40.5–50.7)	37.7%	61.5 (59.2–63.9)	15.4%	54.2 (50.0–58.9)	25.4%	72.7 (72.3–73.1)	
At 20 years:	38.0 (34.2–42.1)	39.3%	51.7 (49.4–54.0)	17.5%	46.8 (43.4–50.4)	25.4%	62.8 (62.4–63.2)	
At 40 years:	22.6 (20.0–25.6)	47.7%	33.0 (31.0–35.1)	23.8%	29.3 (26.8–32.0)	32.3%	43.2 (42.9–43.6)	
Incontinence: Additional years expected to live (95% CI): % life years lost [1]								
At 10 years:	48.6 (44.2–53.5)	33.6%	60.1 (57.5–62.8)	17.9%	64.1 (62.3–65.9)	12.4%	73.2 (72.8–73.7)	
At 20 years:	39.5 (35.5–43.9)	37.3%	50.8 (48.4–53.4)	19.6%	54.3 (52.5–56.0)	14.2%	63.3 (62.9–63.8)	
At 40 years:	23.2 (20.4–26.3)	47.2%	32.8 (30.6–35.1)	25.2%	35.3 (33.9–36.8)	19.4%	43.8 (43.4–44.2)	
Severe visual loss: Additional years expected to live (95% CI): % life years lost [1]								
At 10 years:	47.6 (39.2–57.9)	34.3%	58.5 (56.2–60.9)	19.3%	59.8 (53.9–66.3)	17.5%	72.5 (72.1–73.0)	
At 20 years:	42.1 (37.1–47.8)	32.8%	49.0 (46.8–51.3)	21.5%	51.6 (46.9–56.8)	17.6%	62.7 (62.3–63.0)	
At 40 years:	27.6 (24.2–31.5)	36.0%	30.7 (28.8–32.7)	28.9%	34.7 (31.5–38.3)	19.5%	43.1 (42.8–43.5)	
Severe hearing impairment: Additional years expected to live (95% CI): % life years lost [1]								
At 10 years:	60.3 (54.4–66.8)	16.5%	56.7 (54.4–59.1)	21.5%	73.8 (72.2–75.4)	−2.2%	72.2 (71.8–72.6)	
At 20 years:	50.3 (44.5–56.9)	19.0%	47.5 (45.4–49.7)	23.5%	63.8 (62.2–65.4)	−2.4%	62.3 (61.9–62.7)	
At 40 years:	31.1 (25.8–37.4)	27.5%	29.7 (27.9–31.6)	30.6%	44.0 (42.5–45.5)	−2.7%	42.8 (42.5–43.2)	

Table 2. Cont.

	Intellectual Disability (11,631 Person-Years)				No Intellectual Disability (296,324 Person-Years)			
	Health Need Present		Health Need Absent		Health Need Present		Health Need Absent	
	Epilepsy: Additional years expected to live (95% CI): % life years lost [1]							
	Severe mobility difficulties: Additional years expected to live (95% CI): % life years lost [1]							
At 10 years:	40.9 (35.0–47.8)	44.4%	61.8 (59.4–64.3)	15.9%	43.1 (37.7–49.3)	41.4%	73.5 (73.0–73.9)	
At 20 years:	33.2 (28.8–38.3)	47.4%	52.3 (50.0–54.7)	17.5%	34.7 (30.5–39.6)	44.9%	63.6 (63.2–64.0)	
At 40 years:	18.8 (16.2–21.7)	57.4%	34.0 (32.0–36.1)	22.8%	18.9 (16.5–21.7)	57.0%	44.1 (43.7–44.4)	
	Cerebral palsy: Additional years expected to live (95% CI): % life years lost [1]							
At 10 years:	41.5 (33.3–51.7)	42.6%	59.3 (57.2–61.4)	18.0%	69.2 (52.2–91.9)	4.3%	72.3 (71.9–72.7)	
At 20 years:	35.0 (28.0–43.8)	44.0%	49.6 (47.6–51.6)	20.3%	60.6 (44.6–82.3)	3.2%	62.5 (62.1–62.8)	
At 40 years:	25.8 (19.9–33.3)	40.0%	30.4 (28.9–32.5)	28.6%	44.9 (32.4–62.3)	−4.7%	42.9 (42.6–43.3)	
	PEG [2] feeding: Additional years expected to live (95% CI): % life years lost [1]							
At 10 years:	23.0 (17.1–31.0)	68.3%	58.3 (56.2–60.5)	19.6%	25.7 (18.3–36.0)	64.6%	72.5 (72.1–72.9)	
At 20 years:	14.0 (9.0–22.0)	76.8%	48.6 (46.6–50.7)	22.2%	17.1 (11.0–26.6)	72.0%	62.6 (62.3–63.0)	
At 40 years:	8.5 (4.0–18.2)	80.2%	30.9 (29.2–32.7)	28.3%	9.9 (6.0–16.3)	77.0%	43.1 (42.8–43.5)	
	None of the health needs: Additional years expected to live (95% CI): % life years lost [1]							
At 10 years:	-		65.5 (60.3–71.1)	12.0%	-		74.3 (73.8–74.7)	
At 20 years:	-		55.5 (50.4–61.2)	13.9%	-		64.4 (63.9–64.8)	
At 40 years:	-		36.5 (31.5–42.3)	19.0%	-		44.8 (44.4–45.3)	

[1] Percentage of life years lost compared with people with neither intellectual disability nor the specified health need. [2] PEG: Percutaneous endoscopic gastrostomy.

4. Discussion

This work deepens our understanding of health inequalities in people with intellectual disabilities. By reaffirming that severe health needs make a significant contribution to the mortality disparities that people with intellectual disabilities are known to experience, our findings also reveal that they only partially explain these. After restricting the study population to those without health needs, life expectancy remained shorter for those with intellectual disabilities, with a loss in life years of 12%. Of those with the specified health needs, life expectancy was generally further shortened if intellectual disability was also present, suggesting combined disadvantages.

4.1. Strengths and Limitations

To the best of our knowledge, this is the first time that life expectancy has been explored by health needs in people with and without intellectual disabilities. The utilisation of flexible parametric methods to estimate life expectancy is also a novel component and supports previous methodological findings that borrowing strength from larger covariate samples can be an effective way of increasing statistical precision for small samples [24]. However, we recognise that life expectancy is only a crude measure of health inequalities that does not encapsulate other social determinants of health, such as deprivation, or factors that may contribute towards inequalities, such as access to and quality of healthcare provision. We are also unable to comment on other equally important health indicators, including quality of life and well-being.

As with all electronic health record data of this nature which rely on Read code and ICD diagnoses, we are unable to capture variability in the severity of health needs between people with intellectual disabilities and the general population. A particular concern is incontinence, which is likely to be less severe in the general population if it occurred and was resolved during certain life events, such as post-pregnancy [25]; it is noteworthy that almost three-quarters (73.3%) of the people in the general population with incontinence were female, compared with only half (53.2%) in the intellectual disability population (Supplementary Table S3). Moreover, both incontinence and PEG feeding may be indicative of additional comorbidities (e.g., frailty or dysphagia) rather than directly causing mortality [26,27]. Our findings nonetheless support their relationship (even if indirect) with life expectancy. Another limitation of GP health record data is that they do not provide complete information on the severity of intellectual disabilities; we are also likely to have missed people with mild intellectual disabilities who do not have significant support needs and may also be more vulnerable to abuse, discrimination and high-risk behaviours. We also recognise that many of these health needs co-occur and that they are more likely to do so if the individual also has intellectual disabilities, as is reflected in the larger proportion of individuals with at least one health need (46% vs. 10%) and high prevalence of co-occurring health needs, particularly for individuals with cerebral palsy (53% of individuals with intellectual disabilities also had epilepsy; 56% had severe mobility difficulties) and PEG feeding tubes (55% had cerebral palsy; 65% epilepsy and 70% severe mobility difficulties) (Table S3). This descriptive study does not look in more depth at the co-occurring health needs, nor does it adjust for additional clinically relevant comorbidities, such as dementia, or other social determinants of health which all contribute to the mortality disadvantages that people with intellectual disabilities experience [28]. Such issues could be explored further using propensity score methodologies or multiple logistic regression/time-to-event analyses, which are recommended to further develop the work described here.

This study took place before the COVID-19 pandemic, during which people with intellectual disabilities have been adversely affected owing to increased risk of transmission (e.g., through residential homes and community-based support) and increased risk of respiratory deaths [29–31]. People with severe health needs have also been disproportionately affected by COVID-19 [32]. In the current climate, the recommendations made here are, therefore, likely to be more relevant.

4.2. Comparison with Existing Literature

The prevalence of severe health needs found at baseline in this study is largely similar to that found in previous research carried out in the UK and internationally. The prevalence of epilepsy was 18.7% (vs. 1.1% in the general population), which corresponds with previous population-based studies from England (18.5% vs. 0.7% (matched age/gender/practice population sample) [19]) and Scotland (18.8% vs. 0.8% [10]). The prevalence of incontinence in the intellectual disability population (13.3%) was lower than previous UK estimates using the CPRD (20.5% [19]), which we attribute to the exclusion of 'H/O incontinence' and incontinence diagnoses within 10 years of cohort entry for the current study. The baseline prevalence of 3.8% found in the general population is at the lower end of the estimates of international figures of 3–18% for severe incontinence (urinary only) in adult women (about half of this for men) [33], given that many do not seek support from a healthcare provider [34]. The prevalence of PEG feeding (1.9% vs. 0.1%) also falls within the 5-year incidence rate (1.3%) of PEG procedures in England based on 17,000 per year [35].

In our study, prevalence of severe visual impairment among people with intellectual disabilities (13.0%) was lower than previous estimates in the Netherlands for visual impairment and blindness (13.8% and 5.0%, respectively) but, of the latter population, 40.6% were undiagnosed prior to study commencement [36]. We did not find a relationship between severe hearing impairment and life expectancy, which differs from previous (albeit not statistically significant) work in the general population [37].

The prevalence of cerebral palsy we reported here (8.4% vs. 0.1%) can be interpreted using information from the random general population sample. Given that this sample was drawn from 6.2 million individuals (Supplementary Figure S1) and that 0.5% of the general population sample had intellectual disabilities, and assuming a representative random sample draw, the prevalence of cerebral palsy in our study was approximately 1.42 per 1000 population, which is similar to birth estimates reported of 2.11 per 1000 population [38] conditional on surviving to 10 years. We would also expect there to be 2276 (i.e., 6.2 times as many) people with cerebral palsy in the entire population sample, which would equate to 29% of people with cerebral palsy having intellectual disabilities. This is within the range reported in the literature, which cites 22–40% of individuals with cerebral palsy having cognitive impairment (IQ < 70) [39], although some studies report figures closer to one-half [40]. It is worth emphasising, however, that many—if not most—people with cerebral palsy do not have intellectual disabilities and it is important to make sure that their needs are adequately met. The prevalence of severe mobility difficulties (10.5%) in people with intellectual disabilities is similar to previous estimates of 9.2% for being 'non-mobile' [41], but it is hard to determine the prevalence in the general population owing to the recognised variation in thresholds for reporting mobility disabilities [42].

4.3. Recommendations

Given that this descriptive study did not seek to control for other contributing factors, we are nonetheless able to make some broad recommendations. First, it is clear from our findings that health needs are a significant problem for people with intellectual disabilities and that, with the exception of severe hearing impairments, they play a key role in shortening life expectancy. More effective management and treatment of these health needs, including regular assessment of associated care requirements, have the potential to improve outcomes and quality of life for those affected. Many of these health needs are relatively rare in the general population, so the development of tailored care pathways for people with intellectual disabilities, based on national guidelines and policies where available, is likely to be a priority. Such pathways may include monitoring medication (e.g., epilepsy—with a focus on epilepsy syndromes and tuberous sclerosis), provision of specialist support (e.g., visual impairment and hearing impairment), communication plans (e.g., cerebral palsy), pain management (e.g., severe mobility difficulties), prevention strategies (e.g., incontinence) and oral care (e.g., PEG feeding). All pathways should include mechanisms for the provision of coordinated care between health, social care and voluntary services so that unnecessary burden is not placed on carers. They should also be adequately flexible to allow for individuals' differences and needs.

5. Conclusions

We conclude that differential life expectancy in people living with intellectual disabilities compared to the general population is not wholly attributable to increased prevalence of severe health needs. Our findings highlight the need to continue to find ways to improve health outcomes and quality of life for people living with intellectual disabilities so that they can be supported to lead long and fulfilling lives.

Supplementary Materials: The following supplementary information can be downloaded at https://www.mdpi.com/article/10.3390/ijerph19116602/s1, Table S1: RECORD checklist; Table S2: Diagnostic and classification codes for intellectual disabilities, ethnicity and severe health needs investigated; Figure S1: Data flow diagram of individuals included in the study population from original extracted data; Table S3: Characteristics of individuals with specific health needs under investigation.

Author Contributions: Conceptualisation, F.T. and M.J.R.; data curation, F.T. and M.J.R.; methodology, F.T., M.J.R., R.M., R.K. and S.K.G.; validation, M.J.R.; formal analysis, F.T.; investigation, F.T., M.J.R., R.M., R.K., H.K. and S.K.G.; resources, F.T. and M.J.R.; writing—original draft preparation, F.T.; writing—review and editing, F.T., M.J.R., R.M., R.K., H.K. and S.K.G.; visualisation, F.T. and M.J.R.; supervision, M.J.R. and R.M.; project administration, F.T. and M.J.R.; funding acquisition, F.T. and M.J.R. All authors have read and agreed to the published version of the manuscript.

Funding: This research was funded from a Baily Thomas Doctoral Fellowship award (TRUST/VC/AC/SG/5366-8393). The funders had no role in study design, data collection and analysis, the decision to publish or the preparation of the manuscript. The study is based in part on data from the CPRD GOLD database obtained under licence from the UK Medicines and Healthcare products Regulatory Agency. The provision of CPRD and linked data was through Leicester Real World Evidence (LRWE)

Unit, which is funded by University of Leicester, National Institute for Health Research (NIHR) Applied Research Collaboration (ARC) East Midlands and Leicester NIHR Biomedical Research Centre. The interpretation and conclusions contained in this article are those of the authors alone and not necessarily those of the LRWE Unit, the NHS, the NIHR or the Department of Health and Social Care.

Institutional Review Board Statement: The CPRD has Health Research Authority (HRA) approval for all studies using anonymised data for observational research (East Midlands Research Ethics Committee [REC] No. 05/MRE04/87). Research using the CPRD is also subject to regulatory approval from the UK Medicines and Healthcare products Regulatory Agency (MHRA) Independent Scientific Advisory Committee (ISAC); the approved protocol reference no. for this study is: 19/267RA3.

Informed Consent Statement: The CPRD has Health Research Authority (HRA) approval for all studies using anonymised data for observational research (East Midlands Research Ethics Committee [REC] No. 05/MRE04/87). Consent was not obtained for the use of anonymised data—approval for the use of the CPRD (data controller) was through the UK MHRA Independent Scientific Advisory Committee (ISAC) (approved protocol no. 19/267RA3).

Data Availability Statement: Data for this study were obtained from the Clinical Practice Research Datalink (CPRD), provided by the UK MRHA. The authors' licence for using these data does not allow sharing of raw data with third parties. Information about access to CPRD data is available here: https://www.cprd.com/research-applications (accessed on 20 May 2022). Researchers should contact the ISAC Secretariat at isac@cprd.com for further details.

Acknowledgments: The authors gratefully acknowledge support from people with intellectual disabilities and their family carers for relating their own health-related experiences, health needs and support that they received with their health and social care. In particular, we would like to thank: the Talk & Listen group (Leicester, UK), ably facilitated by Pauline Ndigirwa; the Charnwood Action Group (Leicestershire, UK); Gill Huddleston (Carers' UK); Sarah Stanyer; Amy Stanway and Kate Dolan.

Conflicts of Interest: The authors declare no conflict of interest.

References

1. World Health Organization Commission on Social Determinants of Health. Closing the Gap in a Generation: Health Equity through Action on the Social Determinants of Health. 2008. Available online: https://www.who.int/social_determinants/thecommission/finalreport/en/ (accessed on 22 April 2021).
2. United Nations General Assembly. Political Declaration of the High-Level Meeting on Universal Health Coverage: "Universal Health Coverage: Moving Together to Build a Healthier World" [A/RES/74/]. 2019. Available online: https://www.un.org/en/ga/74/resolutions.shtml (accessed on 22 April 2021).
3. Department of Health and Social Care. Advancing Our Health: Prevention in the 2020s—Consultation Document. 2019. Available online: https://www.gov.uk/government/consultations/advancing-our-health-prevention-in-the-2020s/advancing-our-health-prevention-in-the-2020s-consultation-document (accessed on 27 July 2020).
4. European Commission. The European Pillar of Social Rights in 20 Principles. 2017. Available online: https://ec.europa.eu/info/sites/default/files/social-summit-european-pillar-social-rights-booklet_en.pdf (accessed on 2 December 2021).
5. European Commission. Union of Equality. Strategy for the Rights of Persons with Disabilities 2021–2030. 2021. Available online: https://ec.europa.eu/social/BlobServlet?docId=23707&langId=en (accessed on 30 November 2021).
6. Office of Disease Prevention and Health Promotion; U.S. Department of Health and Human Services. Secretary's Advisory Committee for Healthy People 2030. Report 7: Reviewing and Assessing the Set of Proposed Objectives for Healthy People 2030. 2019. Available online: https://www.healthypeople.gov/sites/default/files/Report%207_Reviewing%20Assessing%20Set%20of%20HP2030%20Objectives_Formatted%20EO_508_05.21.pdf (accessed on 30 November 2021).
7. World Health Organization Regional Office for Europe. Better Health, Better Lives: Research Priorities. 2012. Available online: https://apps.who.int/iris/handle/10665/107303 (accessed on 3 December 2021).
8. Australian Civil Society CRPD Shadow Report Working Group. Disability Rights Now. Australian Civil Society Shadow Report to the United Nations Committee on the Rights of Persons with Disabilities: UN CRPD Review. 2019. Available online: https://tbinternet.ohchr.org/Treaties/CRPD/Shared%20Documents/AUS/INT_CRPD_CSS_AUS_35639_E.pdf (accessed on 14 January 2022).
9. Emerson, E.; Hatton, C. *Health Inequalities and People with Intellectual Disabilities*; Cambridge University Press: Cambridge, UK, 2014.

10. Cooper, S.-A.; McLean, G.; Guthrie, B.; McConnachie, A.; Mercer, S.; Sullivan, F.; Morrison, J. Multiple physical and mental health comorbidity in adults with intellectual disabilities: Population-based cross-sectional analysis. *BMC Fam. Pract.* **2015**, *16*, 110. [CrossRef] [PubMed]
11. Robertson, J.; Hatton, C.; Emerson, E.; Baines, S. The impact of health checks for people with intellectual disabilities: An updated systematic review of evidence. *Res. Dev. Disabil.* **2014**, *35*, 2450–2462. [CrossRef] [PubMed]
12. Tyrer, F.; Morriss, R.; Kiani, R.; Gangadharan, S.K.; Rutherford, M.J. Mortality disparities and deprivation among people with intellectual disabilities in England: 2000–2019. *J. Epidemiol. Community Health* **2022**, *76*, 168–174. [CrossRef] [PubMed]
13. Heslop, P.; Blair, P.; Fleming, P.; Hoghton, M.; Marriott, A.; Russ, L. Confidential Inquiry into Premature Deaths of People with Learning Disabilities (CIPOLD). Norah Fry Research Centre, University of Bristol. 2013. Available online: http://www.bristol.ac.uk/media-library/sites/cipold/migrated/documents/fullfinalreport.pdf (accessed on 14 January 2022).
14. Trollor, J.; Srasuebkul, P.; Xu, H.; Howlett, S. Cause of death and potentially avoidable deaths in Australian adults with intellectual disability using retrospective linked data. *BMJ Open* **2017**, *7*, e013489. [CrossRef]
15. Carey, I.M.; Hosking, F.J.; Harris, T.; DeWilde, S.; Beighton, C.; Cook, D.G. An evaluation of the effectiveness of annual health checks and quality of health care for adults with intellectual disability: An observational study using a primary care database. *NIHR J. Libr.* **2017**, *9*, 9. [CrossRef]
16. Benchimol, E.I.; Smeeth, L.; Guttmann, A.; Harron, K.; Moher, D.; Petersen, I.; Sørensen, H.T.; von Elm, E.; Langan, S.M. The REporting of studies Conducted using Observational Routinely-collected health Data (RECORD) statement. *PLoS Med.* **2015**, *12*, e1001885. [CrossRef]
17. Herrett, E.; Gallagher, A.M.; Bhaskaran, K.; Forbes, H.; Mathur, R.; van Staa, T.; Smeeth, L. Data resource profile: Clinical Practice Research Datalink (CPRD). *Int. J. Epidemiol.* **2015**, *44*, 827–836. [CrossRef]
18. Florio, T.; Trollor, J. Mortality among a cohort of persons with an intellectual disability in New South Wales, Australia. *J. Appl. Res. Intellect. Disabil.* **2015**, *28*, 383–393. [CrossRef]
19. Carey, I.M.; Shah, S.M.; Hosking, F.J.; DeWilde, S.; Harris, T.; Beighton, C.; Cook, D.G. Health characteristics and consultation patterns of people with intellectual disability: A cross-sectional database study in English general practice. *Br. J. Gen. Pract.* **2016**, *66*, e264. [CrossRef]
20. Aaberg, K.M.; Gunnes, N.; Bakken, I.J.; Lund Søraas, C.; Berntsen, A.; Magnus, P.; Lossius, M.I.; Stoltenberg, C.; Chin, R.; Surén, P. Incidence and Prevalence of Childhood Epilepsy: A Nationwide Cohort Study. *Pediatrics* **2017**, *139*, e20163908. [CrossRef]
21. National Institute for Health and Care Excellence (NICE). Epilepsies: Diagnosis and Management, Clinical Guideline [CG137] [updated May 2021]. 2012. Available online: https://www.nice.org.uk/guidance/cg137 (accessed on 18 March 2022).
22. Blair, E.; Langdon, K.; McIntyre, S.; Lawrence, D.; Watson, L. Survival and mortality in cerebral palsy: Observations to the sixth decade from a data linkage study of a total population register and National Death Index. *BMC Neurol.* **2019**, *19*, 111. [CrossRef] [PubMed]
23. Tyrer, F.; Bhaskaran, K.; Rutherford, M.J. Immortal time bias for life-long conditions in retrospective observational studies using electronic health records. *BMC Med. Res. Methodol.* **2022**, *22*, 86. [CrossRef] [PubMed]
24. Tyrer, F.; Chudasama, Y.; Lambert, P.C.; Rutherford, M.J. Flexible Parametric Methods for Calculating Life Expectancy in Small Populations. 2022; under review.
25. Chang, S.-R.; Lin, W.-A.; Lin, H.-H.; Lee, C.-N.; Chang, T.-C.; Lin, M.-I. Cumulative incidence of urinary incontinence and associated factors during pregnancy and after childbirth: A cohort study. *Int. Urogynecology J.* **2021**. (online ahead of print). [CrossRef] [PubMed]
26. Matta, R.; Hird, A.E.; Saskin, R.; Radomski, S.B.; Carr, L.; Kodama, R.T.; Nam, R.K.; Herschorn, S. Is There an Association between Urinary Incontinence and Mortality? A Retrospective Cohort Study. *J. Urol.* **2020**, *203*, 591–597. [CrossRef] [PubMed]
27. Becker, R.; Nieczaj, R.; Egge, K.; Moll, A.; Meinhardt, M.; Schulz, R.J. Functional dysphagia therapy and PEG treatment in a clinical geriatric setting. *Dysphagia* **2011**, *26*, 108–116. [CrossRef]
28. Tyrer, F.; Kiani, R.; Rutherford, M.J. Mortality, predictors and causes among people with intellectual disabilities: A systematic narrative review supplemented by machine learning. *J. Intellect. Dev. Disabil.* **2021**, *46*, 102–114. [CrossRef]
29. Glasson, E.J.; Jacques, A.; Wong, K.; Bourke, J.; Leonard, H. Improved survival in Down syndrome over the last 60 years and the impact of perinatal Factors in recent decades. *J. Pediatrics* **2016**, *169*, 214–220. [CrossRef]
30. Day, S.M.; Wu, Y.W.; Strauss, D.J.; Shavelle, R.M.; Reynolds, R.J. Causes of death in remote symptomatic epilepsy. *Neurology* **2005**, *65*, 216–222. [CrossRef]
31. Public Health England. *COVID-19 Deaths of People Identified as Having Learning Disabilities: Report*; Public Health England: London, UK, 2020. Available online: https://www.gov.uk/government/publications/covid-19-deaths-of-people-with-learning-disabilities/covid-19-deaths-of-people-identified-as-having-learning-disabilities-summary (accessed on 23 February 2021).
32. Read, J.M.; Green, C.A.; Harrison, E.M.; Docherty, A.B.; Funk, S.; Harrison, J.; Girvan, M.; Hardwick, H.E.; Turtle, L.; Dunning, J.; et al. Hospital-acquired SARS-CoV-2 infection in the UK's first COVID-19 pandemic wave. *Lancet* **2021**, *398*, 1037–1038. [CrossRef]
33. Hunskaar, S.; Arnold, E.P.; Burgio, K.; Diokno, A.C.; Herzog, A.R.; Mallett, V.T. Epidemiology and natural history of urinary incontinence. *Int. Urogynecology J. Pelvic Floor Dysfunct.* **2000**, *11*, 301–319. [CrossRef]

34. Duralde, E.R.; Walter, L.C.; Van Den Eeden, S.K.; Nakagawa, S.; Subak, L.L.; Brown, J.S.; Thom, D.H.; Huang, A.J. Bridging the gap: Determinants of undiagnosed or untreated urinary incontinence in women. *Am. J. Obstet. Gynecol.* **2016**, *214*, e261–e266. [CrossRef] [PubMed]
35. Sanders, D.S.; Carter, M.J.; D'Silva, J.; James, G.; Bolton, R.P.; Willemse, P.J.; Bardhan, K.D. Percutaneous endoscopic gastrostomy: A prospective audit of the impact of guidelines in two district general hospitals in the United Kingdom. *Am. J. Gastroenterol.* **2002**, *97*, 2239–2245. [CrossRef] [PubMed]
36. van Splunder, J.; Stilma, J.S.; Bernsen, R.M.; Evenhuis, H.M. Prevalence of visual impairment in adults with intellectual disabilities in the Netherlands: Cross-sectional study. *Eye* **2006**, *20*, 1004–1010. [CrossRef] [PubMed]
37. Contrera, K.J.; Betz, J.; Genther, D.J.; Lin, F.R. Association of Hearing Impairment and Mortality in the National Health and Nutrition Examination Survey. *JAMA Otolaryngol. Head Neck Surg.* **2015**, *141*, 944–946. [CrossRef] [PubMed]
38. Oskoui, M.; Coutinho, F.; Dykeman, J.; Jetté, N.; Pringsheim, T. An update on the prevalence of cerebral palsy: A systematic review and meta-analysis. *Dev. Med. Child Neurol.* **2013**, *55*, 509–519. [CrossRef] [PubMed]
39. Odding, E.; Roebroeck, M.E.; Stam, H.J. The epidemiology of cerebral palsy: Incidence, impairments and risk factors. *Disabil. Rehabil.* **2006**, *28*, 183–191. [CrossRef] [PubMed]
40. Reid, S.M.; Meehan, E.M.; Arnup, S.J.; Reddihough, D.S. Intellectual disability in cerebral palsy: A population-based retrospective study. *Dev. Med. Child Neurol.* **2018**, *60*, 687–694. [CrossRef]
41. Tyrer, F.; Ling, S.; Bhaumik, S.; Gangadharan, S.K.; Khunti, K.; Gray, L.J.; Dunkley, A.J. Diabetes in adults with intellectual disability: Prevalence and associated demographic, lifestyle, independence and health factors. *J. Intellect. Disabil. Res.* **2020**, *64*, 287–295. [CrossRef]
42. Melzer, D.; Lan, T.-Y.; Tom, B.D.M.; Deeg, D.J.H.; Guralnik, J.M. Variation in Thresholds for Reporting Mobility Disability Between National Population Subgroups and Studies. *J. Gerontol. Ser. A* **2004**, *59*, 1295–1303. [CrossRef]

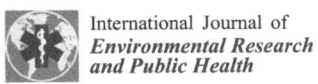

Review

The Association between Physical Environment and Externalising Problems in Typically Developing and Neurodiverse Children and Young People: A Narrative Review

Alister Baird [1,*], Bridget Candy [1], Eirini Flouri [2], Nick Tyler [3] and Angela Hassiotis [1]

1. Division of Psychiatry, University College London, London W1T 7BN, UK
2. Institute of Education, Psychology and Human Development, University College London, London WC1H 0AL, UK
3. Department of Civil, Environmental and Geomatic Engineering, Faculty of Engineering Science, University College London, London WC1E 6DE, UK
* Correspondence: alister.baird.19@ucl.ac.uk

Abstract: The physical environment is of critical importance to child development. Understanding how exposure to physical environmental domains such as greenspace, urbanicity, air pollution or noise affects aggressive behaviours in typical and neurodiverse children is of particular importance given the significant long-term impact of those problems. In this narrative review, we investigated the evidence for domains of the physical environment that may ameliorate or contribute to the display of aggressive behaviours. We have considered a broad range of study designs that include typically developing and neurodiverse children and young people aged 0–18 years. We used the GRADE system to appraise the evidence. Searches were performed in eight databases in July 2020 and updated in June 2022. Additional articles were further identified by hand-searching reference lists of included papers. The protocol for the review was preregistered with PROSPERO. Results: We retrieved 7174 studies of which 67 are included in this review. The studies reported on green space, environmental noise and music, air pollution, meteorological effects, spatial density, urban or rural setting, and interior home elements (e.g., damp/sensory aspects/colour). They all used well validated parent and child reported measures of aggressive behaviour. Most of the studies were rated as having low or unclear risk of bias. As expected, noise, air pollution, urbanicity, spatial density, colour and humidity appeared to increase the display of aggressive behaviours. There was a dearth of studies on the role of the physical environment in neurodiverse children. The studies were heterogeneous and measured a range of aggressive behaviours from symptoms to full syndromes. Greenspace exposure was the most common domain studied but certainty of evidence for the association between environmental exposures and aggression problems in the child or young person was low across all domains. We found a large knowledge gap in the literature concerning neurodiverse children, which suggests that future studies should focus on these children, who are also more likely to experience adverse early life experiences including living in more deprived environments as well as being highly vulnerable to the onset of mental ill health. Such research should also aim to dis-aggregate the underlying aetiological mechanisms for environmental influences on aggression, the results of which may point to pathways for public health interventions and policy development to address inequities that can be relevant to ill health in neurodiverse young people.

Keywords: physical environment; conduct disorders; intellectual disabilities; aggression; review

Citation: Baird, A.; Candy, B.; Flouri, E.; Tyler, N.; Hassiotis, A. The Association between Physical Environment and Externalising Problems in Typically Developing and Neurodiverse Children and Young People: A Narrative Review. *Int. J. Environ. Res. Public Health* **2023**, *20*, 2549. https://doi.org/10.3390/ijerph20032549

Academic Editor: Shoumitro Deb

Received: 21 November 2022
Revised: 28 January 2023
Accepted: 28 January 2023
Published: 31 January 2023

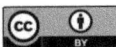

Copyright: © 2023 by the authors. Licensee MDPI, Basel, Switzerland. This article is an open access article distributed under the terms and conditions of the Creative Commons Attribution (CC BY) license (https://creativecommons.org/licenses/by/4.0/).

1. Introduction

The physical environment encompasses all aspects of a child's physical world and may be defined as objective characteristics of the physical context in which children spend their time (e.g., home, neighbourhood, school). The influence of children's physical exposures has been summarised differentially by various models, theorems, and theorists over the previous century. Notably, these include the physical environmental elements of children's exposome (a term introduced by Wild [1,2] regarding the non-genetic influences on outcomes across the lifespan) and Bronfenbrenner's bioecological model [3–5], proposing that children develop within an environmental milieu of five interconnected systems, spanning aspects from urban design (e.g., presence and structure of sidewalks), traffic density, and design of venues for physical activity (e.g., playgrounds, parks, and school yards), to biologically active chemicals, radiation, the internal chemical environment, and psychosocial aspects [6]. The difficulty with these conceptualisations of child development is that they include both physical environmental and (psycho)social influences. As exemplified in a review of the influence of interior hospital environmental interior conditions, Harris [7] segmented the environment into distinct physical exposure categories: ambient, architectural, and interior design.

In this work, an operationalised definition of "physical environment" was incorporated to identify eligible environmental exposures. This classification was derived from a coalescence of Harris's [7], Bronfenbrenner's [3–5] and Wild's [1,2] theorems. This resulted in the inclusion of a diverse array of domains, from ambient exposures (sunlight, sound, meteorology), interior design elements (colour, lighting), architectural features (space/spatial crowding), and biological active agents (i.e., air particulate pollutants), to physical aspects of children's microsystem (i.e., home, school, and neighbourhood characteristics).

A variety of theories have attempted to explain the mechanisms via which environmental domains influence physical and mental health. Although none of these mechanistic models have been fully proven, there are suggestions that positive effects may be the end product of pathways that link several elements, such as mitigation (reduction in air pollution or traffic noise), restoration (stress reduction and attention restoration in alignment with what the Attention Restoration Theory posits) and instoration, whereby attributes of the physical environment, such as greenness in particular, may promote physical activity and social capital and cohesion [8–10].

Previous theories have primarily focused on the stress-reducing effects of greenspace, either via a protective influence from harmful environmental stimuli (noise and air pollution) [11–13], or via the restoration of attentional resources [14,15]. Recently, it has been posited that greenspaces may provide more direct physiological benefits via increased exposure to phytoncides (plant-derived antimicrobial volatile organic compounds) [16]. Whilst preliminary research into the effects of phytoncide exposure is positive, it is currently inconclusive and additional studies are required [17]. Neuroimaging studies are also shedding insight into potential mechanisms for greenspace exposures potential mechanisms, with one study [18] showing that it can beneficially deactivate the prefrontal cortex in regions linked to depression and rumination.

The literature also indicates that aspects such as ambient air particulate matter exposure may negatively impact development via neuroinflammatory pathways [19–24]. Noise pollution may also have detrimental effects via contributions to subjective annoyance and irritation; whilst not necessarily directly causing aggression, noise exposure in those with low threshold for expressing anger may increase its severity [25,26] via draining of attentional and cognitive resources and subsequently leading to increased self-regulatory difficulties [27]. Social-behavioural mechanisms may explain the relationship between behaviour and fluctuations in meteorological effects (such as temperature), e.g., the routine activity theory that proposes that warmer temperatures facilitate more frequent social interaction, increasing opportunity for aggression [28] or that heat increases hostility and physiological arousal and consequently to aggressive behaviour [29]. Theories have posited that high spatial density triggers perceptions of crowding and a subsequent physiological stress arousal response [30–32]. Why proximity elicits these responses is still unclear and has been linked to competition for resources and invasion of personal space [33]. Baird et al. [34] reported a beneficial association between household crowding and reduced conduct problems in children with intellectual disabilities. The authors propose several theories about these potentially counterintuitive findings, suggesting that increased availability of and proximity to family members, in intergenerational households, and parental habituation to problematic conduct behaviours are all potential mechanisms underpinning this finding. Using a sensory room unaccompanied may be associated with a sense of autonomy in children and young people which in turn reduces distress [35]. Other pathways may contribute to the impact that music listening has on a broad range of psychological and physiological benefits [36–41].

As discussed, social-behavioural mechanisms may explain the relationship between aggression and climate effects, for example the routine activity theory proposes that warmer temperatures facilitate more frequent social interaction, increasing opportunity for aggression [28]. Alternatively, the general aggression model (GAM) is more grounded in a physiological aetiology of aggression, suggesting that heat increases hostility and physiological arousal and consequently aggressive behaviours [29].

From the evidence presented so far, it appears that both physical and social environments, in addition to genetic and epigenetic influences, shape the developmental trajectories of children [42–46]. However, in the main, published research is focused on typically developing rather than neurodiverse children [47]. Previous work has evidenced disproportionate influence of children's early environmental milieu in shaping a range of socio-emotional and cognitive developmental outcomes. Specifically, learning disabled children are more likely to be affected by social adversity, poor housing, and poverty [48]. These children are also exponentially more likely to be exposed to negative environmental exposures such as air pollution [49]. To address failings in supporting these children and their families, an important element is to reduce socioeconomic inequality and improve residential conditions [50]. Furthermore, children with complex neurodisabilities have increased barriers to accessing potentially therapeutic aspects of both the physical and social early environments [51]. Disabled child access to urban greenspaces, for example, is not only infrequent in comparison to their typically developing peers [52], but when significant resources are employed to facilitate access for neurodisabled children, the high-risk nature of visiting these spaces requires rigid structure, impacting on the quality of nature experiences when they do occur [53]. This is one example of the health inequities and disparities experienced by neurodiverse children in comparison to their peers, exemplifying the need for additional research in these domains.

Externalising disorders are characterised by display of a range of behaviours which are associated with poor impulse-control, and include rule breaking, impulsivity, and inattention; in addition, a core component of these conditions is the presence of heightened aggression.

Specific child and adolescent externalising disorders include conduct disorder (CD), oppositional defiant disorder (ODD), and attention- deficit-hyperactivity disorder (ADHD). Of particular concern is this repeated presence of aggressive behaviour in these disorders as it is often associated with referral to services and application of a range of restrictive practices, most commonly antipsychotic medications but also inpatient admissions.

Aggressive behaviours and general behavioural problems such as destructive behaviours have an overall negative influence on carers due to stress and negative interactions between carers and the person they care for, likely resulting in a deterioration of the quality of care [54]. Moreover, behavioural problems are associated with increased service costs because of the impact of behaviours on staff and need for high support levels [55]. Aggressive episodes also provoke concerns about threat to personal safety as well as cause panic and upset [56,57].

These behaviours in both typically developing and neurodiverse children compound societal and educational limitations [58–61]. They reduce life satisfaction via degradation of social and familial relationships [62], increase economic costs [63], require higher use of physical restraints [64] and restrictive environmental placements [65,66], limit access to support services [67], impair caregiver functioning [68,69], reduce educational opportunities due to teacher burnout [70] and encourage use of restrictive practices including psychotropic medication use [71,72].

Neurodevelopmental disorders (NDDs) are a category of "etiologically diverse conditions" with onset during the developmental period and are characterised by below average intellectual functioning and adaptive behaviour [73]. This classification includes disorders such as intellectual disability (also called learning disability in the UK), autism spectrum disorders (ASD), and other developmental delays (DD). Whilst we appreciate the nuances of the definitions for brevity and clarity, we will refer to those children with NDDs as neurodiversity in this context.

About one in one hundred individuals has a neurodevelopmental disorder and there are about 351,000 children with intellectual disability in the UK, often coexisting with other neurodevelopmental disorders [74]. Prevalence of aggressive behaviours in NDDs appears to fluctuate depending on sampling methods and assessment strategies, ranging from 8.3% in community samples [75] to 64% in inpatient care [76,77]. Children with intellectual disability were six times more likely to have conduct disorder measured by the Strengths and Difficulties Questionnaire compared to their typically developing peers [78]. Aggressive behaviours are persistent over time [79], with displays of aggression being consistently linked with neurodiversity [57,80–85] though prevalence rates reported can be inconsistent.

Whilst previous research has examined predictors of broadly defined challenging behaviour in children with intellectual disability [86–88], none of the studies has included examination of the influence of the physical environment specifically on such behaviours to date. Here, we build on previous work examining the influence of single domains of the physical environment on aggressive behaviour of typically developing and neurodiverse children by including (1) children across the spectrum of ability and (2) all available objective domains of the physical environment.

Therefore, in this narrative review, we examine the certainty of evidence of the impact of the physical environment on typically developing and neurodiverse children's aggressive behaviours. The outcome of interest was either psychological or biological proxies of aggressive behaviour, annoyance and irritability measured by validated psychometric questionnaires (measures or outcomes which have been empirically evaluated for reliability) or biological markers such as blood pressure, heart rate and skin conductance. The findings are presented by environmental domain (Greenspace, noise pollution, air pollution, meteorology, spatial density, rurality of residence, interior design, and music) and separately for typically developing and neurodiverse children.

2. Materials and Methods

2.1. Search Strategy

We adhered to the Preferred Reporting Items of Systematic reviews and Meta-analyses (PRISMA) statement checklist [89] in conducting the review, as well as guidance from the Synthesis Without Meta-analysis [90], and the Meta-analysis of Observational Studies in Epidemiology [91] to improve the precision of our reporting. The study protocol was preregistered on PROSPERO (CRD42020160251). Because of the heterogeneity in outcome used and the variation in exposure measures, we were unable to perform a meta-analysis. Instead, we reported the degree of certainty of the evidence available in terms of protective/detrimental, inconclusivity, or no association for each outcome and exposure metric across each domain of the physical environment.

The electronic search strategy comprised 8 bibliographic databases (MEDLINE, PsychINFO, Web of Science, CHINAHLplus, Embase, Cochrane library, EThOS and ProQeust dissertations and theses) and two grey literature sources (NICE evidence search and Google scholar). The inclusion of the latter sources facilitated the retrieval of additional studies from a more diverse range of sources (including policy and public health), whilst mitigating publication bias and increasing the comprehensiveness of the review [92,93]. The search was carried out in July 2020, and replicated in the update to June 2022 with no year of publication limit. Bibliographies of retrieved articles were searched to maximise retrieval of relevant articles. The search strategy was overseen by a specialist librarian (see Supplementary Materials).

2.2. Selection Criteria

Studies were included if they (a) reported primary research, (b) were written in English, French, German, Mandarin Chinese and Spanish which were languages spoken by fellow researchers and therefore could be translated, (c) included human participants aged between 0–18 years, (d) contained a psychometrically valid parent or child reported outcome measure of aggressive behaviours or physiological measures of arousal (identified as a proxy measure of aggressive behaviour) and (e) examined exposure to domains of the physical environment.

2.3. Screening and Appraisal Process

All retrieved articles were screened by the first author (A.B.). A sub-sample of titles and abstracts (10%) were co-screened by a senior researcher (A.H.) and a post-doctoral researcher (R.R.). Inter-rater reliability for this initial screening was 87% (0.868). Full text data extraction was conducted by the main author (A.B.) using a modified flexible data extraction template used for non-Cochrane reviews [94] with co-screening conducted for a proportion of studies (59%) by independent researchers (see acknowledgments). Substantial agreement between the primary author and co-screeners was reported (83%, κ = 0.6126) with disagreements resolved by the senior researcher (A.H.) who also crosschecked the extraction table for any inconsistencies.

Risk of bias assessment (RoB) and GRADE protocol were adapted from a systematic review by Clark, Crumpler, and Notley [95] on the evidence relating to effects of environmental noise pollution on mental and physical health outcomes. Four items from this review were used to assess the bias for each paper:

- Evaluation of the quality and validity of the exposure: whether the paper used established or validated environment metrics.
- Bias due to confounding: whether studies included adjustment for potential confounding variables.
- Bias due to sampling methodology and reporting of attrition rate.
- Outcome assessment leading to information bias: whether studies were using validated aggressive behavioural outcome measure(s).

One measure of RoB that was not included in this review was "due to blinding to exposure outcome" as it was not considered appropriate for the methodology of the majority of the retrieved studies which infrequently blind outcome assessors. Overall RoB ratings for each study were aggregates of high, low or unclear across the four domains. We adopted a conservative rating strategy where studies that had equal reports of low and high risk of bias were classified as high.

The GRADE system [96] is a widely used tool recommended by The Cochrane collaboration [97] which provides a ranking of quality for evidence on interventions and relevant outcomes. The modified GRADE approach assigns a priori the highest quality of evidence to longitudinal or intervention studies, and the lowest to cross-sectional studies, subsequently up- or down-grading evidence dependent upon various methodological factors such as RoB, studies not comparing the same variables, inconsistency of findings between studies, imprecision (effect estimate confidence interval containing 25% harm or benefit), publication bias of funnel plot reported, and other considerations (large effect RR > 2, adjustment for all plausible confounding, dose response gradient). As we did not carry out a meta-analysis assessment of GRADE criteria such as precision or publication bias was not possible.

2.4. Measures of Environmental Exposure

- Greenspace was measured by land use data percentage of natural space in the neighbourhood (e.g., for the UK, a census output area such as LSOA) or measured within a set distance of the child's residence. Other indices included satellite derived neighbourhood greenspace (e.g., *normalised difference vegetation index (NDVI)*) and percentage of neighbourhood greenspace.
- Blue space was measured by parents reporting on number of days taking their children to a beach.
- Environmental noise pollution included road traffic, construction noise, and aircraft noise.
- Air pollution was measured by particulate matter, tobacco smoke (nitrogen dioxide: NO_2), and elemental carbon attributed to traffic (ECAT).
- Meteorological variables included seasons, hot or cold weather, humidity and sunlight.
- Spatial density and interior home/facility design included space per child in square metres (high/low density), wall paint, sensory room, presence of damp.
- Urbanicity and rurality were described by the location of the child's residence or school.

2.5. Measures of Aggressive Behaviours

The studies utilised a number of psychometrically valid parent and child reported measures of aggressive behaviour, as well as observer ratings. These comprised the full instrument or conduct, aggression, and externalising behaviour domains as follows:

- Strengths and Difficulties Questionnaire (SDQ) [98]
- Age-appropriate Behaviour Assessment System for Children, Second Edition (BASC-2) [99]
- Child Behaviour Checklist (CBCL) [100]
- Health Related Quality of Life in Children (KINDL-R) [101,102]
- WHO Global School-based Student Health Survey [103]
- National Institute of Mental Health Diagnostic Interview Schedule for Children 4th version (NIMH DISC-IV) [104]
- State-Trait Anger Expression Inventory-2 (STAXI-2) [105]
- Other outcomes used were observer rated frequency of aggressive behaviour

3. Results

The two searches retrieved 7434 records. After deduplication, 7174 were screened of which 257 underwent full-text assessment, resulting in the inclusion of 67 papers (details are shown in the PRISMA flow diagram, Figure 1). Six of which reported on the physical environment and aggressive behaviours in neurodiverse participants.

We report RoB separately for studies carried out with typically developing (Table 1) and neurodiverse populations (Table 2). We follow the same format for the GRADE evidence summaries for the environmental exposures on outcomes of aggressive behaviours for typically developing and neurodiverse children (Tables 3 and 4).

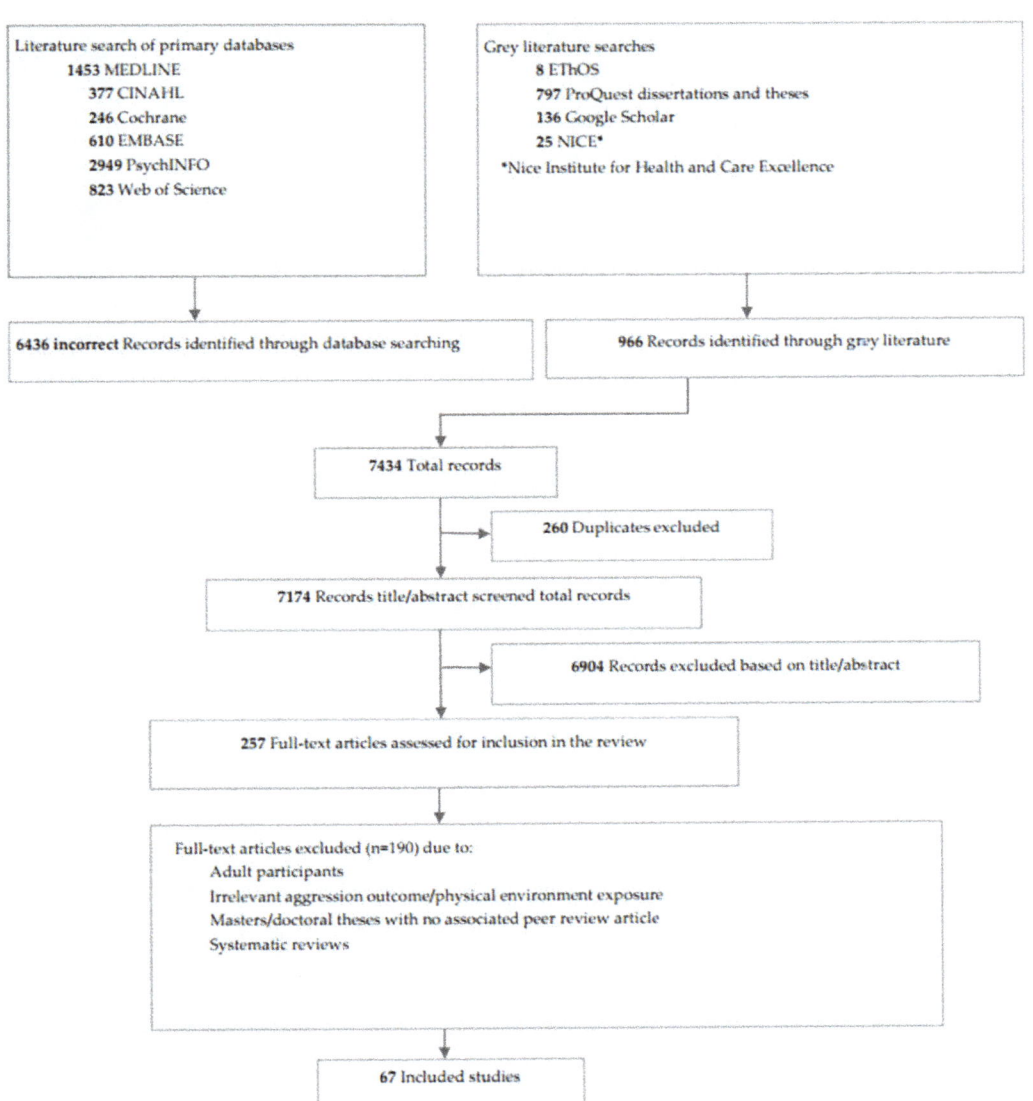

Figure 1. PRISMA flow diagram of the included studies.

Table 1. Risk of Bias (RoB) summary for studies reporting on the association between environmental domains and aggressive behaviours in typically developing children.

Author, Year	Country	Setting	Study Design	N	Age (Years)	Follow Up (Years)	Environmental Exposure	Aggression Outcome	RoB	Association
							Greenspace			
Amoly et al., 2014 [14]	Spain	n.a.	Cross-sectional	2111	7–10	n.a.	**Residential greenspace:** Greenspace surrounding homes in buffer zones measured using the NDVI. **Greenspace playing time:** child's weekly average time spent playing in greenspaces (hours). **Residential proximity to major green spaces:** if home address was within 300 m of available greenspace. **School greenness and combined home-school greenness:** Average weighted NDVI in a 100 m buffer around school and home locations. **Blue space:** Parental report of how many days they accompanied their children to the beach annually.	Parent-completed Strengths and Difficulties Questionnaire (SDQ) [68] conduct problems subscale.	Low	**Beneficial association:** residential greenspace increased greenspace (NDVI) in 100 m and 250 m buffer radii around child's residence was significantly associated with decreased conduct problem scores. **No association:** between greenspace playing time, residential proximity to greenspaces, blue space attendance, and combined school and home greenspace (NDVI) and conduct problems.
Andrusaityte et al., 2020 [10]	Lithuania	n.a.	Cross-sectional	1489	4–6	n.a.	Greenspace (NDVI) in a buffer of 100 m around participants home residence.	Parent-completed Lithuanian version of the Strengths and Difficulties Questionnaire (SDQ) [68].	Low	**No association:** between 100 m NDVI greenspace and risk for conduct problems was reported.
Baird et al., 2022 [4]	UK	n.a.	Longitudinal	8168	3–11	n.a.	**Ward level residential greenspace:** Deciles of the percentage of greenspace within the family's UK ward. **Access to private garden space:** Parent reported child access to private garden space.	Parent-completed Strengths and Difficulties Questionnaire (SDQ) [68] conduct problems subscale.	Low	**No association:** between ward-level greenspace and conduct problem trajectories over time. no association between child access to private garden space and conduct problem trajectories was reported.
Balseviciene et al., [1]	Lithuania	n.a.	Cross-sectional	1468	4–6	n.a.	**Proximity to city parks:** Proximity of residence to nearest park. **Residential greenness:** Greenspace (NDVI) in a buffer of 300 m around participants home residence.	Parent-completed Conduct problems subscale of the Strengths and Difficulties Questionnaire (SDQ) 3.	Low	**Beneficial association:** children whose mothers reported low educational attainment reported significantly more conduct problems as the distance of home residence to closest greenspace (parks) increased. **Harmful association:** increased residential greenspace was associated with increased conduct problems in the high maternal education group and approaching significance in the low education group.
Bijnens et al., 2020 [6]	Belgium	n.a.	Longitudinal	7–15	442	n.a.	Seminatural, forested, blue, and urban green areas (green space) in several radius distances (500, 1000, 2000, 3000, and 500 m) around residential addresses were calculated.	Parent-completed Achenbach Child Behaviour Checklist (CBCL) [101].	Low	**Beneficial association:** for children living in an urban environment, a 1 inter-quartile range increase in greenspace was significantly associated with lower externalising behavioural scores. **No association:** for children residing in rural or suburban areas, no association was reported between greenspace and externalising behaviours.
Feng and Astell-Burt, 2017 [13]	Australia	n.a.	Longitudinal	4968	4	9	Greenspace measured as the percentage of land-use classified as parkland (domestic gardens not included).	Parent-completed externalising behavioural sub-scale (conduct problems and hyperactivity scale combined) of the Strengths and Difficulties Questionnaire (SDQ) [68].	Low	**Beneficial association:** a non-linear association between increased local greenspace and reductions in children's SDQ scores was reported, proportional to local land use classified as greenspace.

Table 1. *Cont.*

Author, Year	Country	Setting	Study Design	N	Age (Years)	Follow Up (Years)	Environmental Exposure	Aggression Outcome	RoB	Association
Flouri et al., 2014 [14]	UK	n.a.	Longitudinal	6384	3	4	Neighbourhood greenspace was defined as the percentage of natural space within groups of census output areas (LSOAs). Private garden access.	Parent-completed conduct problems subscale scores of the Strengths and Difficulties Questionnaire (SDQ) [66].	Low	**No association:** between neighbourhood greenspace and conduct problems was reported. **Beneficial association:** children's access to a private garden was associated with significantly decreased parent reported SDQ conduct scores.
Jimenez et al., 2021 [15]	USA	n.a.	Longitudinal	908	0–13	13	Greenspace (NDVI) in buffers zones of 90 m, 270 m, and 1230 m centred on participants residence.	Parent and teacher completed externalising subscale of the Strengths and Difficulties Questionnaire (SDQ) [66].	Low	**No association:** persistent exposure to maximum (vs. minimum) greenspace exposure during development was not associated with child externalising behaviours.
Madzia et al., 2019 [13]	USA	n.a.	Longitudinal	313	7	5	Varying spatial buffer zones of greenspace surrounding children's residence (NDVI) at ages 7 and 12.	Parent-completed externalising subscale scores of the Behavioural Assessment System for Children, Parent Rating Scale, Second Edition (BASC-2) [71]. Scores $\geq$ 60 classify children as "at risk" for conduct disorder in clinical settings.	Low	**Beneficial association:** greenspace at age 7 was significantly associated with decreased conduct scores at the 200 m buffer radius only. **No association:** no associations were reported between greenspace and conduct scores or aggression scores at age 12 at any buffer radius. **Beneficial association:** increased NDVI at 200 m and 800 m buffers at age 7 was significantly associated with lower probability of being "at risk" of conduct problems.
Markevych et al., 2014 [16]	Germany	n.a.	Longitudinal	1932	9–12	10	Residential proximity to urban greenspace.	Parent-completed conduct problems subscale of the Strengths and Difficulties Questionnaire (SDQ) [4].	Low	**No association.**
McEachan et al., 2018 [5]	UK	n.a.	Longitudinal	2594	4,5	4	Varying buffer zones of green space around participants' home addresses and distance to major green spaces was computed with the normalised difference vegetation index (NDVI).	Parent-completed conduct and hyperactivity subscales (combined in externalising behavioural scores) of the Strengths and Difficulties Questionnaire (SDQ) [66].	Low	**No association:** between NDVI and parent-reported externalising behaviours in White British or South Asian participants.
Mueller et al., 2019 [14]	UK	n.a.	Cross-sectional	3683	10–15	n.a.	Greenspace was measured using land use data, which reports percentage of greenspace in the family's ward (excluding gardens).	Self-completed conduct problems subscale of the Strengths and Difficulties Questionnaire (SDQ) [66].	Low	**No association:** between greenspace and conduct problem scores.
Liao et al., 2020 [17]	China	n.a.	Cross-sectional	6039	5–6	n.a.	Greenspace (NDVI ^{1}) in a 100 m buffer zone was measured and weighted assuming that children spent 16 h per day at home and 8 h at kindergarten.	Parent-completed aggressive behaviour subscale of the Child Behavioural Checklist (CBCL) [100].	Low	**Beneficial association:** increased residence-kindergarten-weighted greenspace was significantly associated with decreased aggressive behaviour scores.
Lee et al., 2019 [18]	Korea	Residence	Cross-sectional	1817	6–18	n.a.	Modified soil-adjusted vegetation index (MSAVI) values were categorised into tertiles (low, moderate, high greenness) and each child was assigned the mean MSAVI within a 1.6 km radius of residence.	Parent-completed externalising subscale of the Child Behavior Checklist (Rule-breaking Behaviour and Aggressive Behaviour combined) of the Child Behavioural Checklist (CBCL) [101].	Low	**Beneficial association:** children residing in highest tertile of average greenness for the 1600 m areas around their homes had significantly lower Externalising Behaviour scores.
Lee and Movassaghi, 2021 [19]	USA	Schools	Cross-sectional	n.a.	5–18	n.a.	Greenspace (NDVI ^{1}) in a 100 m buffer zone surrounding schools	Incidence rates of attacks or threats with and without weapons in schools.	Low	**Harmful association:** increased school greenness was associated with increased incidence of threats and attacks (with or without weapons).

Table 1. Cont.

Author, Year	Country	Setting	Study Design	N	Age (Years)	Follow Up (Years)	Environmental Exposure	Aggression Outcome	RoB	Association
Richardson et al., 2017 [20]	UK	n.a.	Longitudinal	2909	4	2	Greenspace defined as the % area of total natural space [5] and parks within 500 m of the child's residence. Private garden access.	Primary caregiver-completed conduct problems subscale of the Strengths and Difficulties Questionnaire (SDQ) [68].	Low	**No association:** between total green space and children's conduct problem scores. **Beneficial association:** between children not having access to private garden and increased SDQ conduct scores was reported.
Van Aart et al., 2018 [21]	Belgium	n.a.	Longitudinal	172	6–12	6	Semi-natural, forested, and agricultural areas (greenness) and residential and industrial areas in a 5000, 4000, 3000, 2000, 1000, 500, 300 and 100 m buffer from the residential address	Primary caregiver-completed conduct problems subscale of the Strengths and Difficulties Questionnaire (SDQ) [68].	Low	**No association:** between landscape surrounding child's residence and conduct problems were reported.
Younan et al., 2016 [22]	USA	n.a.	Longitudinal	1287	9	9	Greenspace (NDVI [1]) was measured in multiple spatial buffers zones for various periods preceding CBCL assessment.	Parent-completed aggressive behaviour subscale of the Child Behaviour Checklist (CBCL) [2].	Low	**Beneficial association:** increased greenspace (1000 m NDVI) was associated with significant decreases in aggression.
							Noise pollution			
Bao et al., 2022 [23]	China	Residence	Longitudinal	3236	7–13	6	Residential road traffic noise was assessed using modelling different periods of the day, including daytime (Lday), nighttime (Lnight), and weighted 24 h (Ldn).	Parental completed conduct problems subscale of the Strengths and Difficulties Questionnaire (SDQ) [68].	Low	**Harmful association:** weighted 24 h (Ldn) noise exposure was associated with increased conduct problems.
Crombie et al., 2011 [24]	UK/Spain/Netherlands	Schools	Cross-sectional	1900	9–10	n.a.	A continuous noise from aircraft and road traffic measure calculated in dB for each school.	Parental completed conduct problems subscale of the Strengths and Difficulties Questionnaire (SDQ) [68].	Low	**No association:** no association between air traffic noise and conduct problems. **Beneficial association:** between increasing road traffic noise and decreasing SDQ problem scores was reported.
Essers et al., 2022 [25]	Spain/Netherlands	Residence	Longitudinal	7958	18 m–9 years	7.5	Average 24 h noise exposure at the participants' home address during childhood was estimated using EU maps from road traffic noise and total noise (road, aircraft, railway, and industry).	Parental completed Strengths and Difficulties Questionnaire (SDQ) and Child Behavioural Checklist 6–18 (CBCL 6–18) [69,130].	Low	**No association:** between noise exposure and conduct problems or aggressive behaviours was reported.
Geelat et al., 2016 [26]	France	Not reported	Cross-sectional	517	7–11	n.a.	Noise indices were calculated from the front and most exposed façade of the child bedrooms using a noise map.	Child self-report questionnaire on annoyance from various traffic and ambient noise sources.	Unclear	**Harmful association:** increased road and general transport noise exposure was significantly associated with increased child annoyance.
Haines et al., 2001a [27]	UK	Schools	Cross-sectional	340	10	n.a.	Exposure of schools to high and low aircraft noise.	Parent-completed conduct problems subscale of the Strengths and Difficulties Questionnaire (SDQ) [68]. Child self-report questionnaire on annoyance due to aircraft, train, road and neighbour noise.	Low	**No association:** between aircraft noise exposure at school and SDQ conduct problems was reported. **Harmful association:** increased aircraft noise exposure was significantly associated with increased annoyance.
Haines et al., 2001b [28]	United Kingdom	Schools	Longitudinal	275	8–11	1	Exposure of schools to high and low aircraft noise.	Child self-report questionnaire on aircraft, train, road, and neighbour noise annoyance.	Low	**Harmful association:** higher levels of aircraft noise were associated with significantly elevated levels of annoyance.
Haines et al., 2001c [29]	UK	Schools	Cross-sectional	451	9	n.a.	Exposure of schools to high and low aircraft noise.	Parent-completed conduct problems subscale of the Strengths and Difficulties Questionnaire (SDQ) [68]. Child self-report questionnaire on noise annoyance.	Low	**Harmful association:** increased aircraft noise exposure at school was significantly associated with increased annoyance. **No association:** between aircraft noise and SDQ conduct scores were reported.

Table 1. *Cont.*

Author, Year	Country	Setting	Study Design	N	Age (Years)	Follow Up (Years)	Environmental Exposure	Aggression Outcome	RoB	Association
Spilski et al., 2019 [30]	Germany	Not reported	Cross-sectional	1243	8	n.a.	Residential aircraft noise over the preceding 12 months (FANOMOS).	Child self-reported annoyance questionnaire.	Unclear	**Harmful association:** between increased aircraft noise and increased child annoyance.
Stansfeld et al., 2005 [31]	UK/Spain/ Netherlands	Schools	Cross-sectional	2844	9–10	n.a.	Exposure to external aircraft and road traffic noise was predicted from noise contour maps, modelling, and on-site measurements.	Child self-report questionnaire on noise annoyance.	Low	**Harmful association:** increased aircraft and road traffic noise was significantly associated with elevated child annoyance.
Stansfeld et al., 2009 [32]	UK/Spain/ Netherlands	Schools	Cross-sectional	2844	9–10	n.a.	School exposure to high or low road traffic and aircraft noise.	Parent-completed conduct problems subscale of the Strengths and Difficulties Questionnaire (SDQ) [68].	Low	**No association:** between aircraft noise and conduct problems was reported. **Harmful association:** between increased road traffic noise and higher conduct problem scores.
Tiesler et al., 2013 [33]	Germany	Residence	Cross-sectional	872	10	n.a.	Night (L_{night}) and day (L_{den}) indicators of road traffic noise at child's residence were created using weighted long-term annual average sound levels.	Parental completed conduct problems subscale of the Strengths and Difficulties Questionnaire (SDQ) 4	Low	**No association:** between day or night noise exposure and conduct problems was reported.
							Air pollution			
Andrusaityte et al., 2020 [10]	Lithuania	n.a.	Cross-sectional	1489	4–6	n.a.	Ambient air pollution: Modelled annual mean NO_2 and $PM_{2.5}$	Parental completed Lithuanian version of the Strengths and Difficulties Questionnaire (SDQ) [34].	Low	**No association:** between NO_2 and $PM_{2.5}$ and risk for conduct problems was reported.
Baird et al., 2022 [7]	UK	n.a.	Longitudinal	8168	3–11	n.a.	Annual concentrations of neighbourhood (LSOA) level NO_2.	Parent-completed conduct problems subscale of the Strengths and Difficulties Questionnaire (SDQ) [68].	Low	**No association:** between NO_2 exposure and conduct problems was reported.
Bandiera et al., 2011 [35]	USA	Not reported	Cross-sectional	2901	8–15	n.a.	Serum cotinine (a metabolite of nicotine) as a proxy of cigarette smoke exposure.	Parental reported DSM-IV conduct disorder symptoms obtained via The National Institute of Mental Health's Diagnostic Interview Schedule for Children Version IV (DISC-IV) [104].	Low	**Harmful association:** increased smoke exposure was significantly associated with increased conduct disorder symptoms.
Bao et al., 2022 [2]	China	Residence	Longitudinal	3236	7–13	n.a.	Annual mean concentration of nitrogen dioxide (NO_2).	Parent-completed conduct problems subscale of the Strengths and Difficulties Questionnaire (SDQ) [68].	Low	**No association:** between annual mean concentration of NO_2 and child conduct problem scores.
Bauer et al., 2015 [36]	USA	Community paediatric clinics	Cross-sectional	2441	0–6	n.a.	Self-reported cigarette smoke exposure (screening questionnaire asking families if anyone in the household smoked).	Diagnosis of Disruptive Behaviour Disorder (DBD) was gained from child's electronic health record. Diagnoses were identified using International Classification of Diseases-ninth revision (ICD-9) [37].	Unclear	**Harmful association:** childhood smoke exposure increased risk of disruptive behaviour disorder.
Cattke-Kopp et al., 2020 [38]	USA	Residence	Longitudinal	1096	0.5	6.5	Child salivary cotinine (a metabolite of nicotine) was measured as a proxy for exposure to cigarette smoke.	Primary caregiver-completed conduct problems subscale (SDQ) [68] and the Disruptive Behaviours Rating Scale (DBRS) [105]. These scores were combined to create a composite conduct problems score. Teachers completed the conduct problems subscale (SDQ) [68] and Teacher Observation of Child Adaptation-Revised (TOCA-R) [106].	Low	**Harmful association:** increased cotinine levels associated with increases in a multi-informant latent factor of conduct problems.
Karamanos et al., 2021 [11]	UK	Schools	Longitudinal	4775	11–16	5	Ambient air pollution: Modelled annual mean NO_2 and $PM_{2.5}$	Child self-report Strengths and Difficulties Questionnaire (SDQ) [68].	Low	**Beneficial association:** NO_2 and $PM_{2.5}$ were both associated with reduced trajectories of conduct problems over time.

Table 1. Cont.

Author, Year	Country	Setting	Study Design	N	Age (Years)	Follow Up (Years)	Environmental Exposure	Aggression Outcome	RoB	Association
Kelishadi et al., 2015 [42]	Iran	Not reported	Cross-sectional	13,486	6–18	n.a.	Self-reported active, passive, combined or non-smoker status.	Self-reported information on anger and violent behaviours (World Health Organization Global School-based Student Health Survey: WHO-GSHS) [43].	Low	**Harmful association:** increased anger and risk of violent behaviour was associated with any smoker status.
Loftus et al., 2020 [44]	USA	n.a.	Cross-sectional	975	4–6	n.a.	NO_2 and particulate matter less than 10 microns (PM_{10}) at participants' residences was calculated using a national annual average universal kriging model. Proximity to nearest road.	Parental completed Child Behaviour Checklist (CBCL ages 1.5–5 years of age) [10].	Low	**Harmful association:** in fully adjusted models, NO_2 exposure was positively associated with odds of externalising child behaviours. **No association:** was reported for PM_{10} or proximity to nearest road with child externalising behaviours.
Mueller et al., 2019 [16]	UK	Not reported	Cross-sectional	3683	10–15	n.a.	Annual concentrations of neighbourhood level (LSOAs) Nitrogen Dioxide (NO_2).	Self-completed conduct problems subscale of the strengths and Difficulties Questionnaire (SDQ) [15].	Low	**No association:** between NO_2 exposure and conduct problem scores were reported.
Newman et al., 2013 [45]	USA	Not reported	Longitudinal	576	1	6	The average daily concentrations of elemental carbon attributed to traffic pollution (ECAT) measured over the child's first year of life.	Parent-completed aggression and conduct problems subscales from the Behavioural Assessment System for Children, Parent Rating Scale, 2nd Edition (BASC-2) [9].	Low	**No association:** between ECAT exposure and BASC-2 aggression or conduct subscale scores were reported.
Pagani et al., 2017 [46]	Canada	n.a.	Longitudinal	2055	1.5	10.5	Primary caregiver reported household smoking status.	At age 12 children completed questionnaires asking about their antecedent proactive, reactive and conduct problems.	High	**Harmful association:** early exposure to second-hand smoke was significantly associated with increased, conduct problems, proactive, and reactive aggression at age 12.
Park et al., 2020 [47]	Korea	n.a.	Longitudinal	179	5–9	4	Urinary cotinine levels.	Parental completed Korean version of the Child Behaviour Checklist (CBCL).	Low	**Harmful association:** high cotinine levels were significantly associated with increased externalising problems at age 5, but not at ages 7 and 9.
Ramick et al., 2021 [48]	USA	n.a.	Cross-sectional	263	12	n.a.	Ambient concentrations of lead as a constituent of particulate matter of size 2.5 μm or smaller ($PM_{2.5}$).	Parent-completed Behavioural Assessment System for Children, 2nd edition (BASC-2) [9].	Low	**Harmful association:** birth to 7 months was identified as a sensitive window for lead exposure and aggressive behavioural outcomes.
Roberts et al., 2019 [49]	UK	Home residence	Longitudinal	284	12	6	Exposure to annualised particulate matter less than 2.5 microns ($PM_{2.5}$) and NO_2 concentrations were estimated at address-level.	Age 12: Conduct disorder symptoms were self-reported and assessed in reference to DSM-IV [50] conduct disorder criteria. Age 18: DSM-IV [53] Conduct disorder diagnoses.	Low	**Harmful association:** increased $PM_{2.5}$ and NO_2 at age 12 was significantly associated with increased odds for conduct disorders at age 18.
Meteorological effects										
Ciucci et al., 2013 [51]	Italy	Day-care centres	Longitudinal	61	2	9 months	Air temperature (°C), relative humidity (%), solar radiation (Jm^{-2}) and rain (mm) data.	Teacher-completed Daily Behavioural and Emotional Questionnaire (DBEQ) [51].	Low	**Harmful association:** between increased humidity during winter and increased aggression. **No association:** between other meteorological variables and aggression.

Table 1. Cont.

Author, Year	Country	Setting	Study Design	N	Age (Years)	Follow Up (Years)	Environmental Exposure	Aggression Outcome	RoB	Association
Klimstra et al., 2011 [52]	The Netherlands	Not reported	Cross-sectional	415	Age not reported	n.a.	Sunshine, average temperature, and hours of precipitation.	Self-report anger measured via the Daily Mood Scale [6].	Low	**Beneficial association:** between average temperature and anger scores. **No association:** between other meteorological variables and anger.
Lochman et al., 2021 [53]	USA	n.a.	Longitudinal	188	9–13	4	Parent reported tornado exposure measured using the Tornado-Related Traumatic Experiences (TORTE) questionnaire [7].	Parent Rating Scale (PRS) of the Behaviour Assessment System for Children (BASC) [8].	Low	**Harmful association:** greater parent reported tornado exposure scores was positively associated with parent reported child externalising behaviours.
Jones and Molano, 2016 [54]	USA	School	Longitudinal	3330	8	2	Development of children during the first two school years, contrasted with scores during summer recess.	Average aggression score from the Teacher Checklist [55].	Low	**Beneficial association:** a significant decrease in aggression was reported during the summer break in comparison to the academic school years.
Lagacé-Séguin and d'Entremont, 2005 [56]	Canada	School	Cross-sectional	33	4	Daily over 30 days.	Humidity, sunshine hours, and temperature (°C).	Externalising behaviours measured via the Teacher-completed Preschool Behaviour Questionnaire (PBQ) [57].	Low	**Harmful association:** increased humidity was significantly correlated with increased externalising behaviours. **Beneficial association:** increased sunshine was significantly correlated with decreased externalising behaviours. **No association:** temperature was not correlated with externalising behaviours.
Munoz-Reyes et al., 2014 [58]	Chile	Schools	Longitudinal	~1000	14–18	1	Cold season (autumn/winter) contrasted to warm season (spring/summer), temperature and humidity.	Observational recordings of school yard aggressive behaviours over an academic year used to construct an aggression intensity index for each participant.	High	**Harmful association:** frequency of aggression was significantly increased during the warm season. **Beneficial association:** increased temperature and humidity were associated with significantly decreased frequency of aggressive events.
Younan et al., 2018 [59]	USA	Residence	Longitudinal	1287	9–10	8	A monthly time-series of average ambient temperature was constructed, and temperature was further aggregated for the periods 1, 2, and 3 years preceding each CBCL assessment.	Parental completed Child Behaviour Checklist (CBCL) [60].	Low	**Harmful association:** between ambient residential temperature 2 and 3 years prior to assessment and externalising behaviours was reported (this effect remained when controlling for urbanicity, humidity, traffic density and proximity to roads or freeways).
Spatial density										
Baird et al., 2022 [61]	UK	n.a.	Longitudinal	8168	3–11	n.a.	Household crowding (calculated as the total number of rooms in a residence/total occupants)	Parent-completed Strengths and Difficulties Questionnaire (SDQ) [62] conduct problems subscale.	Low	**Harmful association:** household crowding was significantly positively associated with conduct problems across development.

Table 1. Cont.

Author, Year	Country	Setting	Study Design	N	Age (Years)	Follow Up (Years)	Environmental Exposure	Aggression Outcome	RoB	Association
Ginsburg et al., 1977 [66]	USA	School playground	Observational	28–34	8–11	n.a.	Playground area size (small vs. large).	Observed frequency and duration of aggressive behaviours in the playground.	High	**Harmful association:** smaller play area size was significantly associated with increased physical aggression. **Beneficial association:** duration of aggressive behaviours were significantly shorter in the small play area.
Loo and Kennelly, 1979 [61]	USA	Experimentally designed rooms	Observational	72	5	n.a.	Low-density condition (32.70 ft² per child) and high-density condition (16.35 ft² per child).	Observed frequency of physically aggressive behaviours and anger.	High	**Harmful association:** a significant increase in aggression and anger was reported in the high-density condition.
Loo and Smetana, 1978 [63]	USA	Experimentally designed rooms.	Observational	80	10	n.a.	Low-density condition (52.1 ft² per person) and high-density condition (13.6 ft² per person).	Observed frequency of physically aggressive behaviours and anger.	High	**No association:** between density condition, anger or aggression was observed.
Supplee et al., 2007 [65]	USA	Residence	Longitudinal	120	2	4	Overcrowding of Home (number of rooms divided by total number of people per household).	Maternal completed Child Behaviour Checklist (CBCL) [13] at age 4. Teacher completed Teacher Report Form (TRF) [16] between ages 5.5–6.	Unclear	**No association:** between overcrowding in the home (at age 3) and age 4 maternal reported externalising behaviours. **Harmful association:** overcrowding in the home (at age 3) was significantly associated with increased teacher reported externalising behaviours at age 5.
Neill, 1982 [62]	UK	Nursery	Observational	~100	3–5	n.a.	Playroom openness (POP ratio), space per child and room group size.	Observed frequencies of aggression defined as "causing distress by any means".	High	**Beneficial association:** aggression appeared to be higher in more open nursery environments, however due to poor study methodology, associations are unclear.
							Urbanicity and rurality (reference category urban where applicable)			
Baird et al., 2022 [4]	UK	n.a.	Longitudinal	8168	3–11	n.a.	Data from the Office for National Statistics (ONS) was used to assess urbanicity or rurality of children's residence.	Parent-completed Strengths and Difficulties Questionnaire (SDQ) [55] conduct problems subscale.	Low	**No association:** between geographic location of children's residence and conduct problem trajectories.
Evans et al., 2018 [64]	The Netherlands	Schools	Longitudinal	895	8–12	4	Neighbourhood urbanicity: mean number of addresses within a circle of 1 km radius around a participant's residential address.	Teachers completed the Problem Behaviour at School Interview (2000) [67]. Oppositional defiant and conduct disorder subscales were combined into a behavioural problems measure.	Low	**Harmful association:** between urbanicity and behavioural problems was reported (even after full adjustment).
Handal and Hopper, 1985 [68]	USA	Head start and day centres.	Cross-sectional	679	4–5	n.a.	Rural and urban children recruited from Head start centres.	The aggressive subscale of the AML: a behavioural teacher rating tool [69].	High	**No association:** between geography and aggression scores was reported.
Hope and Bierman, 1998 [53]	USA	Residence/schools	Cross-sectional	310	Not reported	n.a.	Schools recruited from urban and rural areas.	Teacher completed Child Behaviour Checklist–Teacher Rating Form (CBCL–TRF) [17]. Parent-completed Child Behaviour Checklist–Parent Rating Form (CBCL–PRF) [17].	Low	**No association:** between parent reported externalising behaviours and children residing in urban and rural environments. **Beneficial association:** urban schoolteachers reported significantly more externalising behaviours than rural teachers.

Table 1. *Cont.*

Author, Year	Country	Setting	Study Design	N	Age (Years)	Follow Up (Years)	Environmental Exposure	Aggression Outcome	RoB	Association
Sheridan et al., 2014 [172]	USA	Residence	Longitudinal	6550	3	2	Urban or rural classification based on zip code; city, suburban, town, or rural.	Preschool and Kindergarten Behaviour Scales–Second Edition [173]; Social Skills Rating System [174]; Family and Child Experiences Survey [175].	Low	**No association:** between geographical location of residence and teacher reported externalising behaviours. **Harmful association:** parents reported higher externalising behaviour in rural children in comparison to city and suburban children but not children residing in towns.
Wongsonglarm et al., 2016 [176]	Thailand	Colleges	Cross-sectional	1028	17	n.a.	Participants were recruited from either Rural (Nakhon) or Urban (Bangkok) Thai provinces.	Self-reported violent behaviour: modified from the Pittsburg Youth Study's measure of serious violence [177]. Violent offences: self-reported via a modified version of the Overt Victimisation subscale of the Problem Behaviour Frequency Scale [178]. Anger expression (internal/external): Frequency of anger was recorded via The State–Trait Anger Expression Inventory–2 (STAXI-2) [105].	Low	**No association:** in self-reported violent behaviour between rural and urban participants was reported. **Beneficial association:** two violent behaviours; "chased with weapons" and "injured someone with weapons" was significantly more frequently reported by urban adolescents. Anger out and in was significantly elevated in the rural condition.
							Interior design			
Baird et al., 2022 [4]	UK	n.a.	Longitudinal	8168	3–11	n.a.	Parental completed questionnaire on damp problems inside the home.	Parent-completed Strengths and Difficulties Questionnaire (SDQ) [68] conduct problems subscale.	Low	**Harmful association:** parental reported damp problems were significantly associated with increased conduct problems trajectories across development.
Glod et al., 1994 [179]	USA	Inpatient psychiatric ward	Single blind within-groups repeated measures	19 [8]	10	n.a.	Sensory room modification.	Observer rated aggression using a modified version of the Overt aggression scale [180] in modified and non-modified sensory rooms.	Unclear	**Beneficial association:** aggression after modified sensory room use was significantly decreased in comparison to non-modified room use.
Vakili et al., 2019 [181]	Iran	Classroom	Case-control pre-post design	70	Not reported	12 weeks	Red painted classroom walls vs. a control condition of white walls.	Buss Perry aggression questionnaire [182].	Unclear	**Harmful association:** red classroom walls significantly increased aggression in comparison to the white wall control condition.
							Music			
Coyne and Padilla-Walker, 2015 [183]	USA	Residence	Longitudinal	548	15	1	Independent assessors rated the physical aggression content of adolescent's favourite music artists at time 5 (T5).	Self-completed 5-item questionnaire on physical aggressive behaviour at T5 and T6.	High	**Harmful association:** preference for artists with aggressive music content was associated with increased self-report aggressive behaviour.
Hinds, 1980 [184]	USA	Mental health clinic	Within-group repeated measures	10	8–10	n.a.	Alternating 15 min periods of silence and slow Instrumental music.	Observer rated aggressive behaviours.	High	**No association:** between music and no-music conditions in relation to frequency of aggressive behaviour.

[1] Normalised difference vegetation index (NDVI). [2] CBCL Version used: 6–18 years [100]. [3] Lithuanian version of the SDQ was used [134]. [4] The German version of the Strengths and Difficulties Questionnaire (SDQ) was used in this study [185]. [5] The authors use "natural space" and "greenspace" interchangeably. [6] An Internet version of the Electronic Mood Device [186]. [7] Tornado exposure was measured using the Tornado-Related Traumatic Experiences (TORTE) questionnaire [187]. [8] Participants were described as comorbid for a "wide range of diagnoses" however no additional information on psychiatric diagnoses was reported.

Table 2. Risk of bias (RoB) summary for studies reporting on environmental domains and aggressive behaviours in neurodiverse children.

Author, Year	Country	Setting	NDD	Study Design	N	Age (Years)	Follow Up (Years)	Physical Environmental Measure(s)	Aggression Outcome	RoB	Association
Baird et al., 2022 [54]	UK	n.a.	ID	Longitudinal	155	3–11	8	Neighbourhood greenspace (NDVI), access to a private garden, Air pollution (NO$_2$) exposure, Urbanicity of residence, household crowding, household damp exposure.	Parent-completed Strengths and Difficulties Questionnaire (SDQ) [68] conduct problems subscale.	Low	**No association:** between ID diagnosis, conduct problems, and environmental measures (except household crowding) were reported. **Beneficial association:** an interaction effect was reported between ID, home crowding, and conduct problems, reporting that children with ID reported lower conduct problems overtime in more spatially crowded homes.
Barger et al., 2020 [58]	USA	Not reported	ASD	Cross-sectional	70,927	6–17	n.a.	Greenspace (tree canopy percentage).	Frequency of conduct disorder diagnosis and severity of conduct problems via The National Survey of Child Health (NSCH, 2012) [89].	Low	**No association:** % of tree canopy was not associated with diagnosis of conduct disorder. **Beneficial association:** caretakers residing in lower % tree canopy areas, reported more severe conduct problems in children with ASD.
Durand and Mapstone, 1997 [63]	USA	Not reported	ID + Cerebral Palsy + Seizure disorder	Quasi-experimental pre-post design	1	7	n.a.	Non-lyrical fast beat or slow beat music.	Observer rated frequency of challenging behaviours.	High	**Harmful association:** slow beat music was associated with increased challenging behaviours. **Beneficial association:** inversely fast beat music was associated with decreased challenging behaviours.
Gul et al., 2019 [91]	Pakistan	School	ID	RCT	40	6–16	6 months	Music (background new age and classical music).	Child-completed Buss Perry aggression questionnaire total scores [82].	Low	**Beneficial association:** background music was associated with a significant reduction in post-test aggression scores.
Oliver et al., 2001 [92]	UK	Therapy room	ID	Observational case study	1	14	n.a.	Distance of therapist to participant: close (0.067 m) and far distance (2 m).	Mean percentage of time the participant enacted aggressive behaviour.	High	**Harmful association:** increased proximity of the therapist was associated with increased duration of aggressive behaviour.
West et al., 2017 [93]	Australia	Psychiatric inpatient unit	NDDs (not specified)	Pre and post open trial.	112	12–18	Follow up post sensory room use.	Sensory room modification.	History of aggression/The Stepping Stones Sensory Room Questionnaire (SSSRQ) [93] measured distress levels pre- and post-sensory room use.	Unclear	**Beneficial association:** between reductions in client-reported stress following modified sensory room use and history of aggression was reported.

Table 3. GRADE summary of quality of evidence for typically developing children.

	Greenspace					
	Satellite Derived Neighbourhood Greenspace (NDVI)	Percentage of Land-Use Classified as Natural	Proximity of Child's Residence (m) to Nearest GREENSPACE	Percentage of Neighbourhood Greenspace	Access to Private Garden	Greenness Surrounding Residence (msavi)
Child self-reported aggression and conduct symptoms	Very Low quality 2 —Inconsistent effect b,c,d,e,f,g (8)	n.a.	n.a.	Very Low quality 1 —No effect a (1)	n.a.	n.a.
Parent reported child aggression and conduct symptoms		High quality—Beneficial effect h,i (2)	Very Low quality 3 —Inconsistent effect j (3)	High quality—No effect a (3)	Moderate quality 4 —Inconsistent effect k (3)	Very Low quality 5 —Beneficial effect L (1)

	Noise pollution		
	Residential aircraft noise exposure	Residential noise exposure	Predicted aircraft and road traffic noise exposure	High and low aircraft noise exposed schools	Predicted road traffic noise exposure
Child self-reported aggression and conduct symptoms	Very Low quality 1 —Harmful effect a (1)	Low quality 2 —Harmful effect b (1)	n.a.	Very Low quality 4 —Harmful effect d (3)	n.a.
Parent reported child aggression and conduct symptoms	Low 5 quality—No effect e (2)	n.a.	n.a.	Very Low quality 6 —Inconsistent effect f (2)	Very Low quality 7 —Inconsistent effect e,g,h,i (5)

( ) Number of studies included in each GRADE summary is denoted by numeric value inside of parentheses.

a Mueller et al., 2019 [134]: self-completed Strengths and Difficulties Questionnaire conduct problems subscale (SDQ) [96].
b Madzia et al., 2019 [111]: Parent-completed externalising subscale of the Behavioural Assessment System for Children, Parent Rating Scale, Second Edition (BASC-2) [99].
c Liao et al., 2020 [111]: Child Behavioural Checklist (CBCL) [100].
d Amoly et al., 2014 [106]: Parent-reported Strengths and Difficulties Questionnaire conduct problems subscale scores (SDQ) [96]/Parental Lithuanian version of the Strengths and Difficulties Questionnaire (SDQ) [134].
e Andrušaitytė et al., 2020 [112]: Parent-completed Lithuanian version of the Strengths and Difficulties Questionnaire (SDQ) [96].
f Jimenez et al., 2021 [113]: Parent and teacher completed externalising subscale of the Strengths and Difficulties Questionnaire (SDQ) [96].
g Lee and Movassaghi, 2021 [138]: Incidence rates of attacks or threats with or without weapons in schools
h Feng and Astell-Burt, 2017 [110]: Parent-completed externalising behaviour subscale scores (hyperactivity and conduct subscales combined) of the Strengths and Difficulties Questionnaire (SDQ) [96].
i Bijnens et al., 2020 [109]: Parent-completed Achenbach Child Behaviour Checklist (CBCL) [100].
j Markevych et al., 2014 [114], Balsevičienė et al., 2014 [108]: German parental version of the Strengths and Difficulties Questionnaire (SDQ) [85]), parent-reported Strengths and Difficulties Questionnaire (SDQ) [96] conduct problems subscale scores, parental Lithuanian version of the Strengths and Difficulties Questionnaire (SDQ) [134].
k Flouri et al., 2014 [111], Richardson et al., 2017 [120], Baird et al., 2022 [94]: Parent-reported Strengths and Difficulties Questionnaire (SDQ) conduct problems subscale scores [96].
L Lee et al., 2019 [116]: Parent-completed externalising subscale (Rule-breaking Behaviour and Aggressive Behaviour combined) of the Childhood Behavioural Checklist (CBCL) [103].

1 Downgraded due to inclusion of cross-sectional study design and inability to assess consistency.
2 Downgraded due to inclusion of cross-sectional study design and inconsistency.
3 Downgraded due to inclusion of cross-sectional study design and inconsistency.
4 Downgraded due to inconsistency.
5 Downgraded due to the inclusion of cross-sectional study design and inability to assess consistency.

1 Downgraded due to unclear risk of bias and inability to assess consistency.
2 Downgraded due inclusion of cross-sectional study design and inability to measure consistency—upgraded 1 level due to large effect size.
3 Downgraded due inclusion of cross-sectional study design and inability to measure consistency.
4 Downgraded due inclusion of cross-sectional study design and inconsistency.
5 Downgraded due inclusion of cross-sectional study design and inability to measure consistency.
6 Downgraded due to inclusion of cross-sectional study design and inconsistency.
7 Downgraded due to inclusion of cross-sectional study design and inconsistency.

a Spilski et al., 2019 [134]: Child self-reported annoyance questionnaire (KINDL-R) [101,102].
b Grelat et al., 2016 [126]: Child self-reported questionnaire on annoyance.
c Stansfeld et al., 2005 [131]: Child self-reported questionnaire on noise annoyance.
d Haines et al., 2001a [127], Haines et al., 2001b [128], Haines et al., 2001c [129]: Child self-report questionnaire on noise annoyance.
e Haines et al., 2001a [127], Crombie et al., 2011 [123]: Parent-completed conduct problems subscale of the Strengths and Difficulties Questionnaire (SDQ) [96].
f Haines et al., 2001a [127], Haines et al., 2001c [129]: Parent-completed conduct problems subscale of the Strengths and Difficulties Questionnaire (SDQ) [96].
g Tiesler et al., 2013 [130]: The conduct problems subscale of the German version of the Strengths and Difficulties Questionnaire (SDQ) [85].
h Bao et al., 2022 [122]: Parent-completed conduct problems subscale of the Strengths and Difficulties Questionnaire (SDQ) [96].
i Essers et al., 2022 [125]: Parent-completed conduct problems subscale of the Strengths and Difficulties Questionnaire (SDQ) [96] and Child Behavioural Checklist 6–18 (CBCL 6-18) [100].

Table 3. Cont.

	Air pollution							
	Active or passive tobacco smoke exposure	Nitrogen Dioxide (NO₂) exposure	Second-hand tobacco smoke exposure	Elemental carbon attributed to traffic (ECAT)	Particulate matter less than 2.5 microns (PM$_{2.5}$) exposure	Particulate matter less than 10 microns (PM$_{10}$) exposure	Ambient lead less than 2.5 microns (PM$_{2.5}$) exposure
Child self-reported aggression and conduct symptoms	Very Low quality 1—Harmful effect ᵃ (1)	n.a.	n.a.	n.a.	n.a.	n.a.	n.a.
Parent reported child aggression and conduct symptoms	n.a.	Very Low quality 2—Inconsistent effect ᵇ,ᶜ,ᵈ (3)	Very Low quality 3—Harmful effect ᵉ (1)	Moderate quality 5—No effect ᶠ (1)	Moderate quality 6—Inconsistent effect ᶜ,ᵈ (2)	n.a.	n.a.
Parent reported aggression and conduct symptoms	n.a.	Very Low quality 9—Inconsistent effects ᵏ,ˡ,ᵐ,ⁿ (4)	Low quality 4—Harmful effect ᶠ,ᵍ,ʰ (3)		Very Low quality 8—No effect ᵏ (1)	Very Low quality 10—No effect ⁿ (1)	Very Low quality 11—Harmful effect ᵒ (1)
Clinician derived aggressive behavioural disorder diagnosis	n.a.	n.a.	Very Low quality 7—Harmful effect ⁱ (1)	n.a.	n.a.	n.a.	n.a.

ᵃ Kolishadi et al., 2015 [42]: Self-reported information on anger and violent behaviours (World Health Organization Global School-based Student Health Survey: WHO-GSHS) [43].
ᵇ Mueller et al., 2019 [44]: Self-completed conduct problems subscale of the Strengths and Difficulties Questionnaire (SDQ) [45].
ᶜ Roberts et al., 2019 [46]: Child disorder symptoms were self-reported with reference to DSM-IV conduct disorder criteria [36].
ᵈ Karamanos et al., 2021 [44]: Child self-reported Strengths and Difficulties Questionnaire (SDQ) [45].
ᵉ Pagani et al., 2017 [46]: Child-completed proactive, reactive and conduct problem questionnaire.
ᶠ Bandiera et al., 2011 [35]: Parental reported DSM-IV conduct disorder symptoms via The National Institute of Mental Health's Diagnostic Interview Schedule for Children Version IV (DISC-IV) [36] and the Disruptive Behaviours Rating Scale (DBDRS) [37]; teachers completed the Teacher Observation of Child Adaptation-Revised (TOCA-R) [48].
ᵍ Gatzke-Kopp et al., 2020 [45]: Primary caregiver-completed conduct problems subscale of the Strengths and Difficulties Questionnaire (SDQ) [45].
ʰ Park et al., 2020 [47]: Parental completed Korean version of the Child Behaviour Checklist (CBCL).
ⁱ Newman et al., 2013 [48]: Parent-completed externalising subscale scores of the Behavioural Assessment System for Children, Parent Rating Scale, Second Edition (BASC-2) [49].
ʲ Bauer et al., 2015 [50]: Diagnosis of Disruptive Behaviour Disorder (DBD) identified using International Classification of Diseases-ninth revision (ICD-9) [51].
ᵏ Andrusaityte et al., 2020: Parent-completed Lithuanian version of the Strengths and Difficulties Questionnaire (SDQ) [45].
ˡ Baird et al., 2022 [52]: Parent-reported Strengths and Difficulties Questionnaire (SDQ) conduct problems subscale scores [45].
ᵐ Bao et al., 2022 [53]: Parent-reported Strengths and Difficulties Questionnaire (SDQ) conduct problems subscale scores [45].
ⁿ Loftus et al., 2020 [54]: Parent-completed Child Behaviour Checklist (CBCL; ages 1.5–5 years of age) [10].
ᵒ Rasnick et al., 2021 [55]: Parent-completed Behavioural Assessment System for Children, 2nd edition (BASC-2) [49].

	Meteorological effects					
	Summer seasonality	Humidity	Sunlight	Temperature (°C)	Student aggression during summer recess	Hours of precipitation per day	Tornado exposure
Observer rated child aggression	Very Low quality 1—Harmful effect ᵃ (1)	n.a.	n.a.	n.a.	n.a.	n.a.	n.a.
Teacher reported child aggression and conduct symptoms	n.a.	Low quality 2—Harmful effect ᵇ,ᶜ (2)	Very Low quality 3—Inconsistent effect ᵇ,ᶜ (2)	Low quality 4—Harmful effect ᵇ,ᶜ (2)	Low quality 5—Beneficial effect ᵈ (1)	n.a.	n.a.
Child self-reported aggression and conduct symptoms	n.a.	n.a.	Very Low quality 6—No effect ᵉ (1)	Very Low quality 6—Beneficial effect ᵉ (1)	n.a.	n.a.	n.a.
Parent reported child aggression and conduct symptoms	n.a.	n.a.	n.a.	Moderate quality 7—Harmful effect ᶠ (1)	n.a.	Very Low quality 6—No effect ᵉ (1)	Moderate quality 8—Harmful effect ᵍ (1)

ᵃ Munoz-Reyes et al., 2014 [56]: Observational recordings of school yard aggressive behaviours over an academic year used to construct an aggression intensity index.
ᵇ Lagacé-Séguin and d'Entremont, 2005 [40]: Teachers completed the Preschool Behaviour Questionnaire (PBQ) [57].
ᶜ Ciucci et al., 2013 [51]: Teacher-completed DBHQ questionnaire items derived from the Child Behaviour Checklist (CBCL/2-3) and Early Childhood Behaviour Questionnaire (ECBQ).
ᵈ Jones and Molano. 2016 [53]: Teacher Checklist [53]: Beneficial effect of summer recess in comparison to aggression during the school year.
ᵉ Klimstra et al., 2011 [53]: Self-report anger measured via the Daily Mood Scale, an Internet version of the Electronic Mood Device [58].
ᶠ Younan et al., 2018 [59]: Aggressive behaviour subscale of the parental completed Child Behaviour Checklist (CBCL) [10].
ᵍ Lochman et al., 2021 [53]: Parent Rating Scale (PRS) of the Behaviour Assessment System for Children (BASC) [49].

1 Downgraded due to high risk of bias, indirect measure of physical environment, and inability to assess consistency.
2 Downgraded due to inclusion of cross-sectional study design.
3 Downgraded due to inclusion of cross-sectional study design and inconsistency.
4 Downgraded due to inclusion of cross-sectional study design.
5 Downgraded due to indirectness and inability to assess consistency.
6 Downgraded due to inclusion of cross-sectional studies and inability to assess consistency.
7 Downgraded due to inability to assess consistency.
8 Downgraded due to inability to assess consistency.

1 Downgraded due to inclusion of cross-sectional study design and inability to assess consistency.
2 Downgraded due to inclusion of cross-sectional study design and inconsistency.
3 Downgraded due to high risk of bias, indirect physical environmental exposure metric, and inability to assess consistency.
4 Downgraded due to inclusion of cross-sectional study design.
5 Downgraded due to inability to measure consistency.
6 Downgraded due to inconsistency.
7 Downgraded due to inclusion of cross-sectional study design and inability to assess consistency.
8 Downgraded due to inclusion of cross-sectional study design and inability to assess consistency.
9 Downgraded due to inclusion of cross-sectional study design and inconsistency.
10 Downgraded due to inclusion of cross-sectional study design and inability to assess consistency.
11 Downgraded due to inclusion of cross-sectional study design and inability to assess consistency.

Table 3. Cont.

	Spatial density				
	Increased playroom openness (POP)	Space per child	Room group size	High density playrooms	Overcrowding of the home
Observer rated child aggression	Low quality [1]—Beneficial effect [a] (1)	Low quality [2]—No effect [a] (1)	Low quality [3]—No effect [a] (1)	Low quality [4]—Inconsistent effect [b,c] (3)	n.a.
Parent reported child aggression and conduct symptoms	n.a.	n.a.	n.a.	n.a.	Moderate quality [5]—Inconsistent effect [e,f] (2)
Teacher reported child aggression and conduct symptoms	n.a.	n.a.	n.a.	n.a.	Moderate quality [6]—Beneficial effect [g] (1)

[a] Neill, 1982 [163]: Observed frequencies of aggressive behaviour.
[b] Loo and Smetana, 1978 [162]: Observed frequencies of physically aggressive behaviours and anger.
[c] Loo and Kennelly, 1979 [161]: Observed frequency of physically aggressive behaviours and anger.
[d] Ginsburg et al., 1977 [164]: Observed frequency and duration of aggressive behaviours in the playground.
[e] Supplee et al., 2007 [165]: Mother-completed Child Behaviour Checklist (CBCL) [100].
[f] Baird et al., 2022 [4]: Parent-reported Strengths and difficulties questionnaire conduct problems subscale scores (SDQ) [64].
[g] Supplee et al., 2007 [165]: Teacher completed Teacher Report Form (TRF) [166].

	Urbanicity (Reference category urban)				
	Urban vs. rural residence			Urbanicity (density of residences surrounding address)	
Child self-reported aggression and conduct symptoms	Very Low quality [1]—Inconsistent effect [a,b,c] (1)	Schools recruited from urban and rural areas	Rural and urban children recruited from Head start centres.		
Parent reported child aggression and conduct symptoms	Moderate quality [2]—Inconsistent effects [d,e] (2)	Very Low quality [3]—No effect [f] (1)	n.a.	n.a.	
Teacher reported child aggression and conduct symptoms	Moderate quality [4]—No effect [g] (1)	Very Low quality [5]—Harmful effect [h] (1)	Very Low quality [6]—No effect [i] (1)	Low quality [7]—Harmful effect [j] (1)	

[a] Wongtongkam et al., 2016 [176]: Questionnaire modified from the Pittsburgh Youth Study's measure of serious violence [177].
[b] Wongtongkam et al., 2016 [176]: Frequency of anger was recorded via The State–Trait Anger Expression Inventory–2 (STAXI-2) [101].
[c] Wongtongkam et al., 2016 [176]: Self-reported violent offences obtained via a modified version of the Overt Victimisation subscale of the Problem Behaviour Frequency Scale [178].
[d] Sheridan et al., 2014 [172]: Parental questionnaire comprised of: the Preschool and Kindergarten Behaviour Scales [173], Social Skills Rating System [174], and Child Experiences Survey [175].
[e] Baird et al., 2022 [4]: Parent-reported Strengths and difficulties questionnaire conduct problems subscale scores (SDQ) [64].
[f] Hope and Bierman, 1998 [170]: Parent-completed Child Behaviour Checklist–Parent Rating Form (CBCL–PRF) [137].
[g] Sheridan et al., 2014 [172]: Teacher questionnaire comprised of: Preschool and Kindergarten Behaviour Scales [173], Social Skills Rating System [174], Child Experiences Survey [175].
[h] Hope and Bierman, 1998 [170]: Teacher completed Child Behaviour Checklist–Teacher Rating Form (CBCL–TRF) [71].
[i] Handal and Hopper, 1985 [168]: Teacher completed The AML Behaviour Rating Scale [167].
[j] Evans et al., 2018 [166]: The Problem Behaviour at School Interview (PBSI) [17].

1 Downgraded due to high risk of bias and inability to assess consistency.
2 Downgraded due to high risk of bias and inability to assess consistency.
3 Downgraded due to high risk of bias and inconsistency.
4 Downgraded due to high risk of bias and inconsistency of results.
5 Downgraded due to inconsistency of results.
6 Downgraded due to inability measure consistency.

1 Downgraded due to inclusion of cross-sectional study design and inconsistency.
2 Downgraded due to inability to assess consistency.
3 Downgraded due to inclusion of cross-sectional study design and inability to assess consistency.
4 Downgraded due to inability to assess consistency.
5 Downgraded due inclusion of cross-sectional study design and inability to assess consistency.
6 Downgraded due to High risk of bias and inability to assess consistency.
7 Downgraded due to High risk of bias and inability to assess consistency.

Table 3. Cont.

	Interior design			Music	
	Red painted classroom walls	Sensory room modification	Household damp problems	Alternating 15 m periods of silence and Instrumental music.	Aggressive content of child's favourite music artists
Child self-reported aggression and conduct symptoms	Low quality [1]—Harmful effect [a] (1)	n.a.	n.a.		
Observer rated child aggression	n.a.	Moderate quality [2]—Beneficial effect [b] (1)	n.a.	Low quality [1]—No effect [a] (1)	
Parent reported child aggression and conduct symptoms	n.a.	n.a.	Moderate quality [3]—Harmful effect [c] (1)		
Child self-reported aggression and conduct symptoms					Very Low quality [2]—Harmful effect [b] (1)

[a] Vakili et al., 2019 [83]: Buss Perry aggression questionnaire [38].
[b] Glod et al., 1994 [79]: Observer rated aggression using a modified version of the Overt aggression scale [38].
[c] Baird et al., 2022 [14]: Parent-reported Strengths and Difficulties Questionnaire (SDQ) conduct problems subscale scores [68]).

[1] Downgraded due to High risk of bias and inability to assess consistency.
[2] Downgraded due inability to assess consistency.
[3] Downgraded due inability to assess consistency.

[a] Hinds, 1980 [84]: Observer rated aggressive behaviours.
[b] Coyne and Padilla-Walker, 2015 [83]: Self-completed 5-item questionnaire on physical aggressive behaviour.

[1] Downgraded due to high risk of bias and inability to assess consistency. [2] Downgraded due to high risk of bias, indirect measure of physical environment, and inability to assess consistency.

Table 4. GRADE summary of quality of evidence for neurodiverse populations.

	Physical Environmental Exposure(s)							
	Satellite Derived Neighbourhood Tree Canopy Percentage	Non-Lyrical Fast Beat Music	Non-Lyrical Slow Beat Music	New Age and Classical Music	High Proximity of Therapist (Compared with Low Proximity)	Sensory Room Modification	Greenspace (NDVI), Air Pollution (NO_2), Private Garden Access, Urban Residence, Household Damp Problems.	Household Crowding
Clinician derived aggressive behaviour disorder	Very Low quality 1—No effect [a] (1)	n.a.	n.a.	n.a.	n.a.	n.a.	n.a.	n.a.
Parent reported child aggression and conduct symptoms	Very Low quality 1—Beneficial effect [b] (1)	n.a.	n.a.	n.a.	n.a.	n.a.	Moderate quality 6—No effect [g] (1)	Moderate quality 7—Beneficial effect [g] (1)
Observer rated child aggression	n.a.	Low quality 2—Beneficial effect [c] (1)	Low quality 2—Harmful effect [c] (1)	n.a.	Very Low quality 3—Harmful effect [d] (1)	n.a.	n.a.	n.a.
Child self-reported aggression and conduct symptoms	n.a.	n.a.	n.a.	Moderate quality 4—Beneficial effect [e] (1)	n.a.	Moderate quality 5—Beneficial effect [f] (1)	n.a.	n.a.

() Number of studies included in each GRADE summary is denoted by numeric value inside of parentheses.

[a] Barger et al., 2020 [88]: Previous clinician diagnosed aggressive behavioural disorder such as: Oppositional Defiant Disorder or Conduct Disorder retrieved from The National Survey of Children's Health (NSCH) [89].
[b] Barger et al., 2020 [88]: Parental reported severity of child's conduct problems retrieved from The National Survey of Children's Health (NSCH) [89].
[c] Durand and Mapstone, 1997 [90]: Observer rated frequency of challenging behaviours.
[d] Oliver et al., 2001 [92]: Mean percentage of time participant enacted aggressive behaviour.
[e] Gal et al., 2019 [91]: Child-completed Buss Perry aggression questionnaire total scores [182].
[f] West et al., 2017 [93]: History of aggression and distress via The Stepping Stones Sensory Room Questionnaire (SSSRQ) [93].
[g] Baird et al., 2022 [14]: Parent-reported Strengths and Difficulties Questionnaire (SDQ) conduct problems subscale scores [98].

1 Downgraded due to inclusion of cross-sectional study design and inability to assess consistency.
2 Downgraded due to high risk of bias and inability to assess consistency.
3 Downgraded due to High risk of bias, Indirectness, and inability to assess consistency.
4 Downgraded due to inability to assess consistency.
5 Downgraded due to inability to assess consistency.
6 Downgraded due to inability to assess consistency.
7 Downgraded due to inability to assess consistency.

3.1. Typically Developing Children

3.1.1. Greenspace

Eleven longitudinal and seven cross-sectional studies (~46,684 participants) examined associations between greenspace exposure and childhood aggression [34,106–122]. Five studies were carried out in the UK, four in the USA, two in Belgium, with the remaining in Australia, Korea, Lithuania, Germany, Spain and China. All greenspace studies were classified as low RoB.

Inconsistent evidence for harms or benefits was reported across eight studies [106–109,112,113,117,121] that examined associations between satellite derived neighbourhood greenspace (NDVI) and parental-reported child aggression related outcomes. Two studies [101,109] examining the association between parental-reported child aggression and conduct problems and percentage of land designated as natural land, reported high-quality evidence. Proximity of the child's residence to greenspace was inconsistently associated with parent reported conduct problems across three studies [106,108,114]. Very low-quality evidence [111,116,120] reported no relationship between percentage of neighbourhood greenspace and both child and parent-reported conduct problems. Moderate-quality evidence from three studies [34,111,120] reported inconsistent beneficial effects of access to private garden space on parent-reported conduct problems.

3.1.2. Environmental Sound and Noise

Three longitudinal and eight cross-sectional studies (n = 23,665) assessed the association between environmental noise pollution including road traffic, construction noise, aircraft noise and aggression outcomes [123–133]. These studies were primarily conducted in the UK, Spain, Germany, and the Netherlands, and one study in China. Three of these studies [124,131,132] used data from the multi-national RANCH study examining the influence of high and low road and aircraft noise on the behaviour of pupils who attended schools that were close to main roads or under flypaths. Two studies were judged to be of unclear RoB [126,130], with the majority being rated as low RoB. A very low-quality evidence for harmful association [130] between residential aircraft noise exposure and increased child annoyance was reported. Similarly, low- and very low-quality evidence was found for associations between increased residential noise [126], predicted air and road traffic noise [131], and heightened self-reported child annoyance. Schools located in areas of high aircraft noise were associated with increased child-reported annoyance [127–129], but inconsistently correlated with parent-reported child conduct problems ([127,129], both very low quality). Two studies [124,132] examining the role of residential aircraft noise on the parent-administered conduct problems subscale of the SDQ reported no association (low quality). Five studies [123–125,133,185] reported very low quality inconsistent evidence for estimated noise exposure effects on parent-reported child aggression.

Two studies (longitudinal and within-group repeated measures) from the USA (n = 658) assessed the association of music on childhood aggression [183,184]. Both studies were rated as high RoB. Aggressive or sexual music content was associated with increased self-reported aggressive behaviour in adolescents ([183], very low quality). Low-quality evidence reported no association between alternating periods of instrumental music and observer rated aggressive behaviours [184]).

3.1.3. Air Pollution

Eight longitudinal and six cross-sectional studies from Lithuania, China, Korea, Iran, Canada, USE, and the UK (n = 45,607) explored the influence of air particulate matter on aggressive behavioural outcomes in typically developing children and young people [34,107,116,123,135,136,138,141,142,144–149]. One study was rated as high RoB [146], one as unclear RoB [136], and the remaining as low RoB.

Five studies [135,136,146,147] provided either low- or very low-quality evidence supporting the harmful influences of tobacco smoke exposure across various aggressive behavioural questionnaires. Very Low-quality evidence for a harmful association [132] between active or passive tobacco exposure and child self-reported anger and aggressive behaviour was found.

Three studies [116,141,149] examined the relationship between Nitrogen Dioxide (NO2) exposure and child self-reported conduct problems symptoms and reported inconsistent evidence for a harmful association (Very Low quality). No effect of Elemental Carbon Attributed to Traffic (ECAT) on parent-reported externalising behaviours (BASC-2) was found ([145], Moderate quality).

In addition, there was inconsistent evidence for an association between exposure to particulate matter less than 2.5 microns (PM2.5), and child self-reported conduct problems [141,149]. No effect was found in a study that examined the influence of PM2.5 on parent reported conduct problem scores [107]. Another study by Loftus et al., 2020 [144] explored the influence of exposure to particulate matter less than 10 microns (PM10) on parent reported child aggressive behaviours but it did not show a significant association (Very Low quality). Ambient air lead exposure (PbA)) was associated with high parent-reported aggressive behaviour ([148], Very Low quality).

3.1.4. Meteorological Exposure

Five longitudinal and two cross-sectional studies (approximately = 6314) from Chile, Canada, the Netherlands, USA, and Italy, assessed associations between meteorological variables and child aggression outcomes [151–159]. One study was rated as high RoB [158] with the remaining studies rated as low RoB.

The study by Muñoz-Reyes et al. [158] contrasted the frequency of observed aggressive behaviours during the warm season (summer/spring) with the frequency of such behaviours during the cold season (autumn/winter), reporting Very Low-quality evidence for harmful effect of warm seasonality. Low-quality evidence associated increased humidity with harmful increases in teacher-reported child aggressive behaviours [151,156]. Studies examining the effects of sunlight exposure on teacher reported [151,156] and child self-assessment [152] behavioural outcomes reported inconsistent or no evidence, respectively (very low quality). Low- and Moderate-quality evidence for the harmful influence of increased temperature on teacher and parent-reported child aggression symptoms was reported in three studies [151,156,159]. However, we found one Very Low-quality study that provided evidence for beneficial effect of temperature on children's self-reported anger [152]. Aggression during summer recess was lower compared with aggression during the school year ([154]; Low quality). No association between hours of precipitation per day and children's self-reported anger was found ([152], Very Low-quality evidence). Finally, a study carried out by Lochman et al. [153] examined longitudinal associations between tornado exposure and externalising symptoms, and reported a harmful associations of Moderate quality.

3.1.5. Spatial Density and Interior Design

Four observational and two longitudinal studies [34,160–163,165] (n = 8568) from the USA and the UK examined spatial density and architectural design in relation to childhood aggression. RoB was judged as high in all studies except one rated as unclear [163] and one rated as low [34]. A study [165] reported a beneficial effect of increased playroom openness, but no effect of space per child or room group size on observed aggressive behaviours. Low-quality evidence assessing the association between high density (in comparison to low density) child playrooms and frequency of aggressive behaviours reported inconsistent results [160–162]. Moderate-quality evidence examining the effect of overcrowding in the home [34,163] reported inconsistent associations with parent-reported conduct problems but was associated with reduced teacher-reported externalising behaviours.

Three studies, two quasi-experimental and one longitudinal (n = 8257) conducted in Iran, the UK, and the USA examined the associations between interior design features and childhood aggression [34,179,181]. Low-quality evidence of association ([181] unclear RoB) between red painted classroom walls and increased self-reported aggression was found. In-patient psychiatric ward sensory room modifications were correlated with beneficial reductions in observer rated aggressive behaviour ([179] unclear RoB Moderate quality). Additionally, presence of damp in the house was associated with elevated trajectories of conduct problems in children ([34], Moderate quality).

3.1.6. Urbanicity and Rurality

Three longitudinal and three cross-sectional studies (n = 17,630) from the USA, the Netherlands, and Thailand explored the influence of urbanicity and rurality of residence on children's aggressive behavioural outcomes [34,164,168,170,172,176]. One study was rated as high RoB [168] with the remaining assessed as low or moderate RoB. One study [176] reported inconsistent associations between the location of the participants and scores across three self-reported aggression outcomes (Very Low quality). Moderate-quality inconsistent evidence [34,172] was reported for the effect of urban residence on child conduct problems and aggressive behaviour in parent-reported questionnaires, whilst evidence for a lack of association was found for teacher-completed aggression outcomes [172]. Another study [170] examined the effects of urban or rural settings on aggressive behaviours in schoolchildren attending schools from either setting. It reported no association of setting with parent-reported behaviours, but a harmful effect of urban school location on teacher-assessed behaviours (both Very Low quality). Very Low-quality evidence reported no association between children recruited from rural or urban Head Start centres and teacher-reported anger ratings ([168]: AML Behaviour Rating Scale). Neighbourhood urbanicity (mean number of addresses within a 1 km radius of participant's residence) was associated with increased teacher-reported child problem behaviours ([166] Low quality).

3.2. Neurodiverse Children

Six studies (n = 79,249) from the USA, Pakistan, the UK, and Australia included neurodiverse participants exclusively [34,188,190–193]. The studies are heterogenous utilising a variety of designs including longitudinal, cross-sectional, quasi-experimental, interventional, including two case studies. Two studies were judged to be of high RoB [190,192], one unclear [193] and the remaining three of low RoB.

Baird et al. [34] explored interaction effects between a sub-sample of children with intellectual disability (assessed via cognitive measures) from the Millennium Cohort Study (MCS) and various physical environmental exposures (neighbourhood greenspace: NDVI, access to a private garden, air pollution: NO_2, urban or rural residence, household density, presence of damp. The authors reported no mediating influence of intellectual disability on the association between environmental exposures and children's conduct problem trajectories, except for household density (beneficial effect, moderate quality). Another study [188] reported no correlation between urban tree canopy coverage and frequency of aggressive behaviours in children with ASD but found an association between residing in lower urban tree canopy areas with increased parent-reported conduct problem severity. However, the evidence was deemed to be of low quality in both studies. The case study by Durand and Mapstone [190] examined the impact of fast and slow beat music on a child with intellectual disability, reporting reductions in observed frequency of aggressive behaviour during the fast beat condition and increases during the slow beat condition in comparison to a no-music baseline (Low quality). Additionally, a clinical trial of new age and classical music [191] provided Moderate-quality evidence for the beneficial effects of music on self-reported aggression in children with intellectual disabilities. A case study [192] assessing the impact of spatial proximity between an adolescent girl with intellectual disability and the therapist, provided a Very Low-quality evidence for a correlation between closer proximity and increased duration of observed aggressive behaviours. Finally, a study [193] examined the efficacy of modified sensory rooms in reducing distress in adolescent psychiatric inpatients, reporting additional benefits for individuals who had a history of aggression (Moderate quality).

4. Discussion

This is the first narrative review that updates previous literature across several environmental domains as well as including neurodiverse children, a previously under reported population in other reviews.

4.1. Physical Environmental Domains

4.1.1. Greenspace

We found evidence that supports the therapeutic benefits of increased natural land and greenness surrounding child residences. Previous reviews have also shown associations between greenspace exposure and reductions in violent behaviours [194,195].

The greenspace evidence synthesised primarily supports the therapeutic influence of neighbourhood nature exposure on child aggressive behavioural outcomes. These effects, at least partially, were also present in NDDs populations. Whilst more epidemiological and experimental research paradigms are required to solidify the evidence for this therapeutic relationship and understand its underlying mechanistic pathways, we provide initial evidence for the role of nature in reducing aggression in neurotypical and diverse children. Initial attempts at establishing guidelines for integration and therapeutic adoption are beginning to be developed [196]. Studies examining socio-cultural barriers to children accessing urban greenspaces [197] are of crucial importance, but these findings need to be communicated to institutions and policy decision makers. We also recommend future experimental studies that aim to elucidate the underlying (neuro)mechanistic pathways via which nature exposure conveys these potential benefits. Advances in this regard would drastically redefine architectural and urban design for physical and mental health.

4.1.2. Noise Pollution

Children appear to consistently self-report higher aggressive and annoyance related behaviours related to environmental noise, whereas parent reported outcomes either show a lack of association or inconsistent associations both for harm and benefit. This may suggest that noise exposure operates on pathways involving subjective annoyance and irritation which may not translate into objective longer-term increases in aggression problems. Additionally, although noise annoyance may not play a direct role in the aetiology of those problems, noise exposure of individuals who experience frustration or irritable mood has been shown to increase its severity [25,26]. Noise pollution, therefore, may not operate as a causal mechanism of aggression, but exacerbate pre-existing manifestation, potentially via draining of attentional and cognitive resources, leading to increased self-regulatory difficulties [27].

4.1.3. Air Pollution

We found absent and inconsistent associations between ECAT, particulate matter less than PM2.5, particulate matter less than PM10 and NO_2 exposure and childhood aggression problems. Tobacco smoke exposure showed a harmful association with aggressive behavioural outcomes irrespective of who was the outcome assessor. We also found this harmful association for childhood exposure to ambient air lead exposure (PbA). The lack of association of PM2.5 and PM10 with these behaviours is potentially anomalous when considering research that has linked air pollution with increased risk of mental health disorders [198]. The harmful effects of tobacco smoke and ambient lead exposure may increase the risk of neuropsychiatric disorders and violent crime, possibly via neuroinflammation [19–24].

Whilst none of the retrieved articles examined the effects of air pollution on neurodiverse children, it was shown that families of these children disproportionately reside in areas of higher particulate concentration than those of typically developing children [49], as well as exhibiting elevated rates of aggressive behaviour [199,200].

4.1.4. Meteorological Effects

Summer seasonality, humidity, temperature, and previous tornado exposure were consistently correlated with increased childhood aggressive behaviours. We found little evidence for either harmful or beneficial effects of ambient temperature and seasonality. Previous studies suggest that humidity compounds the negative effects of heat on mental health [201], as well as being associated with increased emergency department visits for mental health problems [202]. Elevated temperature has also been associated with increased violent crime [203]; however, those associations warrant further examination.

4.1.5. Spatial Density

The negative impact of high spatial density on aggression in young people [204] and inpatients in psychiatric wards has been highlighted previously [205–207]. Notwithstanding the beneficial effects of increased playroom openness, inconsistent influences for other spatial characteristics prevent a firm explanation of findings. Theories have posited that high spatial density triggers perceptions of crowding and a subsequent physiological stress arousal response [30–32]. Further studies on possible mechanistic pathways between high spatial density and aggression in children could lead to therapeutic adaptations in clinical and residential spaces [208].

4.1.6. Urbanicity and Rurality of Residence

Due to the quality of retrieved evidence, we were unable to extricate any definitive conclusions for associations between urban or rural residence and childhood aggressive behaviours. This is potentially anomalous considering that children residing in rural areas are exposed to more greenspace which generally appears to have calming effects [209–214]. Rurality, however, is only one factor in a great number of confounders on childhood aggression. Furthermore, studies do not often use operationalised definitions of "rural" or "rurality" [215], potentially leading to heterogeneity in the underlying conceptual constructs being examined, limiting the replicability and specificity of results.

4.1.7. Interior Design and Housing Quality

Previous work has associated damp problems with increased toxic mould, contributing to poor air quality [216] and/or potential neuroinflammatory and/or neurotoxic responses [20,22]. Damp in a house may also be associated with other adversities such as low socio-economic status and household disruption [217] exemplified by previous research linking poor household conditions to psychological distress [218].

Whilst preliminary evidence from this review supported the positive impact of modified sensory rooms to de-escalate aggression, it is very limited in scope. One study [35] suggested that the increased reduction in distress related to sensory deficits may be attributable to a sense of autonomy children and young people may gain by using the room unaccompanied.

4.1.8. Music

We found preliminary evidence for the therapeutic potential of music in neurodiverse children which is similar with findings reported in adults [219]. Music listening has been associated with a broad range of psychological and physiological benefits [38–40]. Some [36,37] have stated that the therapeutic influences of music may operate mechanistically via enhancing emotional regulation, but such evidence is not yet available [41]. Music is a complex physical phenomenon, which requires additional targeted research to examine its effects on aggressive behaviours in typically developing and neurodiverse young people.

4.2. Strengths and Limitations

This review is comprehensive and has examined the evidence of a wide range of environmental exposures in relation to the display of aggressive behaviours in typical and neurodiverse children. To the best of our knowledge, this is the first review that comparatively examines available research on environmental determinants of aggression in these two groups. The review shows clearly the disproportionately sparse literature relating those children and the physical environment despite the fact that they are more likely to be affected by social adversity, poor housing, air pollutants, and poverty [48–50,220,221].

The incorporation of GRADE to assess the quality of evidence in this review may well be simultaneously both a strength and a limitation. Whilst it facilitated the examination of the certainty of included evidence, the adaptation of GRADE for use in a non-meta-analytic review including epidemiological studies, may, as highlighted previously [95], inadvertently result in downgrading of evidence irrespective of study quality. We also adopted a modified risk of bias protocol which may have impacted the RoB assessments of included studies. There may also have been potential conflicts of interest based on the source of funding which we did not consider in this review.

A final limitation of this evidence synthesis is the inclusion of studies that adopt a diverse range of heterogenous physical environmental exposures and metrics. As has been highlighted previously by experts in physical environmental epidemiological analysis on child socio-cognitive outcomes [116], further research is needed on improving environmental measures of aspects such as air pollution exposure, and access to and quality of children's greenspaces. Developing more holistic, accurate, and reliable measures of environmental exposures will facilitate novel research paradigms (computational, simulatory and experimental) that can elucidate the influences of these aspects, reciprocally informing direction for future research into (neurobiological)mechanistic pathways.

5. Conclusions

Physical environmental exposures sit at the intersection of social, biochemical, and (epi)genetic aetiological influences on the development and progression of a spectrum of physical and mental health outcomes. Further research can support stakeholders, ranging from city planners and environmental legislators to politicians and clinicians, in considering the role of the physical environment in the context of adverse impact on child (neuro)development. Whilst there is obvious need to further examine environmental and climate influences on mental health of all children, particular attention must be paid to neurodiverse children and their families. A recent report recommended that in order to pursue and achieve health parity for those children, we must "reduce poverty and improve living environments" [50]. Research focusing on that population will help to bridge the equity gap that has significant therapeutic and health implications for all citizens.

Supplementary Materials: The following supporting information can be downloaded at: https://www.mdpi.com/article/10.3390/ijerph20032549/s1, Table S1: search strategy.

Author Contributions: Conceptualization: E.F., A.H., N.T. and A.B.; methodology, A.H., A.B. and B.C.; writing—original draft preparation, A.B.; writing—review and editing, N.T., B.C. and A.H. All authors have read and agreed to the published version of the manuscript.

Funding: This research received no external funding.

Institutional Review Board Statement: Not applicable.

Informed Consent Statement: Not applicable.

Data Availability Statement: Not applicable.

Acknowledgments: We thank Nancy Kouroupa, Steven Naughton, Laura Paulauskaite, Peiyao Tang and Rachel Royston for assisting in co-screening studies; Bori Vegh for support with preparation of the manuscript; Louise Marston, for guidance on study heterogeneity and narrative synthesis reporting; Deborah Marletta for assistance with the electronic database protocol development.

Conflicts of Interest: Multiple studies included in this review involved the authorship of Eirini Flouri. Flouri had no influence/involvement in the selection or appraisal of these studies. No other authors report any potential conflict of interest.

References

1. Wild, C.P. Complementing the Genome with an "Exposome": The Outstanding Challenge of Environmental Exposure Measurement in Molecular Epidemiology. *Cancer Epidemiol. Biomark. Prev.* **2005**, *14*, 1847–1850. [CrossRef] [PubMed]
2. Wild, C.P. The exposome: From concept to utility. *Int. J. Epidemiol.* **2012**, *41*, 24–32. [CrossRef] [PubMed]
3. Bronfenbrenner, U. Toward an experimental ecology of human development. *Am. Psychol.* **1977**, *32*, 513–531. [CrossRef]
4. Bronfenbrenner, U. *The Ecology of Human Development: Experiments by Nature and Design*; Harvard University Press: Cambridge, MA, USA, 1949.
5. Bronfenbrenner, U.; Ceci, S.J. Nature-nuture reconceptualized in developmental perspective: A bioecological model. *Psychol. Rev.* **1994**, *101*, 568–586. [CrossRef] [PubMed]
6. Vineis, P.; Robinson, O.; Chadeau-Hyam, M.; Dehghan, A.; Mudway, I.; Dagnino, S. What is new in the exposome? *Environ. Int.* **2020**, *143*, 105887. [CrossRef] [PubMed]
7. Harris, P.B.; McBride, G.; Ross, C.; Curtis, L. A Place to Heal: Environmental Sources of Satisfaction Among Hospital Patients1. *J. Appl. Soc. Psychol.* **2002**, *32*, 1276–1299. [CrossRef]
8. Davison, K.K.; Lawson, C.T. Do attributes in the physical environment influence children's physical activity? A review of the literature. *Int. J. Behav. Nutr. Phys. Act.* **2006**, *3*, 19. [CrossRef]
9. Markevych, I.; Schoierer, J.; Hartig, T.; Chudnovsky, A.; Hystad, P.; Dzhambov, A.M.; de Vries, S.; Triguero-Mas, M.; Brauer, M.; Nieuwenhuijsen, M.J.; et al. Exploring pathways linking greenspace to health: Theoretical and methodological guidance. *Environ. Res.* **2017**, *158*, 301–317. [CrossRef]
10. Luque-García, L.; Corrales, A.; Lertxundi, A.; Díaz, S.; Ibarluzea, J. Does exposure to greenness improve children's neuropsychological development and mental health? A Navigation Guide systematic review of observational evidence for associations. *Environ. Res.* **2022**, *206*, 112599. [CrossRef]
11. Berto, R. The Role of Nature in Coping with Psycho-Physiological Stress: A Literature Review on Restorativeness. *Behav. Sci.* **2014**, *4*, 394–409. [CrossRef]
12. Ulrich, R.S. Natural Versus Urban Scenes: Some Psychophysiological Effects. *Environ. Behav.* **1981**, *13*, 523–556. [CrossRef]
13. Ulrich, R.S.; Simons, R.F.; Losito, B.D.; Fiorito, E.; Miles, M.A.; Zelson, M. Stress recovery during exposure to natural and urban environments. *J. Environ. Psychol.* **1991**, *11*, 201–230. [CrossRef]
14. Kaplan, R.; Kaplan, S. *The Experience of Nature: A Psychological Perspective*; Cambridge University Press: Cambridge, UK, 1989; ISBN 978-0-521-34139-4.
15. Ohly, H.; White, M.P.; Wheeler, B.W.; Bethel, A.; Ukoumunne, O.C.; Nikolaou, V.; Garside, R. Attention Restoration Theory: A systematic review of the attention restoration potential of exposure to natural environments. *J. Toxicol. Environ. Health Part B* **2016**, *19*, 305–343. [CrossRef] [PubMed]
16. Sumitomo, K.; Akutsu, H.; Fukuyama, S.; Minoshima, A.; Kukita, S.; Yamamura, Y.; Sato, Y.; Hayasaka, T.; Osanai, S.; Funakoshi, H.; et al. Conifer-Derived Monoterpenes and Forest Walking. *Mass Spectrom.* **2015**, *4*, A0042. [CrossRef]
17. Pagès, A.B.; Peñuelas, J.; Clarà, J.; Llusià, J.; Campillo i López, F.; Maneja, R. How Should Forests Be Characterized in Regard to Human Health? Evidence from Existing Literature. *Int. J. Environ. Res. Public Health* **2020**, *17*, 1027. [CrossRef]
18. Bratman, G.N.; Hamilton, J.P.; Hahn, K.S.; Daily, G.C.; Gross, J.J. Nature experience reduces rumination and subgenual prefrontal cortex activation. *Proc. Natl. Acad. Sci. USA* **2015**, *112*, 8567–8572. [CrossRef]
19. Bondy, M.; Roth, S.; Sager, L. Crime Is in the Air: The Contemporaneous Relationship between Air Pollution and Crime. *J. Assoc. Environ. Resour. Econ.* **2020**, *7*, 555–585. [CrossRef]
20. Brockmeyer, S.; D'Angiulli, A. How air pollution alters brain development: The role of neuroinflammation. *Transl. Neurosci.* **2016**, *7*, 24–30. [CrossRef]
21. Burkhardt, J.; Bayham, J.; Wilson, A.; Berman, J.D.; O'Dell, K.; Ford, B.; Fischer, E.V.; Pierce, J.R. The relationship between monthly air pollution and violent crime across the United States. *J. Environ. Econ. Policy* **2019**, *9*, 188–205. [CrossRef]
22. Calderón-Garcidueñas, L.; Leray, E.; Heydarpour, P.; Torres-Jardón, R.; Reis, J. Air pollution, a rising environmental risk factor for cognition, neuroinflammation and neurodegeneration: The clinical impact on children and beyond. *Rev. Neurol.* **2016**, *172*, 69–80. [CrossRef]
23. Herrnstadt, E.; Heyes, A.; Muehlegger, E.; Saberian, S. Air Pollution as a Cause of Violent Crime: Evidence from Los Angeles and Chicago. Manuscript in preparation, 2016. Available online: http://www.erichmuehlegger.com/Working%20Papers/crime_and_Pollution_fv.pdf (accessed on 25 March 2021).
24. Lu, J.G. Air pollution: A systematic review of its psychological, economic, and social effects. *Curr. Opin. Psychol.* **2019**, *32*, 52–65. [CrossRef] [PubMed]

25. Donnerstein, E.; Wilson, D.W. Effects of noise and perceived control on ongoing and subsequent aggressive behavior. *J. Pers. Soc. Psychol.* **1976**, *34*, 774–781. [CrossRef] [PubMed]
26. Konecni, V.J. The mediation of aggressive behavior: Arousal level versus anger and cognitive labeling. *J. Pers. Soc. Psychol.* **1975**, *32*, 706–712. [CrossRef] [PubMed]
27. Mueller, M.A.; Flouri, E. Neighbourhood greenspace and children's trajectories of self-regulation: Findings from the UK Millennium Cohort Study. *J. Environ. Psychol.* **2020**, *71*, 101472. [CrossRef]
28. Cohen, L.E.; Felson, M. Social Change and Crime Rate Trends: A Routine Activity Approach. *Am. Sociol. Rev.* **1979**, *44*, 588–608. [CrossRef]
29. Anderson, C.A.; Deuser, W.E.; DeNeve, K.M. Hot temperatures, hostile affect, hostile cognition, and arousal: Tests of a general model of affective externalising behaviours. *Pers. Soc. Psychol. Bull.* **1995**, *21*, 434–448. [CrossRef]
30. Cox, T.; Houdmont, J.; Griffiths, A. Rail passenger crowding, stress, health and safety in Britain. *Transp. Res. Part A Policy Pract.* **2006**, *40*, 244–258. [CrossRef]
31. Aiello, J.R.; Nicosia, G.; Thompson, D.E. Physiological, Social, and Behavioral Consequences of Crowding on Children and Adolescents. *Child Dev.* **1979**, *50*, 195–202. [CrossRef]
32. Walden, T.A.; Forsyth, D.R. Close encounters of the stressful kind: Affective, physiological, and behavioral reactions to the experience of crowding. *J. Nonverbal Behav.* **1981**, *6*, 46–64. [CrossRef]
33. Lawrence, D.L.; Low, S.M. The Built Environment and Spatial Form. *Annu. Rev. Anthropol.* **1990**, *19*, 453–505. [CrossRef]
34. Baird, A.; Papachristou, E.; Hassiotis, A.; Flouri, E. The role of physical environmental characteristics and intellectual disability in conduct problem trajectories across childhood: A population-based Cohort study. *Environ. Res.* **2022**, *209*, 112837. [CrossRef] [PubMed]
35. Lindberg, H.M.; Samuelsson, M.; Perseius, K.-I.; Björkdahl, A. The experiences of patients in using sensory rooms in psychiatric inpatient care. *Int. J. Ment. Health Nurs.* **2019**, *28*, 930–939. [CrossRef] [PubMed]
36. Juslin, P.N.; Sloboda, J. *Handbook of Music and Emotion: Theory, Research, Applications*; Oxford University Press: Oxford, UK, 2011.
37. Saarikallio, S.; Erkkilä, J. The role of music in adolescents' mood regulation. *Psychol. Music.* **2007**, *35*, 88–109. [CrossRef]
38. McKinney, C.H.; Antoni, M.H.; Kumar, M.; Tims, F.C.; McCabe, P.M. Effects of guided imagery and music (GIM) therapy on mood and cortisol in healthy adults. *Health Psychol.* **1997**, *16*, 390–400. [CrossRef]
39. Lai, H.-L.; Good, M. Music improves sleep quality in older adults. *J. Adv. Nurs.* **2006**, *53*, 134–144. [CrossRef]
40. Teng, X.F.; Wong, M.Y.M.; Zhang, Y.T. The Effect of Music on Hypertensive Patients. In Proceedings of the 2007 29th Annual International Conference of the IEEE Engineering in Medicine and Biology Society, Lyon, France, 22–26 August 2007; pp. 4649–4651. [CrossRef]
41. Thoma, M.; Scholz, U.; Ehlert, U.; Nater, U. Listening to music and physiological and psychological functioning: The mediating role of emotion regulation and stress reactivity. *Psychol. Health* **2012**, *27*, 227–241. [CrossRef] [PubMed]
42. Evans, G.W. Child Development and the Physical Environment. *Annu. Rev. Psychol.* **2006**, *57*, 423–451. [CrossRef] [PubMed]
43. Clark, C.; Myron, R.; Stansfeld, S.; Candy, B. A systematic review of the evidence on the effect of the built and physical environment on mental health. *J. Public Ment. Health* **2007**, *6*, 14–27. [CrossRef]
44. Simons, R.L.; Lei, M.K.; Beach, S.R.H.; Brody, G.H.; Philibert, R.; Gibbons, F.X. Social Environment, Genes, and Aggression: Evidence Supporting the Differential Susceptibility Perspective. *Am. Sociol. Rev.* **2011**, *76*, 883–912. [CrossRef]
45. Ferguson, K.T.; Cassells, R.C.; MacAllister, J.W.; Evans, G.W. The physical environment and child development: An international review. *Int. J. Psychol.* **2013**, *48*, 437–468. [CrossRef]
46. Waltes, R.; Chiocchetti, A.G.; Freitag, C.M. The neurobiological basis of human aggression: A review on genetic and epigenetic mechanisms. *Am. J. Med. Genet. Part B Neuropsychiatr. Genet.* **2015**, *171*, 650–675. [CrossRef]
47. Gao, Y.; Zhang, L.; Kc, A.; Wang, Y.; Zou, S.; Chen, C.; Huang, Y.; Mi, X.; Zhou, H. Housing environment and early childhood development in sub-Saharan Africa: A cross-sectional analysis. *PLoS Med.* **2021**, *18*, e1003578. [CrossRef]
48. Blackburn, C.M.; Spencer, N.J.; Read, J.M. Prevalence of childhood disability and the characteristics and circum-stances of disabled children in the UK: Secondary analysis of the Family Resources Survey. *BMC Pediatr.* **2010**, *10*, 21. [CrossRef] [PubMed]
49. Emerson, E.; Robertson, J.; Hatton, C.; Baines, S. Risk of exposure to air pollution among British children with and without intellectual disabilities. *J. Intellect. Disabil. Res.* **2019**, *63*, 161–167. [CrossRef] [PubMed]
50. Rickard, W.; Donkin, A. A Fair, Supportive Society: Summary Report; Institute of Health Equity. 2022. Available online: https://www.instituteofhealthequity.org/resources-reports/a-fair-supportive-society-summary-report/a-fair-supportive-society-summary-report.pdf (accessed on 10 January 2023).
51. Anaby, D.; Hand, C.; Bradley, L.; DiRezze, B.; Forhan, M.; Digiacomo, A.; Law, M. The effect of the environment on participation of children and youth with disabilities: A scoping review. *Disabil. Rehabil.* **2013**, *35*, 1589–1598. [CrossRef]
52. Law, M.; Petrenchik, T.; King, G.; Hurley, P. Perceived environmental barriers to recreational, community, and school participation for children and youth with physical disabilities. *Arch. Phys. Med. Rehabil.* **2007**, *88*, 1636–1642. [CrossRef] [PubMed]
53. von Benzon, N. Discussing Nature, 'Doing' Nature: For an emancipatory approach to conceptualizing young people's access to outdoor green space. *Geoforum* **2018**, *93*, 79–86. [CrossRef]
54. Visser, E.M.; Berger, H.J.C.; Prins, J.B.; Van Schrojenstein Lantman-De Valk, H.M.J.; Teunisse, J.P. Shifting impairment and aggression in intellectual disability and Autism Spectrum Disorder. *Res. Dev. Disabil.* **2014**, *35*, 2137–2147. [CrossRef]

55. Hassiotis, A.; Parkes, C.; Jones, L.; Fitzgerald, B.; Romeo, R. Individual Characteristics and Service Expenditure on Challenging Behaviour for Adults with Intellectual Disabilities. *J. Appl. Res. Intellect. Disabil.* **2008**, *21*, 438–445. [CrossRef]
56. Kiely, J.; Pankhurst, H. Violence faced by staff in a learning disability service. *Disabil. Rehabil.* **1998**, *20*, 81–89. [CrossRef]
57. Brosnan, J.; Healy, O. A review of behavioral interventions for the treatment of aggression in individuals with developmental disabilities. *Res. Dev. Disabil.* **2011**, *32*, 437–446. [CrossRef]
58. Maughan, B.; Rutter, M. Antisocial children grown up. In *Conduct Disorders in Childhood and Adolescence*; Hill, J., Maughan, B., Eds.; Cambridge University Press: Cambridge, UK, 2001; pp. 507–552, ISBN 0521786398(pb).
59. Romeo, R.; Knapp, M.; Scott, S. Economic cost of severe antisocial behaviour in children—And who pays it. *Br. J. Psychiatry* **2006**, *188*, 547–553. [CrossRef] [PubMed]
60. Broidy, L.; Willits, D.; Denman, K.; Schools and neighborhood crime. Prepared for Justice Research Statistics Association 2009. Available online: http://isr.unm.edu/reports/2009/schools-and-crime.pdf (accessed on 14 October 2022).
61. Reef, J.; Diamantopoulou, S.; Van Meurs, I.; Verhulst, F.; Van Der Ende, J. Child to adult continuities of psychopathology: A 24-year follow-up. *Acta Psychiatr. Scand.* **2009**, *120*, 230–238. [CrossRef] [PubMed]
62. White, S.W.; Roberson-Nay, R. Anxiety, Social Deficits, and Loneliness in Youth with Autism Spectrum Disorders. *J. Autism Dev. Disord.* **2009**, *39*, 1006–1013. [CrossRef] [PubMed]
63. Foster, E.M.; Jones, D.E. The Conduct Problems Prevention Research Group The High Costs of Aggression: Public Expenditures Resulting from Conduct Disorder. *Am. J. Public Health* **2005**, *95*, 1767–1772. [CrossRef] [PubMed]
64. Dagnan, D.; Weston, C. Physical Intervention with People with Intellectual Disabilities: The Influence of Cognitive and Emotional Variables. *J. Appl. Res. Intellect. Disabil.* **2006**, *19*, 219–222. [CrossRef]
65. Shoham-Vardi, I.; Davidson, P.W.; Cain, N.N.; Sloane-Reeves, J.E.; Giesow, V.E.; Quijano, L.E.; Houser, K.D. Factors predicting re-referral following crisis intervention for community-based persons with developmental disabilities and behavioral and psychiatric disorders. *Am. J. Ment. Retard.* **1996**, *101*, 109–117.
66. Dryden-Edwards, R.C.; Combrinck-Graham, L. *Developmental Disabilities from Childhood to Adulthood: What Works for Psychiatrists in Community and Institutional Settings*; John Hopkins University Press: Baltimore, MA, USA, 2010; ISBN 10: 0801894182.
67. Hodgetts, S.; Nicholas, D.B.; Zwaigenbaum, L. Home Sweet Home? Families' Experiences with Aggression in Children with Autism Spectrum Disorders. *Focus Autism Other Dev. Disabil.* **2013**, *28*, 166–174. [CrossRef]
68. Raaijmakers, M.A.; Posthumus, J.A.; Van Hout, B.A.; Van Engeland, H.; Matthys, W. Cross-Sectional Study into the Costs and Impact on Family Functioning of 4-Year-Old Children with Aggressive Behavior. *Prev. Sci.* **2011**, *12*, 192–200. [CrossRef]
69. Neece, C.L.; Green, S.A.; Baker, B.L. Parenting Stress and Child Behavior Problems: A Transactional Relationship Across Time. *Am. J. Intellect. Dev. Disabil.* **2012**, *117*, 48–66. [CrossRef]
70. Otero-López, J.M.; Bolaño, C.C.; Mariño, M.J.S.; Pol, E.V. Exploring stress, burnout, and job dissatisfaction in secondary school teachers. *Int. J. Psychol. Psychol. Ther.* **2010**, *10*, 107–123.
71. McLaren, J.L.; Lichtenstein, J.D. The pursuit of the magic pill: The overuse of psychotropic medications in children with intellectual and developmental disabilities in the USA. *Epidemiol. Psychiatr. Sci.* **2018**, *28*, 365–368. [CrossRef] [PubMed]
72. Bassarath, L. Medication Strategies in Childhood Aggression: A Review. *Can. J. Psychiatry* **2003**, *48*, 367–373. [CrossRef] [PubMed]
73. Girimaji, S.C.; Pradeep, A.J.V. Intellectual disability in international classification of Diseases-11: A developmental perspective. *Indian J. Soc. Psychiatry* **2018**, *34*, 68–74. [CrossRef]
74. Maulik, P.K.; Mascarenhas, M.N.; Mathers, C.D.; Dua, T.; Saxena, S. Prevalence of intellectual disability: A meta-analysis of population-based studies. *Res. Dev. Disabil.* **2011**, *32*, 419–436. [CrossRef]
75. Bowring, D.L.; Totsika, V.; Hastings, R.P.; Toogood, S.; Griffith, G.M. Challenging behaviours in adults with an intellectual disability: A total population study and exploration of risk indices. *Br. J. Clin. Psychol.* **2017**, *56*, 16–32. [CrossRef]
76. Crocker, A.G.; Mercier, C.; Lachapelle, Y.; Brunet, A.; Morin, D.; Roy, M.-E. Prevalence and types of aggressive behaviour among adults with intellectual disabilities. *J. Intellect. Disabil. Res.* **2006**, *50*, 652–661. [CrossRef] [PubMed]
77. Lowe, K.; Allen, D.; Jones, E.; Brophy, S.; Moore, K.; James, W. Challenging behaviours: Prevalence and topographies. *J. Intellect. Disabil. Res.* **2007**, *51*, 625–636. [CrossRef]
78. Emerson, E.; Hatton, C. Mental health of children and adolescents with intellectual disabilities in Britain. *Br. J. Psychiatry* **2007**, *191*, 493–499. [CrossRef]
79. Davies, L.; Oliver, C. The age related prevalence of aggression and self-injury in persons with an intellectual disability: A review. *Res. Dev. Disabil.* **2013**, *34*, 764–775. [CrossRef]
80. Matson, J.L.; Mayville, S.B.; Kuhn, D.E.; Sturmey, P.; Laud, R.; Cooper, C. The behavioral function of feeding problems as assessed by the questions about behavioral function (QABF). *Res. Dev. Disabil.* **2005**, *26*, 399–408. [CrossRef] [PubMed]
81. Dominick, K.C.; Davis, N.O.; Lainhart, J.; Tager-Flusberg, H.; Folstein, S. Atypical behaviors in children with autism and children with a history of language impairment. *Res. Dev. Disabil.* **2007**, *28*, 145–162. [CrossRef] [PubMed]
82. Lesch, K.-P.; Waider, J. Serotonin in the Modulation of Neural Plasticity and Networks: Implications for Neurodevelopmental Disorders. *Neuron* **2012**, *76*, 175–191. [CrossRef] [PubMed]
83. Mazurek, M.O.; Kanne, S.M.; Wodka, E.L. Physical aggression in children and adolescents with autism spectrum disorders. *Res. Autism Spectr. Disord.* **2013**, *7*, 455–465. [CrossRef]

84. Fitzpatrick, S.E.; Srivorakiat, L.; Wink, L.K.; Pedapati, E.V.; Erickson, C.A. Aggression in autism spectrum disorder: Presentation and treatment options. *Neuropsychiatr. Dis. Treat.* **2016**, *ume 12*, 1525–1538. [CrossRef]
85. Retz, W.; Rösler, M. The relation of ADHD and violent aggression: What can we learn from epidemiological and genetic studies? *Int. J. Law Psychiatry* **2009**, *32*, 235–243. [CrossRef] [PubMed]
86. McClintock, K.; Hall, S.; Oliver, C. Risk markers associated with challenging behaviours in people with intellectual disabilities: A meta-analytic study. *J. Intellect. Disabil. Res.* **2003**, *47*, 405–416. [CrossRef]
87. Kiernan, C.; Kiernan, D. Challenging behaviour in schools for pupils with severe learning difficulties. *Ment. Handicap. Res.* **1994**, *7*, 177–201. [CrossRef]
88. Oliver, C.; Murphy, G.H.; Corbett, J.A. Self-injurious behaviour in people with learning disabilities: Determinants and interventions. *Int. Rev. Psychiatry* **1987**, *2*, 101–116. [CrossRef]
89. Page, M.J.; McKenzie, J.E.; Bossuyt, P.M.; Boutron, I.; Hoffmann, T.C.; Mulrow, C.D.; Shamseer, L.; Tetzlaff, J.M.; Akl, E.A.; Brennan, S.E.; et al. The PRISMA 2020 statement: An updated guideline for reporting systematic reviews. *Syst. Rev.* **2021**, *10*, 89. [CrossRef]
90. Campbell, M.; McKenzie, J.E.; Sowden, A.; Katikireddi, S.V.; Brennan, S.E.; Ellis, S.; Hartmann-Boyce, J.; Ryan, R.; Shepperd, S.; Thomas, J.; et al. Synthesis without meta-analysis (SWiM) in systematic reviews: Reporting guideline. *BMJ* **2020**, *368*, l6890. [CrossRef] [PubMed]
91. Stroup, D.F.; Berlin, J.A.; Morton, S.C.; Olkin, I.; Williamson, G.D.; Rennie, D.; Moher, D.; Becker, B.J.; Sipe, T.A.; Thacker, S.B. Meta-analysis of observational studies in epidemiology: A proposal for reporting. *JAMA* **2000**, *283*, 2008–2012. [CrossRef] [PubMed]
92. Mahood, Q.; Van Eerd, D.; Irvin, E. Searching for grey literature for systematic reviews: Challenges and benefits. *Res. Synth. Methods* **2013**, *5*, 221–234. [CrossRef] [PubMed]
93. Paez, A. Gray literature: An important resource in systematic reviews. *J. Evid.-Based Med.* **2017**, *10*, 233–240. [CrossRef]
94. Cochrane Effective Practice and Organisation of Care (EPOC). Data Collection Form. *EPOC Resources for Review Authors. 2013 Oslo: Norwegian Knowledge Centre for the Health Services.* Available online: http://epoc.cochrane.org/epoc-specific-resources-review-authors (accessed on 17 October 2022).
95. Clark, C.; Crumpler, C.; Notley, H. Evidence for Environmental Noise Effects on Health for the United Kingdom Policy Context: A Systematic Review of the Effects of Environmental Noise on Mental Health, Wellbeing, Quality of Life, Cancer, Dementia, Birth, Reproductive Outcomes, and Cognition. *Int. J. Environ. Res. Public Health* **2020**, *17*, 393. [CrossRef]
96. Guyatt, G.H.; Oxman, A.D.; Vist, G.E.; Kunz, R.; Falck-Ytter, Y.; Alonso-Coello, P.; Schünemann, H.J. GRADE: An emerging consensus on rating quality of evidence and strength of recommendations. *BMJ* **2008**, *336*, 924–926. [CrossRef] [PubMed]
97. Higgins, J.P.T.; Thomas, J.; Chandler, J.; Cumpston, M.; Li, T.; Page, M.J.; Welch, V.A. (Eds.) Cochrane Handbook for Systematic Reviews of Interventions Version 6.3 (Updated February 2022). Cochrane, 2022. Available online: www.training.cochrane.org/handbook (accessed on 17 October 2022).
98. Goodman, R. The Strengths and Difficulties Questionnaire: A Research Note. *J. Child Psychol. Psychiatry* **1997**, *38*, 581–586. [CrossRef] [PubMed]
99. Reynolds, C.R.; Kamphaus, R.W. *Behavior Assessment System for Children*, 2nd ed.; Pearson Assessments: Bloomington, MN, USA, 2004. Available online: https://pig.bio.ed.ac.uk/pig/sites/sbsweb2.bio.ed.ac.uk.pig/files/pdf/BASC2_Manual.pdf (accessed on 14 October 2022).
100. Achenbach, T.M. The Child Behavior Checklist and related instruments. In *The Use of Psychological Testing for Treatment Planning and Outcomes Assessment*; Maruish, M.E., Ed.; Lawrence Erlbaum Associates Publishers: New York, NY, USA, 1999; pp. 429–466. Available online: https://www.apa.org/depression-guideline/child-behavior-checklist.pdf (accessed on 17 October 2022).
101. Ravens-Sieberer, U.; Bullinger, M. Assessing health-related quality of life in chronically ill children with the German KINDL: First psychometric and content analytical results. *Qual. Life Res.* **1998**, *7*, 399–407. [CrossRef]
102. Ravens-Sieberer, U.; Bullinger, M. News from the KINDL-Questionnaire—A new version for adolescents *Qual. Life Res.* **1998**, *7*, 653.
103. World Health Organization. Global School-Based Student Health Survey (GSHS). 2018. Available online: https://www.who.int/teams/noncommunicable-diseases/surveillance/systems-tools/global-school-based-student-health-survey (accessed on 18 October 2022).
104. Shaffer, D.; Fisher, P.; Lucas, C.P.; Dulcan, M.K.; Schwab-Stone, M.E. NIMH Diagnostic Interview Schedule for Children Version IV (NIMH DISC-IV): Description, Differences from Previous Versions, and Reliability of Some Common Diagnoses. *J. Am. Acad. Child Adolesc. Psychiatry* **2000**, *39*, 28–38. [CrossRef]
105. Spielberger, D.C. *STAXI-2 State Trait Anger Expression Inventory-2, Professional Manual*; Psychological Assessment Resources: Magdalene, FL, USA, 1999. Available online: https://www.parinc.com/Products/Pkey/429 (accessed on 18 October 2022).
106. Amoly, E.; Dadvand, P.; Forns, J.; López-Vicente, M.; Basagaña, X.; Julvez, J.; Alvarez-Pedrerol, M.; Nieuwenhuijsen, M.J.; Sunyer, J. Green and Blue Spaces and Behavioral Development in Barcelona Schoolchildren: The BREATHE Project. *Environ. Health Perspect.* **2014**, *122*, 1351–1358. [CrossRef] [PubMed]
107. Andrusaityte, S.; Grazuleviciene, R.; Dedele, A.; Balseviciene, B. The effect of residential greenness and city park visiting habits on preschool Children's mental and general health in Lithuania: A cross-sectional study. *Int. J. Hyg. Environ. Health* **2020**, *223*, 142–150. [CrossRef] [PubMed]

108. Balseviciene, B.; Sinkariova, L.; Grazuleviciene, R.; Andrusaityte, S.; Uzdanaviciute, I.; Dedele, A.; Nieuwenhuijsen, M.J. Impact of Residential Greenness on Preschool Children's Emotional and Behavioral Problems. *Int. J. Environ. Res. Public Health* **2014**, *11*, 6757–6770. [CrossRef] [PubMed]
109. Bijnens, E.M.; Derom, C.; Thiery, E.; Weyers, S.; Nawrot, T.S. Residential green space and child intelligence and behavior across urban, suburban, and rural areas in Belgium: A longitudinal birth cohort study of twins. *PLoS Med.* **2020**, *17*, e1003213. [CrossRef] [PubMed]
110. Feng, X.; Astell-Burt, T. Residential Green Space Quantity and Quality and Child Well-being: A Longitudinal Study. *Am. J. Prev. Med.* **2017**, *53*, 616–624. [CrossRef]
111. Flouri, E.; Midouhas, E.; Joshi, H. The role of urban neighbourhood green space in children's emotional and behavioural resilience. *J. Environ. Psychol.* **2014**, *40*, 179–186. [CrossRef]
112. Jimenez, M.P.; Aris, I.M.; Rifas-Shiman, S.; Young, J.; Tiemeier, H.; Hivert, M.-F.; Oken, E.; James, P. Early life exposure to greenness and executive function and behavior: An application of inverse probability weighting of marginal structural models. *Environ. Pollut.* **2021**, *291*, 118208. [CrossRef] [PubMed]
113. Madzia, J.; Ryan, P.; Yolton, K.; Percy, Z.; Newman, N.; LeMasters, G.; Brokamp, C. Residential Greenspace Association with Childhood Behavioral Outcomes. *J. Pediatr.* **2019**, *207*, 233–240. [CrossRef]
114. Markevych, I.; Tiesler, C.M.; Fuertes, E.; Romanos, M.; Dadvand, P.; Nieuwenhuijsen, M.J.; Berdel, D.; Koletzko, S.; Heinrich, J. Access to urban green spaces and behavioural problems in children: Results from the GINIplus and LISAplus studies. *Environ. Int.* **2014**, *71*, 29–35. [CrossRef]
115. McEachan, R.R.C.; Yang, T.C.; Roberts, H.; Pickett, K.E.; Arseneau-Powell, D.; Gidlow, C.J.; Wright, J.; Nieuwenhuijsen, M. Availability, use of, and satisfaction with green space, and children's mental wellbeing at age 4 years in a multicultural, deprived, urban area: Results from the Born in Bradford cohort study. *Lancet Planet. Health* **2018**, *2*, e244–e254. [CrossRef]
116. Mueller, M.A.; Flouri, E.; Kokosi, T. The role of the physical environment in adolescent mental health. *Health Place* **2019**, *58*, 102153. [CrossRef] [PubMed]
117. Liao, J.; Yang, S.; Xia, W.; Peng, A.; Zhao, J.; Li, Y.; Zhang, Y.; Qian, Z.; Vaughn, M.G.; Schootman, M.; et al. Associations of exposure to green space with problem behaviours in preschool-aged children. *Int. J. Epidemiol.* **2020**, *49*, 944–953. [CrossRef] [PubMed]
118. Lee, M.; Kim, S.; Ha, M. Community greenness and neurobehavioral health in children and adolescents. *Sci. Total. Environ.* **2019**, *672*, 381–388. [CrossRef] [PubMed]
119. Lee, J.; Movassaghi, K.S. The role of greenness of school grounds in student violence in the Chicago public schools. *Child. Youth Environ.* **2021**, *31*, 54–82. [CrossRef]
120. Richardson, E.A.; Pearce, J.; Shortt, N.K.; Mitchell, R. The role of public and private natural space in children's social, emotional and behavioural development in Scotland: A longitudinal study. *Environ. Res.* **2017**, *158*, 729–736. [CrossRef] [PubMed]
121. Van Aart, C.J.; Michels, N.; Sioen, I.; De Decker, A.; Bijnens, E.M.; Janssen, B.G.; De Henauw, S.; Nawrot, T. Residential landscape as a predictor of psychosocial stress in the life course from childhood to adolescence. *Environ. Int.* **2018**, *120*, 456–463. [CrossRef]
122. Younan, D.; Tuvblad, C.; Li, L.; Wu, J.; Lurmann, F.; Franklin, M.; Berhane, K.; McConnell, R.; Wu, A.H.; Baker, L.A.; et al. Environmental Determinants of Aggression in Adolescents: Role of Urban Neighborhood Greenspace. *J. Am. Acad. Child Adolesc. Psychiatry* **2016**, *55*, 591–601. [CrossRef]
123. Bao, W.-W.; Xue, W.-X.; Jiang, N.; Huang, S.; Zhang, S.-X.; Zhao, Y.; Chen, Y.-C.; Dong, G.-H.; Cai, M.; Chen, Y.-J. Exposure to road traffic noise and behavioral problems in Chinese schoolchildren: A cross-sectional study. *Sci. Total. Environ.* **2022**, *837*, 155806. [CrossRef]
124. Crombie, R.; Clark, C.; Stansfeld, S.A. Environmental noise exposure, early biological risk and mental health in nine to ten year old children: A cross-sectional field study. *Environ. Health* **2011**, *10*, 39. [CrossRef]
125. Essers, E.; Pérez-Crespo, L.; Foraster, M.; Ambrós, A.; Tiemeier, H.; Guxens, M. Environmental noise exposure and emotional, aggressive, and attention-deficit/hyperactivity disorder-related symptoms in children from two European birth cohorts. *Environ. Int.* **2021**, *158*, 106946. [CrossRef]
126. Grelat, N.; Houot, H.; Pujol, S.; Levain, J.-P.; Defrance, J.; Mariet, A.-S.; Mauny, F. Noise Annoyance in Urban Children: A Cross-Sectional Population-Based Study. *Int. J. Environ. Res. Public Health* **2016**, *13*, 1056. [CrossRef] [PubMed]
127. Haines, M.M.; Stansfeld, S.A.; Brentnall, S.; Head, J.; Berry, B.; Jiggins, M.; Hygge, S. The West London Schools Study: The effects of chronic aircraft noise exposure on child health. *Psychol. Med.* **2001**, *31*, 1385–1396. [CrossRef] [PubMed]
128. Haines, M.M.; Stansfeld, S.A.; Job, R.F.S.; Berglund, B.; Head, J. Chronic aircraft noise exposure, stress responses, mental health and cognitive performance in school children. *Psychol. Med.* **2001**, *31*, 265–277. [CrossRef] [PubMed]
129. Haines, M.M.; Stansfeld, S.A.; Job, R.S.; Berglund, B.; Head, J. A follow-up study of effects of chronic aircraft noise exposure on child stress responses and cognition. *Leuk. Res.* **2001**, *30*, 839–845. [CrossRef]
130. Spilski, J.; Rumberg, M.; Berchtold, M.; Bergström, K.; Möhler, U.; Lachmann, T.; Klatte, M. Effects of aircraft noise and living environment on children´s wellbeing and health. In Proceedings of the 23rd International Congress on Acoustics: Integrating 4th EAA Euroregio 2019, Aachen, Germany, 9–13 September 2019; pp. 7080–7087. [CrossRef]
131. Stansfeld, S.; Berglund, B.; Clark, C.; Lopez-Barrio, I.; Fischer, P.; Öhrström, E.; Haines, M.; Head, J.; Hygge, S.; van Kamp, I.; et al. Aircraft and road traffic noise and children's cognition and health: A cross-national study. *Lancet* **2005**, *365*, 1942–1949. [CrossRef]

132. Stansfeld, S.; Clark, C.; Cameron, R.; Alfred, T.; Head, J.; Haines, M.; van Kamp, I.; van Kempen, E.; Lopez-Barrio, I. Aircraft and road traffic noise exposure and children's mental health. *J. Environ. Psychol.* **2009**, *29*, 203–207. [CrossRef]
133. Tiesler, C.M.; Birk, M.; Thiering, E.; Kohlböck, G.; Koletzko, S.; Bauer, C.-P.; Berdel, D.; von Berg, A.; Babisch, W.; Heinrich, J. Exposure to road traffic noise and children's behavioural problems and sleep disturbance: Results from the GINIplus and LISAplus studies. *Environ. Res.* **2013**, *123*, 1–8. [CrossRef]
134. Gintilienė, G.; Černiauskaitė, D.; Povilaitis, R.; Girdzijauskienė, S.; Lesinskienė, S.; Pūras, D. Lietuviskasis SDQ—Standartizuotas mokyklinio amziaus vaikų "Galiu ir sunkumu klausimynas". *Psichologija* **2004**, *2*, 89–105.
135. Bandiera, F.C.; Richardson, A.K.; Lee, D.J.; He, J.-P.; Merikangas, K.R. Secondhand Smoke Exposure and Mental Health Among Children and Adolescents. *Arch. Pediatr. Adolesc. Med.* **2011**, *165*, 332–338. [CrossRef]
136. Bauer, N.S.; Anand, V.; Carroll, A.E.; Downs, S.M. Secondhand Smoke Exposure, Parental Depressive Symptoms and Preschool Behavioral Outcomes. *J. Pediatr. Nurs.* **2014**, *30*, 227–235. [CrossRef]
137. World Health Organization. *International Classification of Diseases: [9th] Ninth Revision, Basic Tabulation List with Alphabetic Index*; World Health Organization: Geneva, Switzerland, 1978. Available online: https://apps.who.int/iris/handle/10665/39473 (accessed on 24 October 2022).
138. Gatzke-Kopp, L.; Willoughby, M.T.; Warkentien, S.; Petrie, D.; Mills-Koonce, R.; Blair, C. Association between environmental tobacco smoke exposure across the first four years of life and manifestation of externalizing behavior problems in school-aged children. *J. Child Psychol. Psychiatry* **2020**, *61*, 1243–1252. [CrossRef] [PubMed]
139. Friedman-Weieneth, J.L.; Doctoroff, G.L.; Harvey, E.A.; Goldstein, L.H. The Disruptive Behavior Rating Scale—Parent Version (DBRS-PV): Factor Analytic Structure and Validity among Young Preschool Children. *J. Atten. Disord.* **2009**, *13*, 42–55. [CrossRef] [PubMed]
140. Koth, C.W.; Bradshaw, C.P.; Leaf, P.J. Teacher Observation of Classroom Adaptation—Checklist: Development and Factor Structure. *Meas. Evaluation Couns. Dev.* **2009**, *42*, 15–30. [CrossRef]
141. Karamanos, A.; Mudway, I.; Kelly, F.; Beevers, S.D.; Dajnak, D.; Elia, C.; Cruickshank, J.K.; Lu, Y.; Tandon, S.; Enayat, E.; et al. Air pollution and trajectories of adolescent conduct problems: The roles of ethnicity and racism; evidence from the DASH longitudinal study. *Soc. Psychiatry Psychiatr. Epidemiol.* **2021**, *56*, 2029–2039. [CrossRef] [PubMed]
142. Kelishadi, R.; Babaki, A.E.S.; Qorbani, M.; Ahadi, Z.; Heshmat, R.; Motlagh, M.E.; Ardalan, G.; Ataie-Jafari, A.; Asayesh, H.; Mohammadi, R. Joint Association of Active and Passive Smoking with Psychiatric Distress and Violence Behaviors in a Representative Sample of Iranian Children and Adolescents: The CASPIAN-IV Study. *Int. J. Behav. Med.* **2015**, *22*, 652–661. [CrossRef] [PubMed]
143. World Health Organization, Regional Office for South-East Asia. *Global School-Based Student Health Survey GSHS: A Tool for Integrated Youth Behavioral Surveillance*; World Health Organization, Regional Office for South-East Asia: New Delhi, India, 2018. Available online: https://apps.who.int/iris/handle/10665/275390 (accessed on 23 October 2022).
144. Loftus, C.T.; Ni, Y.; Szpiro, A.A.; Hazlehurst, M.F.; Tylavsky, F.A.; Bush, N.R.; Sathyanarayana, S.; Carroll, K.N.; Young, M.; Karr, C.J.; et al. Exposure to ambient air pollution and early childhood behavior: A longitudinal cohort study. *Environ. Res.* **2020**, *183*, 109075. [CrossRef]
145. Newman, N.C.; Ryan, P.; LeMasters, G.; Levin, L.; Bernstein, D.; Hershey, G.K.K.; Lockey, J.E.; Villareal, M.; Reponen, T.; Grinshpun, S.; et al. Traffic-Related Air Pollution Exposure in the First Year of Life and Behavioral Scores at 7 Years of Age. *Environ. Health Perspect.* **2013**, *121*, 731–736. [CrossRef]
146. Pagani, L.S.; Lévesque-Seck, F.; Archambault, I.; Janosz, M. Prospective longitudinal associations between household smoke exposure in early childhood and antisocial behavior at age 12. *Indoor Air* **2017**, *27*, 622–630. [CrossRef]
147. Park, B.; Park, B.; Kim, E.-J.; Kim, Y.J.; Lee, H.; Ha, E.-H.; Park, H. Longitudinal association between environmental tobacco smoke exposure and behavioral problems in children from ages 5 to 9. *Sci. Total. Environ.* **2020**, *746*, 141327. [CrossRef]
148. Rasnick, E.; Ryan, P.H.; Bailer, A.J.; Fisher, T.; Parsons, P.J.; Yolton, K.; Newman, N.C.; Lanphear, B.P.; Brokamp, C. Identifying sensitive windows of airborne lead exposure associated with behavioral outcomes at age 12. *Environ. Epidemiol.* **2021**, *5*, e144. [CrossRef]
149. Roberts, S.; Arseneault, L.; Barratt, B.; Beevers, S.; Danese, A.; Odgers, C.L.; Moffitt, T.E.; Reuben, A.; Kelly, F.J.; Fisher, H.L. Exploration of NO2 and PM2.5 air pollution and mental health problems using high-resolution data in London-based children from a UK longitudinal cohort study. *Psychiatry Res.* **2019**, *272*, 8–17. [CrossRef] [PubMed]
150. American Psychiatric Association. *Diagnostic and Statistical Manual of Mental Disorders: DSM 4*, 4th ed.; American Psychiatric Association: Washington, DC, USA, 1994.
151. Ciucci, E.; Calussi, P.; Menesini, E.; Mattei, A.; Petralli, M.; Orlandini, S. Seasonal variation, weather and behavior in day-care children: A multilevel approach. *Int. J. Biometeorol.* **2013**, *57*, 845–856. [CrossRef] [PubMed]
152. Klimstra, T.A.; Frijns, T.; Keijsers, L.; Denissen, J.J.A.; Raaijmakers, Q.A.W.; van Aken, M.A.G.; Koot, H.M.; van Lier, P.A.C.; Meeus, W.H.J. Come rain or come shine: Individual differences in how weather affects mood. *Emotion* **2011**, *11*, 1495–1499. [CrossRef]
153. Lochman, J.E.; Vernberg, E.; Glenn, A.; Jarrett, M.; McDonald, K.; Powell, N.P.; Abel, M.; Boxmeyer, C.L.; Kassing, F.; Qu, L.; et al. Effects of Autonomic Nervous System Functioning and Tornado Exposure on Long-Term Outcomes of Aggressive Children. *Res. Child Adolesc. Psychopathol.* **2021**, *49*, 471–489. [CrossRef]

154. Jones, S.M.; Molano, A. Seasonal and Compositional Effects of Classroom Aggression: A Test of Developmental-Contextual Models. *J. Cogn. Educ. Psychol.* **2016**, *15*, 225–247. [CrossRef]
155. Dodge, K.A.; Coie, J.D. Social-information-processing factors in reactive and proactive aggression in children's peer groups. *J. Pers. Soc. Psychol.* **1987**, *53*, 1146–1158. [CrossRef] [PubMed]
156. Lagacé-Séguin, D.G.; D'Entremont, M.L. Weathering the preschool environment: Affect moderates the relations between meteorology and preschool behaviors. *Early Child Dev. Care* **2005**, *175*, 379–394. [CrossRef]
157. Behar, L.B. The Preschool Behavior Questionnaire. *J. Abnorm. Child Psychol.* **1977**, *5*, 265–275. [CrossRef]
158. Muñoz-Reyes, J.A.; Flores-Prado, L.; Beltrami, M. Seasonal differences of aggressive behavior in Chilean adolescents. *J. Aggress. Confl. Peace Res.* **2014**, *6*, 129–138. [CrossRef]
159. Younan, D.; Li, L.; Tuvblad, C.; Wu, J.; Lurmann, F.; Franklin, M.; Berhane, K.; McConnell, R.; Wu, A.H.; Baker, L.A.; et al. Long-Term Ambient Temperature and Externalizing Behaviors in Adolescents. *Am. J. Epidemiol.* **2018**, *187*, 1931–1941. [CrossRef]
160. Ginsburg, H.J.; Pollman, V.A.; Wauson, M.S.; Hope, M.L. Variation of aggressive interaction among male elementary school children as a function of changes in spatial density. *J. Nonverbal Behav.* **1977**, *2*, 67–75. [CrossRef]
161. Loo, C.; Kennelly, D. Social density: Its effects on behaviors and perceptions of preschoolers. *J. Nonverbal Behav.* **1979**, *3*, 131–146. [CrossRef]
162. Loo, C.; Smetana, J. The effects of crowding on the behavior and perception of 10-year-old boys. *J. Nonverbal Behav.* **1978**, *2*, 226–249. [CrossRef]
163. Supplee, L.H.; Unikel, E.B.; Shaw, D.S. Physical environmental adversity and the protective role of maternal monitoring in relation to early child conduct problems. *J. Appl. Dev. Psychol.* **2007**, *28*, 166–183. [CrossRef]
164. Achenbach, T.M.; Rescorla, L.A. *Manual for the ASEBA School-Age Forms and Profiles*; University of Vermont Research Center for Children, Youth, & Families: Burlington, VT, USA, 2001.
165. Neill, S.R.S.J. Preschool design and child behaviour. *J. Child Psychol. Psychiatry* **1982**, *23*, 309–318. [CrossRef] [PubMed]
166. Evans, B.E.; Buil, J.M.; Burk, W.J.; Cillessen, A.H.N.; van Lier, P.A.C. Urbanicity is Associated with Behavioral and Emotional Problems in Elementary School-Aged Children. *J. Child Fam. Stud.* **2018**, *27*, 2193–2205. [CrossRef]
167. Erasmus, M.C. *Problem Behavior at School Interview*; Department of Child and Adolescent Psychiatry: Rotterdam, The Netherlands, 2000.
168. Handal, P.J.; Hopper, S. Relationship of Sex, Social Class and Rural/Urban Locale to Preschoolers' AML Scores. *Psychol. Rep.* **1985**, *57*, 707–713. [CrossRef]
169. Durlak, J.A.; Stein, M.A.; Mannarino, A.P. Behavioral validity of a brief teacher rating scale (the AML) in identifying high-risk acting-out schoolchildren. *Am. J. Community Psychol.* **1980**, *8*, 101–115. [CrossRef]
170. Hope, T.L.; Bierman, K.L. Patterns of Home and School Behavior Problems in Rural and Urban Settings. *J. Sch. Psychol.* **1998**, *36*, 45–58. [CrossRef] [PubMed]
171. Achenbach, T.M. *Integrative Guide to the 1991 CBCL/4-18, YSR, and TRF Profiles*; University of Vermont, Department of Psychology: Burlington, VT, USA, 1991.
172. Sheridan, S.M.; Koziol, N.A.; Clarke, B.L.; Rispoli, K.M.; Coutts, M.J. The Influence of Rurality and Parental Affect on Kindergarten Children's Social and Behavioral Functioning. *Early Educ. Dev.* **2014**, *25*, 1057–1082. [CrossRef]
173. Merrell, K.W. *Preschool and Kindergarten Behavior Scales*, 2nd ed.; Pro-Ed: Austin, TX, USA, 2003.
174. Gresham, F.M.; Elliott, S.N. *The Social Skills Rating System*; American Guidance Service: Circle Pines, MN, USA, 1990.
175. U.S. Department of Health and Human Services. *Head Start Family and Child Experiences Survey (FACES)*; Administration for Children and Families: Washington, DC, USA, 1997–2013.
176. Wongtongkam, N.; Ward, P.R.; Day, A.; Winefield, A.H. The Relationship Between Exposure to Violence and Anger in Thai Adolescents. *J. Interpers. Violence* **2015**, *31*, 2291–2301. [CrossRef]
177. Loeber, R.; Farrington, D.P.; Stouthamer-Loeber, M.; Moffitt, T.E.; Caspi, A.; White, H.R.; Wei, E.H.; Beyers, J.M. The Development of Male Offending: Key Findings from Fourteen Years of the Pittsburgh Youth Study. In *Taking Stock of Delinquency: An Overview of Findings from Contemporary Longitudinal Studies*; Thornberry, T.P., Krohn, M.D., Eds.; Kluwer Academic/Plenum Publishers: New York, NY, USA, 2003; pp. 93–136.
178. Kelder, S.H.; Orpinas, P.; McAlister, A.; Frankowski, R.; Friday, J. The students for peace project: A comprehensive violence-prevention program for middle school students. *Am. J. Prev. Med.* **1996**, *12*, 22–30. [CrossRef] [PubMed]
179. Glod, C.A.; Teicher, M.H.; Butler, M.; Savino, M.; Harper, D.; Magnus, E.; Pahlavan, K. Modifying Quiet Room Design Enhances Calming of Children and Adolescents. *J. Am. Acad. Child Adolesc. Psychiatry* **1994**, *33*, 558–566. [CrossRef]
180. Yudofsky, S.C.; Silver, J.M.; Jackson, W.; Endicott, J.; Williams, D. The Overt Aggression Scale for the objective rating of verbal and physical aggression. *Am. J. Psychiatry* **1986**, *143*, 35–39. [CrossRef] [PubMed]
181. Vakili, H.; Niakan, M.H.; Najafi, N. The Effect of Classroom Red Walls on the Students' Aggression. *Int. J. Sch. Health* 2019, in press. [CrossRef]
182. Buss, A.H.; Perry, M. The Aggression Questionnaire. *J. Pers. Soc. Psychol.* **1992**, *63*, 452–459. [CrossRef]
183. Coyne, S.M.; Padilla-Walker, L.M. Sex, violence, & rock n' roll: Longitudinal effects of music on aggression, sex, and prosocial behavior during adolescence. *J. Adolesc.* **2015**, *41*, 96–104. [CrossRef]
184. Hinds, P.S. Music: A Milieu Factor with Implications for the Nurse-Therapist. *J. Psychosoc. Nurs. Ment. Health Serv.* **1980**, *18*, 28–33. [CrossRef]

185. Woerner, W.; Fleitlich-Bilyk, B.; Martinussen, R.; Fletcher, J.; Cucchiaro, G.; Dalgalarrondo, P.; Lui, M.; Tannock, R. The Strengths and Difficulties Questionnaire overseas: Evaluations and applications of the SDQ beyond Europe. *Eur. Child Adolesc. Psychiatry* **2004**, *13*, II47–II54. [CrossRef]
186. Hoeksma, J.B.; Sep, S.M.; Vester, F.C.; Groot, P.F.C.; Sijmons, R.; De Vries, J. The electronic mood device: Design, construction, and application. *Behav. Res. Methods Instrum. Comput.* **2000**, *32*, 322–326. [CrossRef]
187. Vernberg, E.M.; University of Kansas, Lawrence, KS, USA; Jacobs, A.K.; University of Kansas, Lawrence, KS, USA. Tornado related traumatic exposure scale. 2005, *unpublished manuscript*.
188. Barger, B.; Larson, L.R.; Ogletree, S.; Torquati, J.; Rosenberg, S.; Gaither, C.J.; Bartz, J.M.; Gardner, A.W.; Moody, E. Tree Canopy Coverage Predicts Lower Conduct Problem Severity in Children with ASD. *J. Ment. Health Res. Intellect. Disabil.* **2020**, *13*, 43–61. [CrossRef]
189. Bramlett, M.D.; Blumberg, S.J.; Zablotsky, B.; George, J.M.; Ormson, A.E.; Frasier, A.M.; Santos, K.B. Design and operation of the National Survey of Children's Health, 2011–2012. *Vital Health Stat.* **2017**, *59*, 1–256.
190. Durand, V.M.; Mapstone, E. Influence of "Mood-Inducing" Music on Challenging Behavior. *Am. J. Ment. Retard.* **1997**, *102*, 367–378. [CrossRef]
191. Gul, N.; Jameel, H.T.; Mohsin, M.N. Effectiveness of background music on aggressive behavior of intellectually disabled children. *Int. J. Incl. Educ.* **2019**, *3*, 49–61.
192. Oliver, C.; Oxener, G.; Hearn, M.; Hall, S. Effects of social proximity on multiple aggressive behaviors. *J. Appl. Behav. Anal.* **2001**, *34*, 85–88. [CrossRef]
193. West, M.; Melvin, G.; McNamara, F.; Gordon, M. An evaluation of the use and efficacy of a sensory room within an adolescent psychiatric inpatient unit. *Aust. Occup. Ther. J.* **2017**, *64*, 253–263. [CrossRef]
194. Bogar, S.; Beyer, K.M. Green Space, Violence, and Crime: A Systematic Review. *Trauma Violence Abus.* **2015**, *17*, 160–171. [CrossRef]
195. Shepley, M.; Sachs, N.; Sadatsafavi, H.; Fournier, C.; Peditto, K. The Impact of Green Space on Violent Crime in Urban Environments: An Evidence Synthesis. *Int. J. Environ. Res. Public Health* **2019**, *16*, 5119. [CrossRef]
196. Barakat, H.A.-E.; Bakr, A.; El-Sayad, Z. Nature as a healer for autistic children. *Alex. Eng. J.* **2019**, *58*, 353–366. [CrossRef]
197. Li, D.; Larsen, L.; Yang, Y.; Wang, L.; Zhai, Y.; Sullivan, W.C. Exposure to nature for children with autism spectrum disorder: Benefits, caveats, and barriers. *Health Place* **2019**, *55*, 71–79. [CrossRef]
198. Hao, G.; Zuo, L.; Xiong, P.; Chen, L.; Liang, X.; Jing, C. Associations of PM2.5 and road traffic noise with mental health: Evidence from UK Biobank. *Environ. Res.* **2022**, *207*, 112221. [CrossRef] [PubMed]
199. Politte, L.C.; Fitzpatrick, S.E.; Erickson, C. Externalising behaviours in autism spectrum disorder and other neurodevelopmental disorders. In *Externalising behaviours: Clinical Features and Treatment Across the Diagnostic Spectrum*; American Psychiatric Association Publishing: Washington, DC, USA, 2018; pp. 53–80.
200. Kanne, S.M.; Mazurek, M. Aggression in Children and Adolescents with ASD: Prevalence and Risk Factors. *J. Autism Dev. Disord.* **2011**, *41*, 926–937. [CrossRef] [PubMed]
201. Ding, N.; Berry, H.L.; Bennett, C.M. The Importance of Humidity in the Relationship between Heat and Population Mental Health: Evidence from Australia. *PLoS ONE* **2016**, *11*, e0164190. [CrossRef] [PubMed]
202. Vida, S.; Durocher, M.; Ouarda, T.B.M.J.; Gosselin, P. Relationship Between Ambient Temperature and Humidity and Visits to Mental Health Emergency Departments in Québec. *Psychiatr. Serv.* **2012**, *63*, 1150–1153. [CrossRef]
203. Tiihonen, J.; Halonen, P.; Tiihonen, L.; Kautiainen, H.; Storvik, M.; Callaway, J. The Association of Ambient Temperature and Violent Crime. *Sci. Rep.* **2017**, *7*, 1–7. [CrossRef] [PubMed]
204. Makinde, O.; Björkqvist, K.; Österman, K. Overcrowding as a risk factor for domestic violence and antisocial behaviour among adolescents in Ejigbo, Lagos, Nigeria. *Glob. Ment. Health* **2016**, *3*, e16. [CrossRef]
205. Aquilina, C. Violence by Psychiatric In-Patients. *Med. Sci. Law* **1991**, *31*, 306–312. [CrossRef]
206. Davis, S. Violence by Psychiatric Inpatients: A Review. *Psychiatr. Serv.* **1991**, *42*, 585–590. [CrossRef]
207. Palmstierna, T.; Huitfeldt, B.; Wistedt, B. The Relationship of Crowding and Aggressive Behavior on a Psychiatric Intensive Care Unit. *Psychiatr. Serv.* **1991**, *42*, 1237–1240. [CrossRef]
208. Nijman, H.L.I.; Rector, G. Crowding and Aggression on Inpatient Psychiatric Wards. *Psychiatr. Serv.* **1999**, *50*, 830–831. [CrossRef]
209. Dzhambov, A.; Dimitrova, D. Urban green spaces' effectiveness as a psychological buffer for the negative health impact of noise pollution: A systematic review. *Noise Health* **2014**, *16*, 157–165. [CrossRef] [PubMed]
210. Zupancic, T.; Westmacott, C.; Bulthuis, M. *The Impact of Green Space on Heat and Air Pollution in Urban Communities: A Meta-Narrative Systematic Review*; David Suzuki Foundation: Vancouver, BC, Canada, 2015. Available online: https://davidsuzuki.org/wp-content/uploads/2017/09/impact-green-space-heat-air-pollution-urban-communities.pdf (accessed on 25 March 2021).
211. Cohen-Cline, H.; Turkheimer, E.; Duncan, G.E. Access to green space, physical activity and mental health: A twin study. *J. Epidemiol. Community Health* **2015**, *69*, 523–529. [CrossRef] [PubMed]
212. Dadvand, P.; Rivas, I.; Basagaña, X.; Alvarez-Pedrerol, M.; Su, J.; De Castro Pascual, M.; Amato, F.; Jerret, M.; Querol, X.; Sunyer, J.; et al. The association between greenness and traffic-related air pollution at schools. *Sci. Total Environ.* **2015**, *523*, 59–63. [CrossRef] [PubMed]
213. McCracken, D.S.; Allen, D.A.; Gow, A.J. Associations between urban greenspace and health-related quality of life in children. *Prev. Med. Rep.* **2016**, *3*, 211–221. [CrossRef]

214. Li, M.; Van Renterghem, T.; Kang, J.; Verheyen, K.; Botteldooren, D. Sound absorption by tree bark. *Appl. Acoust.* **2020**, *165*, 107328. [CrossRef]
215. Gallent, N.; Gkartzios, M. Defining rurality and the scope of rural planning. In *The Routledge Companion to Rural Planning*; Scott, M., Gallent, N., Gkartzios, M., Eds.; Routledge: New York, NY, USA, 2019.
216. Singh, J. Toxic Moulds and Indoor Air Quality. *Indoor Built Environ.* **2005**, *14*, 229–234. [CrossRef]
217. Singh, A.; Daniel, L.; Baker, E.; Bentley, R. Housing Disadvantage and Poor Mental Health: A Systematic Review. *Am. J. Prev. Med.* **2019**, *57*, 262–272. [CrossRef]
218. Evans, G.W. The Built Environment and Mental Health. *J. Urban Health* **2003**, *80*, 536–555. [CrossRef]
219. Bosch, K.A.V.D.; Andringa, T.C.; Peterson, W.; Ruijssenaars, W.A.J.J.M.; Vlaskamp, C. A comparison of natural and non-natural soundscapes on people with severe or profound intellectual and multiple disabilities. *J. Intellect. Dev. Disabil.* **2017**, *42*, 301–307. [CrossRef]
220. Beresford, B.; Oldman, C. *Housing Matters: National Evidence Relating to Disabled Children and Their Housing*; Policy Press: Bristol, UK, 2002.
221. Emerson, E. Deprivation, ethnicity and the prevalence of intellectual and developmental disabilities. *J. Epidemiol. Community Health* **2010**, *66*, 218–224. [CrossRef]

Disclaimer/Publisher's Note: The statements, opinions and data contained in all publications are solely those of the individual author(s) and contributor(s) and not of MDPI and/or the editor(s). MDPI and/or the editor(s) disclaim responsibility for any injury to people or property resulting from any ideas, methods, instructions or products referred to in the content.

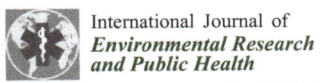

Review

Developmental Delays in Socio-Emotional Brain Functions in Persons with an Intellectual Disability: Impact on Treatment and Support

Tanja Sappok [1,*], Angela Hassiotis [2,3], Marco Bertelli [4], Isabel Dziobek [5] and Paula Sterkenburg [6,7]

1. Berlin Center for Mental Health in Developmental Disabilities, Ev. Krankenhaus Königin Elisabeth Herzberge, 10365 Berlin, Germany
2. Division of Psychiatry, University College London, London W1T 7BN, UK
3. Camden and Islington NHS Foundation Trust, London NW1 0PE, UK
4. CREA (Research and Clinical Centre), San Sebastiano Foundation, Misericordia di Firenze, 50142 Florence, Italy
5. Clinical Psychology of Social Interaction, Humboldt-Universität zu Berlin, 10099 Berlin, Germany
6. Bartiméus, 3941 XM Doorn, The Netherlands
7. Department of Clinical Child and Family Studies, Vrije Universiteit Amsterdam, 1081 BT Amsterdam, The Netherlands
* Correspondence: tanja.sappok@t-online.de

Abstract: Intellectual disability is a neurodevelopmental disorder with a related co-occurrence of mental health issues and challenging behaviors. In addition to purely cognitive functions, socio-emotional competencies may also be affected. In this paper, the lens of developmental social neuroscience is used to better understand the origins of mental disorders and challenging behaviors in people with an intellectual disability. The current concept of intelligence is broadened by socio-emotional brain functions. The emergence of these socio-emotional brain functions is linked to the formation of the respective neuronal networks located within the different parts of the limbic system. Thus, high order networks build on circuits that process more basic information. The socio-emotional skills can be assessed and complement the results of a standardized IQ-test. Disturbances of the brain cytoarchitecture and function that occur at a certain developmental period may increase the susceptibility to certain mental disorders. Insights into the current mental and socio-emotional functioning of a person may support clinicians in the calibration of treatment and support. Acknowledging the trajectories of the socio-emotional brain development may result in a more comprehensive understanding of behaviors and mental health in people with developmental delays and thus underpin supports for promotion of good mental health in this highly vulnerable population.

Keywords: developmental neuroscience; emotional functioning; intellectual disability; intervention mental health; limbic system; social brain network

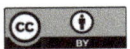

1. Introduction

According to a nationwide US survey, one in six persons has a developmental disability, with most suffering from neurodevelopmental disorders, such as attention-deficit/hyperactivity disorder (ADHD) (9.5%), autism spectrum disorders (2.5%), learning disability (7.9%), or intellectual disability (1.2%) [1]. During the past decade, these prevalence rates have increased, e.g., from 1.1% to 2.5% for autism and from 0.9% to 1.2% for intellectual disability [1,2] as a result of better assessment and diagnosis. According to the WHO Global Health metrics, there are about 100 million people with an intellectual disability world-wide [3].

People with an intellectual disability are more vulnerable to physical or mental disorders [4–7]. According to the recent meta-analysis of Mazza [4], 33,6% suffer from a mental disorder, which is about double of the prevalence rates in the general population. In 2018, one in three persons with a cognitive disability experienced more than 50% physically unhealthy days, and one in two persons reported more than 50% mentally unhealthy days [7]. Furthermore, approximately one in two persons with a cognitive disability slept less than 6 h a night, had experienced depression, and rated their health as fair to poor [7]. Especially these chronic and secondary health conditions decrease the life expectancy of persons with an intellectual disability by around 20 years compared to the general population [8,9]. Factors associated with death in people with an intellectual disability are mental and physical illnesses (e.g., cancer, heard, pulmonary and renal diseases) and physical disabilities such as cerebral palsy and epilepsy [10]. More than a third of those deaths are potentially amenable to healthcare interventions [11,12]. Due to the poorer management of chronic health conditions in primary healthcare, application of reasonable adjustments in services and awareness training have to be expanded to meet the needs of people with developmental disabilities [12].

People with an intellectual disability face various barriers to receiving adequate healthcare. Hence, person-related factors, such as lack of information and health literacy or communication difficulties, and system-related aspects, such as insufficient knowledge or even discriminatory attitudes among practitioners and service providers, have to be considered [10]. Health impairments lead to a significant emotional, social, and financial burden on the patients and on their social networks. In the European Union, intellectual disability was amongst the top ten most expensive diseases of the brain [13], requiring an annual expenditure of 43.3€ billions in 2010. In a Canadian study, adults with an intellectual disability were nearly four times more likely to incur high annual healthcare costs than those without an intellectual disability [14]. An Australian study demonstrated the considerable economic impact of intellectual disability on families, governments, and broader society [15], and a study on health-service use and the costs of Americans with an intellectual disability revealed that the presence of chronic medical conditions and poor mental health status predicted high expenses across various types of healthcare [16]. Taken together, all the evidence points to the urgent need for public health to focus on effective interventions for and the holistic management of secondary disorders in people with an intellectual disability.

The present paper develops five main themes. First, the current understanding of intelligence and the options of broadening the concept by integrating socio-emotional competencies will be outlined. Second, the development of socio-emotional brain functions will be linked to the maturation of the socio-emotional brain networks. Third, options to systematically assess socio-emotional brain functions will be offered. Fourth, the relatedness of developmental neuroscience and mental health in persons with an intellectual disability will be addressed. Finally, the implications of the developmental approach to treatment and support will be posed.

The lens of developmental neuroscience provides insights into the co-regulating processes of emotion regulation, social interaction and adaptation and may serve as a window into general psychological mechanisms. In a translational pathway, the underlying processes may have a broad impact on our understanding of human behavior [17].

2. Intellectual Disability Revisited: About the Current Understanding of Intelligence and Why There Is a Need for Broadening the Concept towards the Social Realm

In Western societies, Descartes [18] laid the foundation for continental rationalism: "Je pense, donc je suis" ['I think therefore I am']. Pioneers such as Damasio [19] overcame the dualistic body-mind distinction and delineated the importance of emotion and the sensorial body within cognitive science approaches. Socio-emotional and cognitive processes have been proposed to be highly intertwined and overtly present in all physiological and pathological mental activities. Ciompi [20] and the RDoC (Research Domain Criteria) framework [21] provided well-known examples. In the International Classification of Diseases, ICD-11, disorders of the intellectual development (also termed "intellectual disability" in DSM-5) are counted among the neurodevelopmental disorders that "arise during the developmental period" and "involve significant difficulties in the acquisition and execution of specific intellectual, motor, language, or social functions" [22]. As such, in addition to poor cognitive functions, social, affective, and adaptive functions are also affected. However, the concept of "intelligence" is still dominated by Descartes' rationalism, and the diagnosis of an intellectual disability is still centred on general IQ measures, academic learning, and complex logical-deductive executive functions, such as working memory, processing speed, attention, encoding, verbal comprehension and expression, abstract reasoning, and problem solving.

However, emotional and social intelligence differ from cognitive intelligence and require different neural circuitries [23]. Socio-emotional brain functions refer to the ability to regulate one's own emotional expression, to identify the emotional expressions of others, to interpret emotional cues, to respond accordingly, and to self-soothe and manage emotional outbursts. Emotional intelligence is therefore essential for the quality of relationships with the self and with other people, the ability to adapt, to cope with stress and to communicate and interact appropriately [24]. A functional account of emotions posits that emotions are mental activities that respond to environmental stimuli, such as a social or physical challenge, and determine in turn physical and behavioral reactions. Emotional brain functions also influence cognitive processes, including perception, attention, learning, memory, reasoning, and problem solving and vice-versa. A detailed knowledge about emotional competencies such as emotional awareness, managing of own emotions and emotions of other people, self-motivation, impulse control and empathy may support caregivers, clinicians, and therapists to get an insight into the mental processes and needs of persons with low cognitive abilities [23,24].

In this theoretical paper, we aim to integrate knowledge from developmental neuroscience to expand our understanding of intellectual disability. As intellectual disability is a disorder of the brain that manifests during the developmental period, the stepwise acquisition of the different emotional and social skills can be depicted alongside the developmental trajectories of typically developing children [25,26], c.f. Table 1.

Table 1. Development of socio-emotional brain functions [26].

Level of Socio-Emotional Development (Reference Age)	Corresponding Level of Intellectual Functioning	Socio-Emotional Developmental Milestones
1. Adaptation 2. (0–6 months of age)	Profound intellectual disability (F73)	Integration of sensory information and external stimuli (place, time and people), processing of stimuli, regulation of physical processes
3. Socialisation 4. (7–18 months of age)	Profound intellectual disability (F73)	Social bonds, object permanence, rough body scheme
5. First Individuation (19–36 months of age)	Severe-profound intellectual disability (F72–F73)	Self-Other differentiation, recognizing and expressing one's own will.
6. Identification 7. (4–7 years of age)	Moderate-severe intellectual disability (F71–F72)	Ego formation, change of perspective (Theory of Mind), interaction with peers, differentiation between fantasy and reality
8. Reality awareness (8–12 years of age)	Mild-moderate intellectual disability (F70–F71)	Moral action, assessment of one's own abilities, self-differentiation, awareness of reality, logical thinking
9. Social Individuation (13–18 years of age)	Borderline-mild intellectual disability, typical intelligence	Abstract thinking skills, sexual identity, self-reflection, independence, responsibility, identity formation, moral self

3. Linking the Socio-Emotional Brain Functions with the Maturation of the Socio-Emotional Brain Networks

Depending on the functionality of the respective brain networks, different ways of thinking and developmental tasks, needs, and skills can be learned [25,26]. Knowledge of the socio-emotional brain network functions may provide the clinician with insights into the "inner world" of people who experience difficulties expressing their own thoughts/feelings, and it could increase the understanding of their behaviors [25–27]. We therefore wish to outline the developmental milestones of brain development and link it to the respective socio-emotional functions. Persons with a developmental delay principally follow the same trajectories as people with a neurotypical development; however, the developmental milestones may be reached later or incompletely.

The brain architecture is scaffolded prenatally and early in life, followed by an extended period of differentiation of the cytoarchitecture by dendritic growth and the formation, pruning, and stabilization of synapses. While short-range connectivity predominates in infancy, there is a shift towards long-range networks in adolescents and adults [25]. The developmental changes of structural brain connectivity result from a sequence of genetic and epigenetic mechanisms at key developmental stages [25,28–30]. Environmental factors and early life experiences in social interactions play a crucial role in the coordination and timing of the specific neuronal patterning [25,31,32].

At birth, the neuronal networks are already at a certain stage of maturity. However, functional magnetic resonance imaging studies showed that local brain activity and functional connectivity differ between neonates and adults. While in the neonatal brain, for example, sensorimotor, visual and auditory areas were most active, other frontal brain regions, the basal ganglia and limbic/paralimbic areas showed lower dynamic connections than adult brains [28]. The emergence of the various socio-emotional skills is linked to the formation of the respective brain networks located within the different parts of the limbic system [33]. Thus, higher order networks build on circuits that process more basic information [25]. The recognition of emotional-communicative signals, for example, is a prerequisite for the proper functioning of the Theory of Mind network, or stress and emotion regulation abilities are necessary for successful impulse control.

The different steps (Figure 1) provide an insight into the stepwise emerging mentalization abilities. Depending on the respective developmental stage, different ways of thinking occur [32]:

- The first step is the action-oriented way of thinking also called the 'teleological thinking'. At this stage, feelings and thoughts cannot be expressed with words but goal-oriented actions. Self-injurious or destructive behaviors can represent a common response to frustration.
- The second step is the 'concrete thinking' stage. In this stage, persons cannot discriminate between their own thoughts and the thoughts of other persons, meaning that thinking is reality to them: "The way I think, the way it is".
- The third step is thinking in the pretend mode of thinking 'pseudomentalization'. In this stage, the inner world (fantasy/imagination) is disconnected from the outside world. The interpretation of a situation is unrelated to the reality of other people. People in the pretend mode of thinking may have problems with feeling emotions in the 'here and now' and use clichés and empty words.
- In a further step, the individual is able to acknowledge that other persons have different feelings, thoughts, intentions, and motivations: The Theory of Mind network is developed and the person is able to mentalize (c.f. Figure 1).

Knowledge of the development of the mentalization abilities is supportive for a proper understanding of a person's mental framework, especially in the case of the non-mentalizing ways of thinking.

Figure 1 exemplifies the stepwise development of the Theory of Mind network.

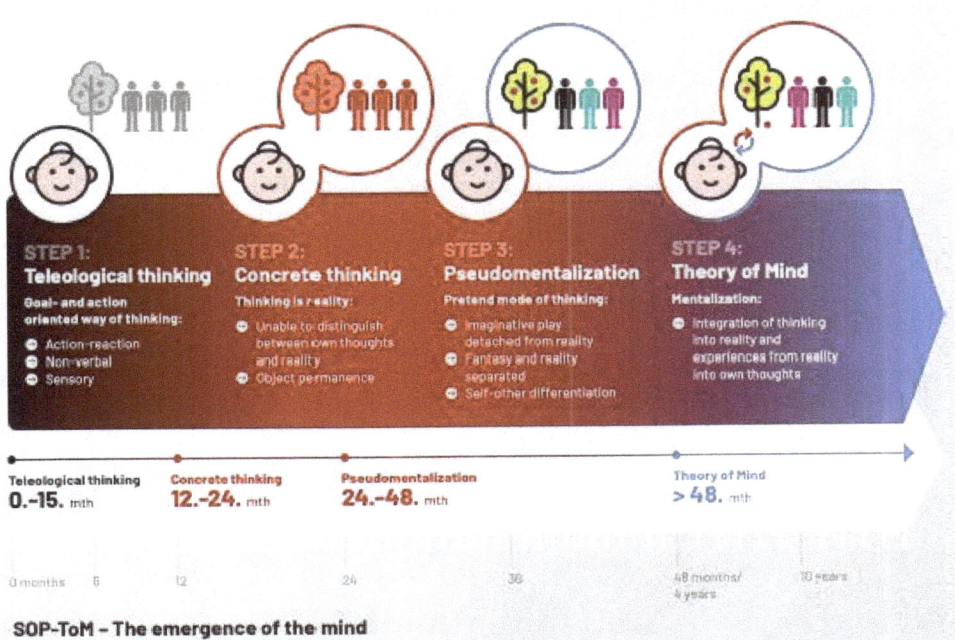

Figure 1. Milestones of development of the Theory of Mind network: Teleological thinking (0–15 months); concrete thinking (15–24 months); Pseudomentalization (24–48 months); Theory of Mind network (>48 months). Details c.f. [32,34].

Depending on a variety of factors, including specific brain alterations and their time course, in persons with an intellectual disability, the formation of the socio-emotional brain networks may differ from the pattern that can be observed in typical development [35,36]. According to the definition in the ICD-11/DSM-5, intellectual disability begins during the developmental period and is associated with impairments of the different brain functions, which will be related to the different neural networks in the following stage.

However, when the developmental delay is severe, the *deep limbic system* drives most emotional and relational acts. This part of the limbic system develops prenatally and during the very first months after birth and includes the central nucleus of the amygdala, the hypothalamus, and parts of the brain stem including the periventricular grey and the vegetative nuclei. This first step of brain development is accompanied by an action-oriented *way* of thinking with an inability to express feelings and thoughts with words [32]. Feelings and thoughts cannot yet be expressed with words but involve goal-oriented actions. The autonomic and the stress-regulation systems process basal functions for survival, such as heart rate and temperature control, feeding, sexuality, territoriality, and stress responses including fight-flight reactions (see Figure 2) [32]. These mostly unconscious processes are genetically-epigenetically determined and influenced by early life experiences [37].

In moderate to severe forms of developmental delay, the functions located within the *mesolimbic system* determine the way of thinking and social interaction. This part of the limbic system is located in the basolateral amygdala, the ventral tegmental area, and the nucleus accumbens/ventral striatum and is the seat of the reward and the reward expectation system where emotional conditioning and emotion regulation are processed. Hence, basic emotional functions, such as fear, sadness, disgust, happiness, and anger, are determined [31,38]. The basic needs are safety and security [25,26]. In this stage of brain development, the person is learning to build up an inner picture of the outside environment (object permanence) and to experience his/her own thoughts as reality (concrete thinking) [39]. This may result in misunderstandings, as facts are not differentiated from convictions [32]. In the next step, accompanied by the ability to differentiate between the self and the other, the pretend mode of thinking 'pseudo-mentalization' arises [32]. This can lead to meaningless conversations, such as repetitive questioning, and in the case of trauma, may result in dissociation [32]. The mesolimbic system develops within the first months and years of life and operates predominantly unconsciously (cf. Figure 2) [33].

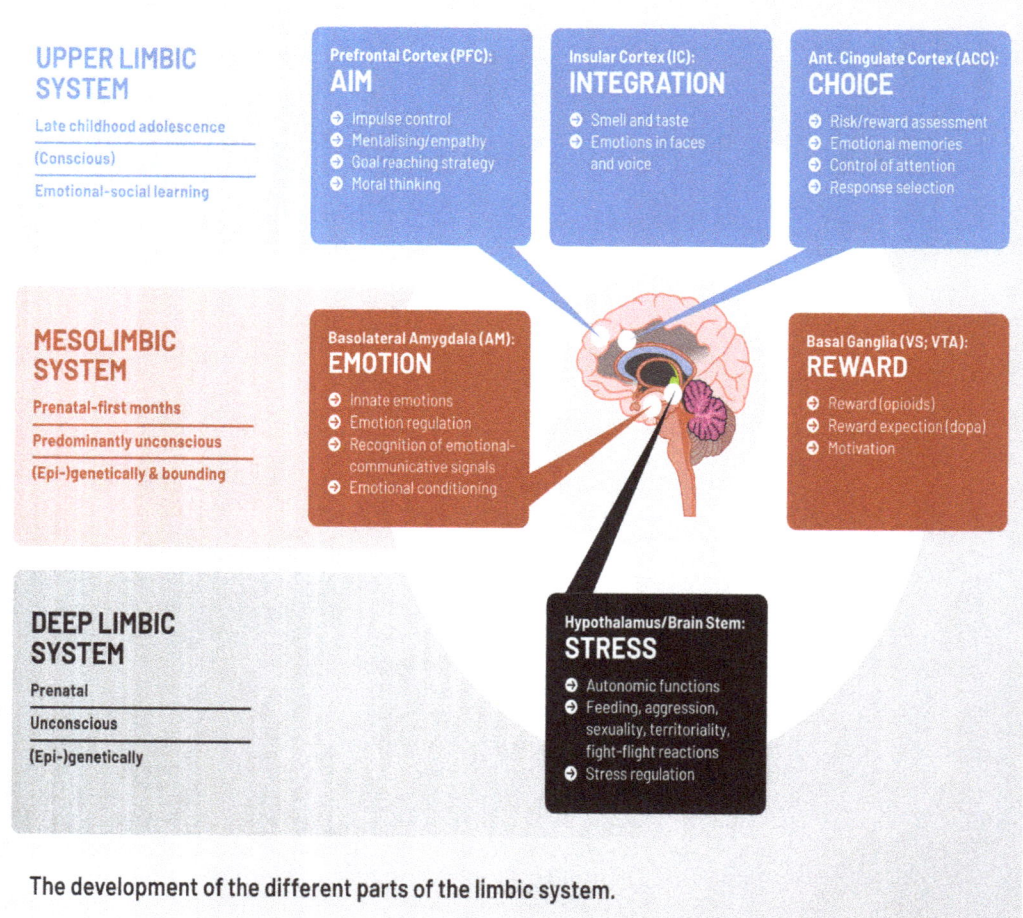

Figure 2. The development of the different parts of socio-emotional brain networks. Details about the different parts and functions of the limbic system c.f. [33]. Socio-emotional brain functions rely on a proper formation of the respective brain areas of the limbic system. Depending on the severity of brain damage, also socio-emotional competencies are affected accordingly. Abbreviations: PFC: Prefrontal Cortex; IC: Insular Cortex; Ant.: Anterior; ACC: Anterior Cingulate Cortex; Bl.: Basolateral; AM: Amygdala; Basal Gang.: Basal Ganglia; VS: Ventral Striatum; VTA: Ventral Tegmental Area.

In milder forms of developmental delays, the *upper limbic system* dominates social cognition and adaptive behaviors. It is composed of a group of tightly interconnected cortical brain areas including the prefrontal, the orbitofrontal, the ventromedial frontal, the anterior cingulate, and the insular cortex. It comprises the neural activity that controls the Theory of Mind, different aspects of executive functions, risk assessment, and reality awareness [40–42]. In a top-down mechanism, these neocortical networks attenuate the emotional responses of the lower-order brain circuits located within the mesolimbic and deep limbic systems [43]. Logical thinking, impulse control, delayed gratification, and affect regulation are important for pro-social behaviors [44]. Concomitantly, emotional states, such as empathy, friendship, loyalty, and moral thinking, may be observed [27,45,46]. The upper limbic system evolves in late childhood and adolescence and can be partly modulated by learning [33].

A variety of conditions associated with an intellectual disability, such as ASD, meningoencephalitis, or genetic syndromes, may cause impairments of the early wiring within the limbic system and the associated brain functions [25,42,45,47,48]. Therefore, the socio-emotional brain functions, e.g., perspective-taking skills, may differ in persons with different syndromes (Cornelia de Lange syndrome vs. William syndrome) or comorbidities such as ASD or attention-deficit-hyperactivity disorders (ADHD) [34,49]. Furthermore, stress and trauma can influence social brain functions in general, and specifically for persons with intellectual disabilities [25,26,50].

So far, there is a lack of assessment instruments for emotional and social competencies. Thus, incorporating structured information about the social, emotional, and practical skills into the assignment to the different levels of intellectual disability may be supportive for clinical care, especially when it comes to the more severe forms where classical IQ-tests cannot be applied.

4. Assessment of Socio-Emotional Functioning

Depending on the individual pattern of developmental delay, also in adults with an intellectual disability, socio-emotional brain functions may be delayed. For a comprehensive evaluation of the mental abilities of a person, we propose integrating the assessment of the different emotional and social skills located in the respective brain network, as these are crucial for perception, the way of thinking, and adaptive behaviors outcomes. Currently, IQ tests focus on logical-deductive academic skills [23,24,51]. However, the IQ score does not always relate to the individual's functioning at a specific point in time, and emotional competences, such as affect regulation, risk assessment, delayed gratification, impulse control, mentalizing abilities, and reality awareness, must also be taken into account [24,46]. Structured assessments addressing these abilities may be helpful to further ascertain this population and support clinicians in the calibration of treatment and support.

Being aware that development is a continuous process, for an assessment of the functional skills, a stepwise model is necessary. Researchers have developed assessment instruments to determine the socio-emotional functioning of a person with an intellectual disability [52,53]. In particular, the Scale of Emotional Development-Short (SED-S) is based on the normative developmental trajectory of the social brain network to define the central characteristic of socio-emotional functioning in a certain age group [35]. The instrument was tested for proof of evidence for criterion validity on item, domain, and scale level by applying the scale to a sample of typically developing children [54]. For the majority of items, the expected response pattern emerged, showing the highest response probabilities in the respective target age groups. Agreement between the classification of the different SED-S domains and the chronological age of children with normative development was high ($\kappa w = 0.95$; exact agreement = 80.6%) [54]. Interrater reliability at domain level ranged from $\kappa w = 0.98$ to 1.00, and internal consistency was high ($\alpha = 0.99$) [54]. The SED-S is applicable and valid in children [55] and adults with ID [34]. Lower levels of socio-emotional development are associated with more severe forms of challenging behaviors [49]. Mentalization abilities can be assessed using the Reflective Functioning Questionnaire–

Mild to Borderline intellectual Disabilities + (RFQ-MBID) [56]. Depending on the pattern of brain alterations, in persons with an intellectual disability, the intellectual reference age is likely to be distinct from the emotional age [49]. Therefore, we argue that the socio-emotional brain functions should be evaluated separately, and specific instruments should be added to those already in use to measure the IQ itself. The utility of the comprehensive assessment of the level of socio-emotional brain functions should be viewed as paramount in supporting clinicians in personalizing treatment and care in the clinical setting. A person's social, emotional, and practical abilities are central for the adaptive behavior, emotional well-being, and mental health.

5. Mental Disorders and Developmental Neuroscience in Persons with an Intellectual Disability

Mental health and emotional functioning in a particular social environment are strongly interrelated. Persons with an intellectual disability are highly vulnerable to mental disorders [4–6]. The conceptualization of psychopathology and mental disorders relies on the grouping of defined symptoms into syndromes that yield a psychiatric diagnosis. The co-occurrence of certain developmental disorders and intellectual disability may suggest a common underlying neurobiology at an early stage of brain development. The increasing evidence for shared genetic etiology across different psychiatric disorders and intellectual disability suggests a continuum of neurodevelopmental causality that includes both the heterogeneity and the overlap of risk factors and disease mechanisms [57]. The developmental miswiring within the social brain networks at sensitive periods may be associated with mental disorders that occur at a certain point of brain development [45,58]. Hence, certain disorders such as autism spectrum disorders (ASD) may be more prevalent in people with more severe forms of intellectual disability while other disorders such as social anxiety disorders may be more often seen in milder forms of intellectual disability.

In ASD, for example, core symptoms, such as perspective-taking skills, are rooted in developmental delays of the brain circuits related to social cognition [59]. In ADHD, widespread alterations of structural and functional brain connectivity are described [60]. Insecure attachment appears to be linked to social experiences that occur during critical periods of development which affect the architecture of the limbic and stress regulation system and have an impact on emotion processing, emotion regulation, and risk assessment [23,25,61]. Alterations in specific neural circuits that develop prenatally or very early in life are also often reported in persons with an intellectual disability, especially when the developmental delay is severe [45,58].

However, other psychiatric disorders, such as social anxiety disorders, dissociative disorders, or personality disorders, may require the maturation of higher-order social brain networks and so cannot be found earlier than age 5 years [62–64]. Social anxiety disorders require perspective-taking skills located in the Theory of Mind network [62]. Dissociative disorders are associated with subcortical white matter alterations within the higher limbic system [63,64]. Conduct disorders may progress to antisocial personality disorders during adolescence/early adulthood [65]. Social anxiety, dissociative disorders, or personality disorder can be linked to disturbances of higher-order brain circuits and typically arise concomitantly to the formation of the respective neural networks during childhood and adolescence. These mental disorders are rarely observed in severe forms of intellectual disability and are more prevalent in persons with borderline intellectual functioning or mild cognitive impairments [5].

Therefore, it can be argued that disturbances of the brain cytoarchitecture and function that occur at a certain developmental period may increase the susceptibility to certain mental disorders. This is supported by research examining emotional intelligence and psychopathy [66,67]. The developmental approach for socio-emotional brain functions in persons with an intellectual disability offers a fundamental perspective in mental health and opens up new treatment options [45].

6. Impact of the Social Brain Development on Treatment and Support

The quantity and quality of studies evaluating the efficacy of psychological therapies in persons with an intellectual disability and mental ill-health are still limited, especially in those with severe to profound intellectual disabilities [68]. Some studies tested commonly used psychosocial interventions, such as cognitive behavioral therapy, and there are valuable efforts to adapt the methods to the level of cognitive functioning; however, treatment manuals for severe and profound levels are still scarce [49,69]. In addition, effectiveness studies often exclude persons with multiple disabilities and comorbidities which is the clinical reality we are faced with [49,68].

With regard to treatment and care, aspects such as the level of socio-emotional functioning and the associated mental competencies and possibilities for reflection may support the decision for or against a certain therapeutic approach. Well-developed perspective-taking skills, for example, may increase the probability of the individual deriving benefit from cognitive behavioral therapy or mentalization-based treatment, while individuals with limited stress regulation abilities may be more likely to respond to bodily and experience-based treatment methods, such as attachment-based behavioral therapy or dance and movement therapy [48,70–72]. Targeting evidence-based treatment programs that are personalized and in line with the individual's abilities and goals is particularly vital in persons with developmental disabilities [49,73]. The 'social information processing model', for example, aims to choose the type of intervention according to the mental state of a person during a social interaction [74]. Moreover, knowledge of the emotional reference age of the individual may enable caregivers to be more attuned to his/her emotional needs and, therefore, promote and maintain good mental health. Finally, the awareness of the socio-emotional functioning of persons with an intellectual disability at that time point may enhance the diagnostic process of ascertaining co-occurrent psychiatric disorders. Externalizing behaviors or observable psychological distress may be interpreted as psychopathological symptoms but could be better explained as a mismatch between the level of individual development expected for the chronological age and the level of actual individual functioning [56,75]. This is particularly useful in persons with low or absent verbal communication skills, in whom key elements of psychiatric disorders, such as delusions, hallucinations, or suicidal ideation, are often very hard to recognize and may only be expressed by changes in behavior [76]. Matson et al. [77] claimed that "accurately identifying the causes of adaptive skill deficits will likely result in more precise and effective treatment" (p. 1317). Therefore, disturbances of the socio-emotional brain networks at a certain developmental period may increase the susceptibility to certain mental disorders. Aligning treatment options according to the level of socio-emotional functioning may strengthen the efficacy and increase the outcome of treatment of certain mental disorders. Furthermore, teaching emotional competencies may further improve skills such as emotional awareness, managing of own emotions and emotions of other people, self-motivation and empathy [78].

7. Discussion

The developmental perspective on the socio-emotional brain network may give insights into their own perspective and experiences, especially in people who experience difficulties expressing their own thoughts and feelings, and it may support clinicians to better understand the shown behaviors [25–27]. Therefore, the linkage of the developmental milestones of brain development with the respective socio-emotional functions may help adapt treatment and support accordingly. We are aware that the staged limbic-structure theory is simplifying the complexity of human brain development [79,80]. This perspective or framework opens up the road for rolling out and promoting early intervention strategies that impact both behavior and adaptive skills as these appear to be likely modifiable factors that can improve longer term outcomes. Further in-depth insights into the perceptual, cognitive, and social-communicative functions in specific syndromes like Downs syndrome or Williams syndrome need to be considered [81,82].

8. Conclusions

The focus of this article is to connect recent knowledge from developmental neuroscience with clinical research in persons with an intellectual disability with the aim of deducing the implications for treatment and support. Despite the given limitations of the broad-brush description of the stepwise development of the brain, specifically of the different parts of the limbic system and its associated functions, a developmental neurobiological basis may offer an additional perspective in our understanding and conceptualization of psychopathology and mental health in persons with developmental delays. The developmental miswiring within the socio-emotional brain networks at sensitive periods may be associated with mental disorders that occur at a certain point of brain development [45,58]. A common underlying neurobiology at an early stage of brain development may cause an association of certain disorders with different severities of intellectual disability. This synthesis offers relevant evidence about the necessity to integrate developmental neuroscience into clinical practice and care for persons with an intellectual disability to further promote mental health in this highly vulnerable population. Knowledge of development of the socio-emotional brain is important in the clinical and daily work context, as it provides insights into the inner world of persons who may have difficulties in reporting about their own thoughts and needs. Accordingly, this article aims to cross the bridge from basic neuroscience to the practical work with persons with developmental disabilities. A comprehensive assessment of intellectual functioning including socio-emotional functioning is important in treatment provision that is personalized and addresses individual goals and deficits. Therapeutic considerations should not only contribute to increased well-being but should also be consistent with the person's emotional status and congruent with the social environment (cf. Figure 1). This extended understanding of how people with intellectual disability function and how they participate in society may enable persons with developmental disabilities to "participate in every aspect of life to the best of their abilities and desires" [7]. We assert that it is only in this way that the person can be supported to fully realize his/her potential and prevent new onset or exacerbations of a mental disorder.

Author Contributions: The article was conceptualized and the original draft written by T.S., A.H., M.B., I.D. and P.S. substantially contributed in discussing the outline, writing certain paragraphs, reviewing and editing the whole manuscript. All authors have read and agreed to the published version of the manuscript.

Funding: This research was supported by funds of the v. Bodelschwinghsche Stiftungen Bethel (c.f. Board Meeting Protocol from 19.1.2016). P.S. was funded by the Bartiméus Fund (reference number P00238).

Institutional Review Board Statement: Not applicable.

Informed Consent Statement: Not applicable.

Data Availability Statement: Not applicable.

Acknowledgments: This analysis of the development of the social brain functions and its impact on the needs of persons with an intellectual disability would not have been possible without the work of the founding father of the dynamic developmental approach, Anton Došen. In 2015, Došen, together with clinicians and scientists of different professions from all over Europe, founded an international working group, the *Network of Europeans on Emotional Development* (NEED), which meets annually in different European cities. The ideas and fruitful discussion of this group contributed greatly to the content of the article. We thank Filip Morisse for his valuable comments and suggestions on the manuscript.

Conflicts of Interest: T.S. receives royalties from different publishers (esp. Hogrefe, Kohlhammer) for various books and funds of the v. Bodelschwinghsche Stiftungen Bethel. No conflict of interest is declared for M.B., A.H., I.D. and P.S. The authors declare that the research was conducted in the absence of any commercial or financial relationships that could be construed as a potential conflict of interest.

References

1. Zablotsky, B.; Black, L.I.; Maenner, M.J.; Schieve, L.A.; Danielson, M.L.; Bitsko, R.H.; Blumberg, S.J.; Kogan, M.D.; Boyle, C.A. Prevalence and Trends of Developmental Disabilities among Children in the United States: 2009–2017. *Pediatrics* **2019**, *144*, e20190811. [CrossRef] [PubMed]
2. McGuire, D.O.; Tian, L.H.; Yeargin-Allsopp, M.; Dowling, N.F.; Christensen, D.L. Prevalence of cerebral palsy, intellectual disability, hearing loss, and blindness, National Health Interview Survey, 2009–2016. *Disabil. Health J.* **2019**, *12*, 443–451. [CrossRef] [PubMed]
3. GBD 2017 Disease and Injury Incidence and Prevalence Collaborators. Global, regional, and national incidence, prevalence, and years lived with disability for 354 diseases and injuries for 195 countries and territories, 1990–2017: A systematic analysis for the Global Burden of Disease Study 2017. *Lancet* **2018**, *392*, 1789–1858. [CrossRef]
4. Mazza, M.G.; Rossetti, A.; Crespi, G.; Clerici, M. Prevalence of co-occurring psychiatric disorders in adults and adolescents with intellectual disability: A systematic review and meta-analysis. *J. Appl. Res. Intellect. Disabil.* **2019**, *33*, 126–138. [CrossRef]
5. Cooper, S.-A.; Smiley, E.; Morrison, J.; Williamson, A.; Allan, L. Mental ill-health in adults with intellectual disabilities: Prevalence and associated factors. *Br. J. Psychiatry* **2007**, *190*, 27–35. [CrossRef] [PubMed]
6. Sheehan, R.; Hassiotis, A.; Walters, K.; Osborn, D.; Strydom, A.; Horsfall, L. Mental illness, challenging behaviour, and psychotropic drug prescribing in people with intellectual disability: UK population based cohort study. *BMJ* **2015**, *351*, h4326. [CrossRef]
7. Centers for Disease Control and Prevention, National Center on Birth Defects and Developmental Disabilities, Division of Human Development and Disability. Disability and Health Data System (DHDS) Data. Available online: https://www.cdc.gov/ncbddd/disabilityandhealth/dhds/index.html (accessed on 2 October 2022).
8. Glover, G.; Williams, R.; Heslop, P.; Oyinlola, J.; Grey, J. Mortality in people with intellectual disabilities in England. *J. Intellect. Disabil. Res.* **2016**, *61*, 62–74. [CrossRef]
9. O'Leary, L.; Cooper, S.; Hughes-McCormack, L. Early death and causes of death of people with intellectual disabilities: A systematic review. *J. Appl. Res. Intellect. Disabil.* **2017**, *31*, 325–342. [CrossRef]
10. Reppermund, S.; Srasuebkul, P.; Dean, K.; Trollor, J.N. Factors associated with death in people with intellectual disability. *J. Appl. Res. Intellect. Disabil.* **2019**, *33*, 420–429. [CrossRef]
11. Hosking, F.J.; Carey, I.M.; Shah, S.M.; Harris, T.; DeWilde, S.; Beighton, C.; Cook, D.G. Mortality Among Adults With Intellectual Disability in England: Comparisons With the General Population. *Am. J. Public Health* **2016**, *106*, 1483–1490. [CrossRef] [PubMed]
12. Cooper, S.-A.; Hughes-McCormack, L.; Greenlaw, N.; McConnachie, A.; Allan, L.; Baltzer, M.; McArthur, L.; Henderson, A.; Melville, C.; McSkimming, P.; et al. Management and prevalence of long-term conditions in primary health care for adults with intellectual disabilities compared with the general population: A population-based cohort study. *J. Appl. Res. Intellect. Disabil.* **2017**, *31*, 68–81. [CrossRef]
13. Gustavsson, A.; Svensson, M.; Jacobi, F.; Allgulander, C.; Alonso, J.; Beghi, E.; Dodel, R.; Ekman, M.; Faravelli, C.; Fratiglioni, L.; et al. CDBE 2010 Study Group. Cost of disorders of the brain in Europe 2010. *Eur. Neuropsychopharmacol. J. Eur. Coll. Neuropsychopharmacol.* **2011**, *21*, 718–779. [CrossRef]
14. Lunsky, Y.; De Oliveira, C.; Wilton, A.; Wodchis, W. High health care costs among adults with intellectual and developmental disabilities: A population-based study. *J. Intellect. Disabil. Res.* **2018**, *63*, 124–137. [CrossRef]
15. Arora, S.; Goodall, S.; Viney, R.; Einfeld, S. Societal cost of childhood intellectual disability in Australia. *J. Intellect. Disabil. Res.* **2020**, *64*, 524–537. [CrossRef]
16. Fujiura, G.T.; Li, H.; Magaña, S. Health Services Use and Costs for Americans With Intellectual and Developmental Disabilities: A National Analysis. *Intellect. Dev. Disabil.* **2018**, *56*, 101–118. [CrossRef]
17. Grawe, K. *Neuropsychotherapie*; Hogrefe: Göttingen, Germany, 2004.
18. Descartes, R. Discours sur la Méthode Pour Bien Conduire sa Raison et Chercher la Vérité dans les Sciences. édition Adam et Tannery. 1902. 1637. Available online: https://zulu-ebooks.com/fachbuecher/discours-de-la-methode (accessed on 2 October 2022).
19. Damasio, A. *Self Comes to Mind. Constructing the Conscious Brain*; Vintage Books: New York, NY, USA, 2012.
20. Ciompi, L. Affects as central organizing and integrating factors: A new psychosocial/biological model of the psyche. *Br. J. Psychiatry* **1991**, *159*, 97–105. [CrossRef]
21. Insel, T.; Cuthbert, B.; Garvey, M.; Heinssen, R.; Pine, D.S.; Quinn, K.; Sanislow, C.; Wang, P. Research Domain Criteria (RDoC): Toward a New Classification Framework for Research on Mental Disorders. *Am. J. Psychiatry* **2010**, *167*, 748–751. [CrossRef]
22. World Health Organization. International Statistical Classification of Diseases and Related Health Problems. 11th ed.; 2019. Available online: https://icd.who.int/browse11/l-m/en (accessed on 2 October 2022).
23. Bar-On, R.; Tranel, D.; Denburg, N.L.; Bechara, A. Exploring the neurological substrate of emotional and social intelligence. *Brain* **2003**, *126*, 1790–1800. [CrossRef]
24. Pisanos, D.E. Emotional Intelligence: It's More Than IQ. *J. Contin. Educ. Nurs.* **2011**, *42*, 439–440. [CrossRef]
25. Fox, S.E.; Levitt, P.; Nelson, C.A., 3rd. How the timing and quality of early experiences influence the development of brain architecture. *Child Dev.* **2010**, *81*, 8–40. [CrossRef]
26. Došen, A. Applying the developmental perspective in the psychiatric assessment and diagnosis of persons with intellectual disability: Part I—Assessment. *J. Intellect. Disabil. Res.* **2005**, *49*, 1–8. [CrossRef]

27. Koenigs, M.; Young, L.; Adolphs, R.; Tranel, D.; Cushman, F.; Hauser, M.; Damasio, A. Damage to the prefrontal cortex increases utilitarian moral judgments. *Nature* **2007**, *19446*, 908–911. [CrossRef]
28. Huang, Z.; Wang, Q.; Zhou, S.; Tang, C.; Yi, F.; Nie, J. Exploring functional brain activity in neonates: A resting-state fMRI study. *Dev. Cogn. Neurosci.* **2020**, *45*, 100850. [CrossRef]
29. Power, J.D.; Fair, D.A.; Schlaggar, B.L.; Petersen, S.E. The Development of Human Functional Brain Networks. *Neuron* **2010**, *67*, 735–748. [CrossRef]
30. Knudsen, E.I. Sensitive Periods in the Development of the Brain and Behavior. *J. Cogn. Neurosci.* **2004**, *16*, 1412–1425. [CrossRef]
31. Diano, M.; Tamietto, M.; Celeghin, A.; Weiskrantz, L.; Tatu, K.; Bagnis, A.; Duca, S.; Geminiani, G.; Cauda, F.; Costa, T. Dynamic Changes in Amygdala Psychophysiological Connectivity Reveal Distinct Neural Networks for Facial Expressions of Basic Emotions. *Sci. Rep.* **2017**, *7*, srep45260. [CrossRef]
32. Fonagy, P.; Bateman, A.W. *Handbook of Mentalizing in Mental Health Practice*; American Psychiatric Publishing: Arlington, TX, USA, 2012.
33. Roth, G. Chapter 2: Gehirn und limbisches System. [engl.: The brain and the limbic system]. In *Wie das Gehirn die Seele Macht. [engl.: How the Brain Forms the Soul]*, 7th ed.; Roth, G., Strüber, N., Eds.; Klett-Cotta: Stuttgart, Germany, 2018; pp. 45–94.
34. Sappok, T.; Heinrich, M.; Böhm, J. Autism Spectrum Disorder, intellectual developmental disabilities, and emotional development: Relatedness and diagnostic impact. *J. Intellect. Disabil. Res.* **2020**, *64*, 946–955. [CrossRef]
35. Sappok, T.; Barrett, B.F.; Vandevelde, S.; Heinrich, M.; Poppe, L.; Sterkenburg, P.; Vonk, J.; Kolb, J.; Claes, C.; Bergmann, T. Scale of emotional development-Short. *Res. Dev. Disabil.* **2016**, *59*, 166–175. [CrossRef]
36. Baurain, C.; Nader-Grosbois, N. Theory of Mind, Socio-Emotional Problem-Solving, Socio-Emotional Regulation in Children with Intellectual Disability and in Typically Developing Children. *J. Autism Dev. Disord.* **2012**, *43*, 1080–1097. [CrossRef]
37. McLaughlin, K.A.; Sheridan, M.A.; Tibu, F.; Fox, N.A.; Zeanah, C.H.; Nelson, C.A. Causal effects of the early caregiving environment on development of stress response systems in children. *Proc. Natl. Acad. Sci. USA* **2015**, *112*, 5637–5642. [CrossRef]
38. Kalin, N.H.; Shelton, S.E.; Davidson, R. The Role of the Central Nucleus of the Amygdala in Mediating Fear and Anxiety in the Primate. *J. Neurosci.* **2004**, *24*, 5506–5515. [CrossRef]
39. Cerniglia, L.; Bartolomeo, L.; Capobianco, M.; Russo, S.L.M.L.; Festucci, F.; Tambelli, R.; Adriani, W.; Cimino, S. Intersections and Divergences Between Empathizing and Mentalizing: Development, Recent Advancements by Neuroimaging and the Future of Animal Modeling. *Front. Behav. Neurosci.* **2019**, *13*, 212. [CrossRef] [PubMed]
40. Bowman, L.C.; Thorpe, S.G.; Cannon, E.N.; Fox, N.A. Action mechanisms for social cognition: Behavioral and neural correlates of developing Theory of Mind. *Dev. Sci.* **2016**, *20*, e12447. [CrossRef]
41. Girgis, F.; Lee, D.J.; Goodarzi, A.; Ditterich, J. Toward a Neuroscience of Adult Cognitive Developmental Theory. *Front. Neurosci.* **2018**, *12*, 4. [CrossRef]
42. Moessnang, C.; the EU-AIMS LEAP group; Baumeister, S.; Tillmann, J.; Goyard, D.; Charman, T.; Ambrosino, S.; Baron-Cohen, S.; Beckmann, C.; Bölte, S.; et al. Social brain activation during mentalizing in a large autism cohort: The Longitudinal European Autism Project. *Mol. Autism* **2020**, *11*, 1–17. [CrossRef]
43. Hariri, A.R. Modulating emotional responses: Effects of a neocortical network on the limbic system. *Neuroreport* **2000**, *11*, 43–48. [CrossRef]
44. Steinbeis, N.; Bernhardt, B.C.; Singer, T. Impulse Control and Underlying Functions of the Left DLPFC Mediate Age-Related and Age-Independent Individual Differences in Strategic Social Behavior. *Neuron* **2012**, *73*, 1040–1051. [CrossRef]
45. Happé, F.; Frith, U. Annual Research Review: Towards a developmental neuroscience of atypical social cognition. *J. Child Psychol. Psychiatry* **2013**, *55*, 553–577. [CrossRef] [PubMed]
46. Sappok, T.; Zepperitz, S.; Hudson, M. *Meeting Emotional Needs in Intellectual Disability: The Developmental Approach*; Hogrefe Publishing: Göttingen, Germany, 2021. [CrossRef]
47. Martínez-Castilla, P.; Burt, M.; Borgatti, R.; Gagliardi, C. Facial emotion recognition in Williams syndrome and Down syndrome: A matching and developmental study. *Child Neuropsychol.* **2014**, *21*, 668–692. [CrossRef]
48. Cicchetti, D.; Ganbian, J. The organization and coherence of developmental processes in infants and children with Down syndrome. In *Issues in the Developmental Approach*; Hodapp, R.M., Burack, J.A., Zigler, E., Eds.; Cambridge University Press: Cambridge, UK, 1990; pp. 169–225.
49. Sappok, T.; Budczies, J.; Dziobek, I.; Bölte, S.; Dosen, A.; Diefenbacher, A. The Missing Link: Delayed Emotional Development Predicts Challenging Behavior in Adults with Intellectual Disability. *J. Autism Dev. Disord.* **2013**, *44*, 786–800. [CrossRef]
50. Dekker-van der Sande, F.; Sterkenburg, P.S. Learning from Mentalization Based Therapy for Mentalization Based Support in Daily Care. *J. Ment. Health Res. Intellect. Disabil.* **2016**, *10*, 104.
51. Wechsler, D. *Wechsler Adult Intelligence Scale, Fourth Edition (WAIS–IV)*; Pearson: London, UK, 2012.
52. Frankish, P. Meeting the emotional needs of handicapped people: A psycho-dynamic approach. *J. Ment. Defic. Res.* **1989**, *33*, 407–414.
53. Hoekman, J.; Miedema, A.; Otten, B.; Gielen, J. De constructie van een schaal voor de bepaling van het sociaal-emotionele ontwikkelingsniveau. Achtergrond, opbouw en betrouwbaarheid van de ESSEON. [engl.: The construction of a scale for determining the level of socio-emotional development. Background, structure and reliability of the ESSEON]. *Ned. Tijdschr. Voor De Zorg Aan Mensen Met Verstand. Beperkingen* **2007**, *33*, 215–232.

54. Sappok, T.; Böhm, J.; Birkner, J.; Roth, G.; Heinrich, M. How is your mind-set? Proof of concept for the measurement of the level of emotional development. *PLoS ONE* **2019**, *14*, e0215474. [CrossRef] [PubMed]
55. Sterkenburg, P.; Kempelmann, G.; Hentrich, J.; Vonk, J.; Zaal, S.; Erlewein, R.; Hudson, M. Scale of emotional development–short: Reliability and validity in two samples of children with an intellectual disability. *Res. Dev. Disabil.* **2020**, *108*, 103821. [CrossRef]
56. Derks, S.; Willemen, A.; Vrijmoedt, C.; Sterkenburg, P. Psychometric Properties of an Adapted, Dutch Version of the Reflective Functioning Questionnaire (RFQ) for People with Mild to Borderline Intellectual Disabilities. submitted.
57. Owen, M.J. Intellectual disability and major psychiatric disorders: A continuum of neurodevelopmental causality. *Br. J. Psychiatry* **2012**, *200*, 268–269. [CrossRef] [PubMed]
58. Di Martino, A.; Fair, D.A.; Kelly, C.; Satterthwaite, T.D.; Castellanos, F.X.; Thomason, M.E.; Craddock, R.C.; Luna, B.; Leventhal, B.L.; Zuo, X.-N.; et al. Unraveling the Miswired Connectome: A Developmental Perspective. *Neuron* **2014**, *83*, 1335–1353. [CrossRef] [PubMed]
59. Samson, A.C.; Phillips, J.M.; Parker, K.J.; Shah, S.; Gross, J.J.; Hardan, A.Y. Emotion Dysregulation and the Core Features of Autism Spectrum Disorder. *J. Autism Dev. Disord.* **2013**, *44*, 1766–1772. [CrossRef] [PubMed]
60. Konrad, K.; Eickhoff, S.B. Is the ADHD brain wired differently? A review on structural and functional connectivity in attention deficit hyperactivity disorder. *Hum. Brain Mapp.* **2010**, *31*, 904–916. [CrossRef] [PubMed]
61. Fairchild, G.; Hawes, D.J.; Frick, P.J.; Copeland, W.E.; Odgers, C.; Franke, B.; Freitag, C.M.; De Brito, S.A. Conduct disorder. *Nat. Rev. Dis. Prim.* **2019**, *5*, 43. [CrossRef] [PubMed]
62. Plana, I.; Lavoie, M.-A.; Battaglia, M.; Achim, A.M. A meta-analysis and scoping review of social cognition performance in social phobia, posttraumatic stress disorder and other anxiety disorders. *J. Anxiety Disord.* **2014**, *28*, 169–177. [CrossRef] [PubMed]
63. Jans, T.; Schneck-Seif, S.; Weigand, T.; Schneider, W.; Ellgring, H.; Wewetzer, C.; Warnke, A. Long-term outcome and prognosis of dissociative disorder with onset in childhood or adolescence. *Child Adolesc. Psychiatry Ment. Health* **2008**, *2*, 19. [CrossRef]
64. Sierk, A.; Manthey, A.; Brakemeier, E.-L.; Walter, H.; Daniels, J.K. The dissociative subtype of posttraumatic stress disorder is associated with subcortical white matter network alterations. *Brain Imaging Behav.* **2020**, *15*, 643–655. [CrossRef]
65. Junewicz, A.; Billick, S.B. Conduct Disorder: Biology and Developmental Trajectories. *Psychiatr. Q.* **2019**, *91*, 77–90. [CrossRef] [PubMed]
66. Varo, C.; Jimenez, E.; Solé, B.; Bonnín, C.M.; Torrent, C.; Valls, E.; Morilla, I.; Lahera, G.; Martínez-Arán, A.; Vieta, E.; et al. Social cognition in bipolar disorder: Focus on emotional intelligence. *J. Affect. Disord.* **2017**, *217*, 210–217. [CrossRef]
67. Copestake, S.; Gray, N.S.; Snowden, R.J. Emotional intelligence and psychopathy: A comparison of trait and ability measures. *Emotion* **2013**, *13*, 691–702. [CrossRef]
68. Vereenooghe, L.; Flynn, S.; Hastings, R.; Adams, D.; Chauhan, U.; Cooper, S.-A.; Gore, N.; Hatton, C.; Hood, K.; Jahoda, A.; et al. Interventions for mental health problems in children and adults with severe intellectual disabilities: A systematic review. *BMJ Open* **2018**, *8*, e021911. [CrossRef]
69. Koslowski, N.; Klein, K.; Arnold, K.; Kösters, M.; Schützwohl, M.; Salize, H.J.; Puschner, B. Effectiveness of interventions for adults with mild to moderate intellectual disabilities and mental health problems: Systematic review and meta-analysis. *Br. J. Psychiatry* **2016**, *209*, 469–474. [CrossRef] [PubMed]
70. Mohamed, A.R.; Mkabile, S. An attachment-focused parent-child intervention for biting behaviour in a child with intellectual disability: A clinical case study. *J. Intellect. Disabil.* **2015**, *19*, 251–265. [CrossRef] [PubMed]
71. Mastrominico, A.; Fuchs, T.; Manders, E.; Steffinger, L.; Hirjak, D.; Sieber, M.; Thomas, E.; Holzinger, A.; Konrad, A.; Bopp, N.; et al. Effects of Dance Movement Therapy on Adult Patients with Autism Spectrum Disorder: A Randomized Controlled Trial. *Behav. Sci.* **2018**, *8*, 61. [CrossRef] [PubMed]
72. Sterkenburg, P.S.; Janssen, C.G.C.; Schuengel, C. The Effect of an Attachment-Based Behaviour Therapy for Children with Visual and Severe Intellectual Disabilities. *J. Appl. Res. Intellect. Disabil.* **2008**, *21*, 126–135. [CrossRef]
73. Lai, M.C.; Anagnostou, E.; Wiznitzer, M.; Allison, C.; Baron-Cohen, S. Evidence-based support for autistic people across the lifespan: Maximising potential, minimising barriers, and optimising the person-environment fit. *Lancet Neurol.* **2020**, *19*, 434–451. [CrossRef]
74. Larkin, P.; Jahoda, A.; MacMahon, K. The Social Information Processing Model as a Framework for Explaining Frequent Aggression in Adults with Mild to Moderate Intellectual Disabilities: A Systematic Review of the Evidence. *J. Appl. Res. Intellect. Disabil.* **2013**, *26*, 447–465. [CrossRef]
75. Cooper, S.A.; Salvador-Carulla, L. Intellectual disabilities. In *Psychiatric Diagnosis: Challenges and Prospects*; Salloum, I.M., Mezzich, J.E., Eds.; John Wiley & Sons: Hoboken, NJ, USA, 2009; pp. 141–146.
76. Bertelli, M.; Scuticchio, D.; Ferrandi, A.; Lassi, S.; Mango, F.; Ciavatta, C.; Porcelli, C.; Bianco, A.; Monchieri, S. Reliability and validity of the SPAID-G checklist for detecting psychiatric disorders in adults with intellectual disability. *Res. Dev. Disabil.* **2012**, *33*, 382–390. [CrossRef]
77. Matson, J.L.; Rivet, T.T.; Fodstad, J.C.; Dempsey, T.; Boisjoli, J.A. Examination of adaptive behavior differences in adults with autism spectrum disorders and intellectual disability. *Res. Dev. Disabil.* **2009**, *30*, 1317–1325. [CrossRef]
78. Tuyakova, U.; Baizhumanova, B.; Mustapaeva, T.; Alekeshova, L.; Otarbaeva, Z. Developing emotional intelligence in student teachers in universities. *Humanit. Soc. Sci. Commun.* **2022**, *9*, 1–6. [CrossRef]

79. Karmiloff-Smith, A. Neuroimaging of the developing brain: Taking "developing" seriously. *Hum. Brain Mapp.* **2010**, *31*, 934–941. [CrossRef]
80. Cao, M.; Wang, J.-H.; Dai, Z.-J.; Cao, X.-Y.; Jiang, L.-L.; Fan, F.-M.; Song, X.-W.; Xia, M.-R.; Shu, N.; Dong, Q.; et al. Topological organization of the human brain functional connectome across the lifespan. *Dev. Cogn. Neurosci.* **2013**, *7*, 76–93. [CrossRef]
81. Lott, I.T.; Dierssen, M. Cognitive deficits and associated neurological complications in individuals with Down's syndrome. *Lancet Neurol.* **2010**, *9*, 623–633. [CrossRef]
82. Donnai, D.; Karmiloff-Smith, A. Williams syndrome: From genotype through to the cognitive phenotype. *Am. J. Med. Genet.* **2000**, *97*, 164–171. [CrossRef]

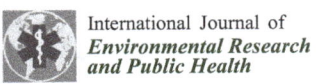

Article

More than a Physical Problem: The Effects of Physical and Sensory Impairments on the Emotional Development of Adults with Intellectual Disabilities

Paula S. Sterkenburg [1,2,*], Marie Ilic [3], Miriam Flachsmeyer [4] and Tanja Sappok [4]

[1] Department of Clinical Child and Family Studies & Amsterdam Public Health, Faculty of Behavioural and Movement Sciences, Vrije Universiteit Amsterdam, Van der Boechorststraat 7, 1081 BT Amsterdam, The Netherlands
[2] Department of Assessment and Treatment, Bartiméus, 3941 XM Doorn, The Netherlands
[3] Diakonische Stiftung Wittekindshof, 32549 Bad Oeynhausen, Germany
[4] Berlin Center for Mental Health in Intellectual Developmental Disabilities, Ev. Krankenhaus Königin Elisabeth Herzberge, 10365 Berlin, Germany
* Correspondence: p.s.sterkenburg@vu.nl; Tel.: +31-(0)20-5988890

Abstract: With the introduction of the ICD-11 and DSM-5, indicators of adaptive behavior, including social–emotional skills, are in focus for a more comprehensive understanding of neurodevelopmental disorders. Emotional skills can be assessed with the Scale of Emotional Development-Short (SED-S). To date, little is known about the effects of physical disorders and sensory impairments on a person's developmental trajectory. The SED-S was applied in 724 adults with intellectual disabilities, of whom 246 persons had an additional physical and/or sensory impairment. Ordinal regression analyses revealed an association of movement disorders with more severe intellectual disability and lower levels of emotional development (ED) on the overall and domain levels (*Others*, *Body*, *Material*, and *Communication*). Visual impairments predicted lower levels of ED in the SED-S domains *Material* and *Body*, but not the overall level of ED. Hearing impairments were not associated with intellectual disability or ED. Epilepsy correlated only with the severity of intellectual disability. Multiple impairments predicted more severe intellectual disabilities and lower levels of overall ED. In conclusion, physical and sensory impairments may not only affect physical development but may also compromise intellectual and emotional development, which should be addressed in early interventions.

Keywords: emotional development; intellectual disability; visual impairment; hearing impairment; physical disability; sensory impairments

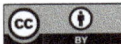

1. Introduction

People with intellectual disabilities have a higher risk of developing psychological stress than people without intellectual disabilities [1]. Possibly contributing to this, people with intellectual disabilities have difficulty assessing and processing information [2], they need predictable environments [3], and they have poor coping mechanisms [4]. Furthermore, due to affected children's limited behavioral repertoires, parents and caregivers need to have a high level of sensitivity and responsiveness to signals and react adequately to the behavior, needs, and wishes of the person with an intellectual disability [4,5]. Consequently, there is a higher risk of disturbed attachment and emotional and behavioral problems [6,7].

According to the American Association on Intellectual and Developmental Disabilities (AAIDD), people are classified as having an intellectual disability when they have an IQ score below 70 and/or a significant limitation in their adaptive behavior [8]. The need for support for conceptual, social, and practical skills starts before the age of 22 [8]. Likewise, the classification systems DSM-5 and ICD-11 also include limitations in adaptive behavior and social skills in the diagnostic criteria for intellectual disability/disorders of intellectual development, respectively. Intellectual disability is often associated with a delay in emotional development [9]. Delayed social–emotional development and associated neglect of basic emotional and support needs result in stress and consequently possibly challenging behavior [7]. To provide adequate care matching the emotional functioning and needs of persons with intellectual disability, the Scale for Emotional Development-Short (SED-S) has been developed and studied in children with and without intellectual disabilities [9–11] as well as in adults [12–15]. The SED-S is based on the Scheme for Appraisal of Emotional Development (SAED) [16], the Scale for Emotional Development–Revised (SED-R) [17], and the SED-R2 [18]. Adequate psychometric properties are reported for the SED-S [9,10].

The prevalence of co-occurring impairments (such as physical, visual, and hearing impairments) is higher among persons with intellectual disability than in those without [19,20]. In studies conducted in the Netherlands among 1598 persons with intellectual disability who were older than 18 years of age, the following prevalence rates were reported: visual impairment, 14%; blindness, 5%; mild hearing loss, 30%; moderate to severe hearing loss, 15%; and dual impairments (visual and hearing impairments), 5% [20–22]. What is more, in a Finnish study among 461 persons with profound to severe intellectual disability, the prevalences of motor impairments and epilepsy were, respectively, 35% and 51% [23]. These impairments in addition to intellectual disability may affect emotional functioning.

Auditory sensory loss is, for example, of interest when studying social–emotional development in people with intellectual disabilities. In studies conducted before the implementation of neonatal hearing screening programs, results indicated that children over the age of 4 with hearing loss had more social–emotional difficulties than did children without hearing loss [24]. An uncompensated hearing impairment also affects communication in a negative way in adulthood [25,26]. However, the results of a study conducted in 18-month-old children with hearing loss found no apparent difficulties in social–emotional functioning [27]. Additionally, Lederberg and Mobley [28] found no difference in the quality of attachment of children with and without hearing impairments. This could be thanks to the ability of parents and children to communicate nonverbally during the child's first years, with children with a hearing impairment being able to adequately imitate facial expressions and hand and body movements, in addition to using gestures and pointing [29]. Moreover, parents put much effort into early communication, such as trying to establish (eye) contact or elicit a response through manifesting exaggerated facial expressions, waving their hands, and moving objects or people into the child's line of sight [29]. Although parents and children have compensatory communication in place, Dirks et al. [30] did report that children with a hearing impairment are at risk for social–emotional difficulties. Adding to this, Sterkenburg et al. [9] reported that children with an intellectual disability and a hearing-and/or visual impairment (n = 9) showed lower emotional functioning than children with intellectual disabilities without these sensory impairments (n = 108). These results were found on the SED-S overall score and on the domain *Others* (meaning "relating to significant others"). However, due to the small sample size in this study, people with visual or hearing impairments were combined into one group. Consequently, it is unclear whether emotional functioning is lowered by the separate sensory impairments.

Regarding the emotional development of persons with visual disabilities, the physical, cognitive, and social development of a child are affected by visual impairment [31]. Urqueta Alfaro et al. [32] confirmed that, compared with children without visual impairment, the overall development of children with visual disabilities is delayed. To be precise, the visual impairment hinders their social development, as social behavior and communication mostly develop through eye contact and observation [31]. Zooming in on the emotional development of children with visual impairment, Fraiberg [33] reported that blind children show more fear of strangers than sighted peers and that their facial expressions are frequently indistinct. Additionally, their nonverbal expressions are sometimes different and very subtle [34]. The findings of Fraiberg [33], suggested that children with a visual impairment do develop mental representations of their attachment figures, but that these representations start at a later age and/or show different characteristics than in sighted peers. This delay may affect their emotional functioning. Furthermore, infants with visual impairments need more help and encouragement to become aware of their range of motion. This help prevents them from remaining in their natural passive state, which could hinder their physical development, including posture and mobility [35], and affect their exploration and social and emotional development.

Next to the influence of a hearing or visual impairment, a child's physical development may also impact their emotional development. Persons with an intellectual disability have an increased risk for physical disabilities and epilepsy [19,36]. Vandesande et al. [37] conducted a study among children with severe and profound intellectual disabilities during a stressful situation, where the child's parents and a stranger were present. Interestingly, the child's differentiated responses to comfort seemed to be related to their fine motor skills [37]. Therefore, to adequately support persons with intellectual and physical disabilities, it is important to examine the effects of the disabilities on the different domains of emotional development.

According to Došen [38], the social–emotional development of a neurotypical child goes through several stages, and these stages are linked to social–emotional developmental milestones [38–40]. For children with intellectual disabilities and sensory, physical, or multiple impairments, reaching these milestones requires more effort than it does for children without these impairments. Up to now, to our knowledge, no studies have been conducted among adults with intellectual disability to examine the effect of visual, hearing, or physical impairments on emotional functioning. Therefore, the aim of this study was to examine whether physical or sensory impairments of adults with intellectual disabilities can predict their level of social–emotional functioning.

2. Materials and Methods

2.1. Setting and Design

The study was conducted from May 2016 to November 2020 in three hospitals and five home care facility centers in Belgium, the Netherlands, and Germany. Inclusion criteria were age >18 years and a diagnosis of intellectual disability. There were no exclusion criteria within this respective population. A sample of 724 adults with intellectual disabilities was recruited, among which 246 persons (34%) had an additional physical disorder and/or sensory impairment such as a hearing and/or visual impairment, movement disorder, and/or epilepsy.

The participating organizations were Tordale in Torhout (Belgium), Cordaan in Amsterdam (Netherlands), ORO in Helmond (Netherlands), De Twentse Zorgcentra in Losser (Netherlands), Bartiméus in Doorn (Netherlands), the Evangelisches Krankenhaus Königin Elisabeth Herzberge in Berlin (Germany), Klinikum München Oberbayern in München (Germany), and St. Lukas-Klink in Liebenau (Germany). The persons themselves or their legal guardians gave their informed consent for participation in this study.

2.2. Participants

The total study sample consisted of 724 participants with intellectual disabilities. Due to missing information about the researched impairments, two persons were omitted from the analyses, leaving a total sample of 722 participants. The average participant age was 37.4 years (18–76 years, $SD = 13.3$) and males were slightly in the majority (56.4%). The degree of intellectual disability ranged from mild (IQ 50–55 to 70: 28.2%), moderate (IQ 35–40 to 50–55: 37.4%), and severe (IQ 20–25 to 35–40: 26.8%), to profound (IQ < 20–25: 7.6%).

The age of the 246 (34%) participants with sensory impairments ranged from 18 to 76 years, and the average age was 39.9 years ($SD = 13.7$). This sample included more males (60.2%) than females. All levels of intellectual disability were represented; most of the participants had moderate intellectual disabilities (38.2%), followed by severe intellectual disabilities (28.5%), mild intellectual disabilities (19.5%), and profound intellectual disabilities (13.8%). In this group with sensory impairments, 44 persons (17.9%) had hearing impairments and 64 persons (26%) had visual impairments. In the sample with sensory impairments, 87 persons (35.4%) had a movement disorder. Epilepsy was reported in 130 persons (52.8%).

2.3. Assessment

The level of emotional development (ED) was assessed using the SED-S [10]. The SED-S is a semi-structured interview consisting of 200 binary items in eight domains, concerning different aspects of daily life behaviors. The scale assesses five developmental stages with reference ages ranging from 0 to 12 years of age. Each level of ED is assessed by five items per domain. The eight domains are: (1) *Body* (Relating to His/Her Own Body), (2) *Others* (Relating to Significant Others), (3) *Object* (Dealing with *Change*: Object Permanence), (4) *Emotions* (Differentiating Emotions), (5) *Peers* (Relating to Peers), (6) *Material* (Engaging with the Material World), (7) *Communication* (Communicating with Others), and (8) *Affect* (Regulating Affect).

Within the SED-S items, behaviors for a certain level of ED are described, which are either typical in the respective person ("yes" answers) or not typical ("no" answers). To determine the level of ED in a certain domain, the number of "yes "answers is counted. The level with the most "yes "answers is the domain-wise level of ED. Estimating the overall level of ED, these domain-specific results are ordered from low to high, and the four lowest domains determine the overall result. Trained psychologists, psychiatrists, developmental psychologists, or ortho-pedagogues conducted the interview with two to five informants, such as family members or close caregivers. The assessment relied on behaviors displayed during the previous 2 weeks.

Expert validity can be taken as given, as the scale is based on a survey of developmental psychology experts and their assessments of behaviors typical for specific levels of development, [10]. Validation against a group of 160 typically developed children showed a high degree of correspondence (81% exact agreement; 0.95 weighted kappa value) [11]. An exploratory factor analysis provided a one-factor model with a good model fit in 724 adults with ID, most of them having additional mental health problems [15,41], in 118 children with ID and mental health problems [9] and in 83 healthy adults with ID [14,41]. Divergent validity was found for chronological age in children with ID [9] and in healthy adults with ID [14,41]. Convergent validity with the Vineland Adaptive Behavior Scale could be seen in the children's sample ($r = 0.642$, $p < 0.001$; [9]). Strong negative associations with the severity of ID could be shown in 327 adults with ID and mental health problems ($r = -0.654$, $p < 0.001$; [11]), in 83 adults with ID without mental health problems (-0.753, $p < 0.001$; [14,41]) and in 118 children with ID ($G = -0.69$; $p < 0.001$; [9]). Inter-rater reliability for 25 typically developed children was 1.0 (Cohen's kappa). Internal consistency as measured by Cronbach's alpha was 0.99 in typically developing children [11], 0.94 in 118 children with ID [9] and 0.92 in 83 adults with ID without mental health problems [14,41].

The degree of intellectual disability was diagnosed using the Disability Assessment Schedule (DAS), which is an informant-based structured interview [41]. It poses several questions about adaptive behaviors in four parts: continence, self-help skills, communication, and (cognitive) skills. Depending on the presence of these behaviors, points are given and summed to a total score (minimum 15 points; maximum 71). The total score corresponds with the levels of ID (mild, moderate, severe, profound). The DAS is a reliable measure when applied by trained professionals [42]. Evidence pertaining to its validity in people with ID is provided by correlation analysis with the Colored Progressive Matrices and the Columbia Mental Maturity Scale [43].

The data regarding hearing and visual impairment, movement disorders, and epilepsy were systematically recorded upon the assessment of the SED-S.

2.4. Statistical Analysis

The statistical analyses were conducted using IBM SPSS 27 Statistics for Windows, USA. Associations of hearing and/or visual impairment, and movement disorder and/or epilepsy, with the severity of the intellectual disability and the level of ED (overall and domain wise) were examined by applying an ordinal logistic regression analysis. The ordinal logistic regression model was chosen because of the dichotomous variable structure of the impairments and because the severity of the intellectual disability and level of ED were ordinal variables [44]. A further key assumption of ordinal logistic regression analysis is that of assumption of proportional odds, which in SPSS is examined with the test of parallel lines. Chi-square was used to determine whether the assumed model with an explanatory variable was improved in comparison with the baseline model without this explanatory variable.

A significant p-value indicates an improved fit to the data. Nagelkerke R^2 is reported as a pseudo R^2 value, indicating the proportion of variation in the outcome that can be accounted for by the explanatory variables. To specifically analyze the relationship between the sensory impairments and the intellectual disability and ED, odds ratios and the Wald χ^2 were calculated to investigate whether a significant impact of the explanatory variables existed.

3. Results

Assumptions of parallel lines were met for all our analyses ($p > 0.05$) with one exception: for the regression of the domain *Others* on the four impairments, it was significant with $p = 0.044$, meaning these results should be interpreted cautiously.

3.1. Number of Impairments as a Predictor of Intellectual Disability and ED

Since many participants had more than one reported impairment, the number of impairments (e.g., visual, hearing) was analyzed as a predictor of the intellectual disability and ED. For intellectual disability, ordinal regression analysis revealed that higher numbers of co-occurrent physical impairments were related to more severe intellectual disability ($\Delta\chi^2 = 37.85$, $df = 4$, $p < 0.001$; Nagelkerke $R^2 = 0.055$). The individual odds ratios were nonsignificant. Additionally, the level of ED improved the model fit of the regression analysis when the number of impairments was used as a predictor to explain the level of ED ($\Delta\chi^2 = 11.56$, $df = 4$, $p < 0.021$; Nagelkerke $R^2 = 0.017$). Again, the individual odds ratios were nonsignificant.

3.2. Different Forms of Impairments as Predictors of Intellectual Disability and ED

Looking at the frequency of the different levels of intellectual disability and ED for the different groups of impairments (reported in Tables 1 and 2), not only the presence or absence of physical or sensory impairments, but also the type of impairment was relevant. For an overview of the results, see Table 3.

Table 1. The Different Impairments and Severities of Intellectual Disability.

Severity of Intellectual Disability	No Additional Impairment ($n = 476$)	Hearing Impairment ($n = 44$)	Visual Impairment ($n = 64$)	Movement Disorder ($n = 87$) *	Epilepsy ($n = 130$) *
Mild ($n = 204$)	153 (32.1)	10 (22.7)	13 (20.3)	11 (12.6)	20 (15.4)
Moderate ($n = 271$)	178 (37.4)	16 (36.4)	24 (37.5)	24 (27.6)	57 (43.8)
Severe ($n = 194$)	124 (26.1)	12 (27.3)	20 (31.3)	30 (34.5)	36 (27.7)
Profound ($n = 55$)	21 (4.4)	6 (13.6)	7 (10.9)	22 (25.3)	17 (13.1)

Note. In parentheses are percentages per column. Regression analyses for the impairments marked with * showed a significant association with the severity of intellectual disability.

Table 2. The Different Impairments and Levels of Emotional Development.

Level of ED	No additional Impairment (n = 473)	Hearing Disorder (n = 44)	Visual Disorder (n = 64)	Movement Disorder * (n = 87)	Epilepsy (n = 129)
SED-S 1	66 (13.9)	10 (22.7)	14 (21.9)	19 (21.8)	21 (16.2)
SED-S 2	112 (23.3)	6 (13.6)	16 (25)	24 (27.6)	36 (27.7)
SED-S 3	164 (34.5)	18 (40.9)	25 (39.1)	33 (37.9)	52 (40.0)
SED-S 4	114 (23.9)	9 (20.5)	8 (12.5)	10 (11.5)	16 (12.3)
SED-S 5	17 (3.6)	1 (2.3)	1 (1.6)	1 (1.1)	4 (3.1)

Note. In parentheses are percentages per column. Regression analyses for the impairments marked with * showed a significant association with level of ED.

Table 3. The associations between sensory impairments, ID, and ED.

Sensory Impairments	Intellectual Disability (ID)	Emotional Development (ED)
Hearing impairment	No association	No association
Visual impairment	No association	No association -except on domain level for the domains *Body* and *Material*
Movement disorder	Relation to more severe forms of ID	Relation to lower levels of ED -on domain level for *Body*, *Others*, *Material*, and *Communication*
Epilepsy	Relation to more severe forms of ID	No association
Accumulation of impairments	Relation to more severe forms of ID	Related to lower levels of ED

Hearing impairment. Hearing impairments were not associated with the severity of intellectual disability or the level of ED in any of the ten analyses (Details for the nonsignificant analyses are available from the authors upon request).

Visual impairment. Having a visual impairment was related neither to the intellectual disability nor to the level of overall ED. However, visual impairments significantly predicted lower levels of ED on the domains of *Body* (odds ratio 1.65, 95% CI 1.022–2.68; Wald $\chi^2(1) = 4.082$, $p = 0.043$) and *Material* (odds ratio 1.71, 95% CI 1.06–2.72, Wald $\chi^2(1) = 4.823$, $p = 0.028$).

Movement disorder. A movement disorder was related to more severe forms of the intellectual disability (odds ratio 0.28, 95% CI 0.18–0.43; Wald $\chi^2(1) = 33.446$, $p < 0.001$). Furthermore, the presence of a movement disorder was related to lower levels of ED in general (odds ratio 1.59, 95% CI 1.05–2.42; Wald $\chi^2(1) = 4.815$, $p = 0.028$) and for the domains of *Body* (odds ratio 2.25, 95% CI 1.47–3.45; Wald $\chi^2(1) = 13.988$, $p < 0.001$), *Others* (odds ratio 1.66, 95% CI 1.06–2.72; Wald $\chi^2(1) = 5.591$, $p = 0.018$), *Material* (odds ratio 1.66, 95% CI 1.10–2.50; Wald $\chi^2(1) = 5.821$, $p = 0.016$), and *Communication* (odds ratio 2.14, 95% CI 1.41–3.24; Wald $\chi^2(1) = 12.964$, $p < 0.001$).

Epilepsy. Epilepsy was associated with more severe forms of intellectual disability (odds ratio 0.65, 95% CI 0.46–0.93; Wald $\chi^2(1) = 5.590$, $p = 0.018$), but not with the level of ED (neither overall nor domain wise).

4. Discussion

The aim of this study was to examine if adults with intellectual disability and physical and/or sensory impairments score lower on the SED-S than adults with intellectual disability but without these additional impairments. At first, the results indicated that an accumulation of impairments predicts lower emotional functioning. This could be explained by one impairment significantly affecting the other. For example, as Fraiberg [35] reported, a visual impairment may influence physical development. This in turn may shape emotional development. What is more, persons with a disability are unable to compensate for the co-occurrent impairment. For instance, Gunther [45] reported that the presence of a visual impairment in addition to an intellectual disability means that vision cannot be used to compensate for the intellectual disability, and vice versa. Therefore, people with visual and intellectual disabilities find it is even more difficult to understand social relationships than do people with only intellectual disabilities [46]. Additionally, as found in this study, in persons with a visual and intellectual disability as well as an added hearing impairment, emotional functioning is significantly lower than it is in adults with intellectual disabilities with either a hearing or a visual impairment (not having both impairments).

A second finding of this study is that hearing impairments seem not to be associated with intellectual disability or emotional development. These findings indicate that although there is a risk for social–emotional difficulties in children [30], the focus on learning to communicate [29] and socially interact may eventually buffer the effect of the hearing impairment on emotional functioning. Early intervention programs focusing on joint engagement and emotional availability can be used for this purpose [47,48].

Third, in this study, no significant effects of visual impairment and intellectual disability on the total score for emotional development were found. However, it is important to note that there were domain-specific outcomes, namely in the domains *Relating to His/Her Own Body* and *Engaging with the Material World*. Zooming in on the items of these domains, the hindering effect of the visual impairment becomes more clear: for example, in the use of tactile senses to explore the world, the need to feel safe in an open space, and requiring more time to explore materials, while contact with others is less evident. This may confirm what Fraiberg [33] suggested, namely that emotional development could be delayed and/or show different characteristics than it does in sighted peers. These outcomes are presumably of great importance for (early) intervention programs, which it seems should be more focused on these aspects of socio-emotional development. Additionally, as for all persons, disharmonious emotional development may affect well-being, and therefore should be noticed [49].

A fourth finding of this study is that having a physical disability was associated with more severe forms of intellectual disability and lower levels of emotional functioning. These results indicate that a tailored approach is needed for these persons. Due to the severe or profound disability, repetition, patience, and interaction are needed for emotional development. Nowadays, technology can also be used in daily care to support emotional development [50] and communication. The results of this study stress the importance of addressing these caregiving and assistive technology needs in interventions.

Fifth, epilepsy was related to intellectual disability but could not be linked to emotional development. Thus, epilepsy does not seem to directly obstruct emotional functioning, although adequate care and support for emotional and physical needs is required.

Sterkenburg et al. [9] found a significant relation between visual and hearing senses and emotional development in children. However, in this study the focus was on adults with a mean age of 37.4 years and less-significant links were found. Matching the findings reported by Fraiberg [33] for children with a visual impairment, there was a delay in development, but there seems to be a catching up later in life. However, accumulated impairments did show significant relations with emotional development. Thus, (early) intervention programs are essential and should consider the different co-occurring impairments. There are programs such as: "Development of an attachment relationship" [51]; "Learning together" [52]; "Little room" [53]; "Barti-mat" [54], and the Light Curtain [55]. These results may encourage the application of early interventional strategies that impact both physical and social–emotional skills in people with intellectual and additional disabilities. Hereby, longer-term outcomes, quality of life, and social participation may be improved substantially. Therefore, we recommend continued investment in and provision of (early) intervention programs for parents of infants with intellectual disability and sensory impairment. Additionally, there is a need for more projects focusing on parent–child interaction and the use of technology in supporting the social and emotional development of persons with intellectual disability and sensory impairment.

Limitations

During the assessment, the data regarding visual and hearing impairments, physical disabilities, and epilepsy were reported based on participants' records. However, on-the-spot assessments were not conducted. Thus, the data may be incomplete or not adequately reported in the records and may, therefore, be biased. However, comparing the prevalence of the impairments reported in this study to the prevalence mentioned in the literature [20–23], this does not seem to be the case.

The reported results are based on cross-sectional data, so causal interpretations need to be made with caution. A longitudinal study that follows the development of children with and without intellectual disabilities and physical impairments would be required to be able to fully understand how these factors influence each other and social–emotional development.

The study was conducted in three Western European countries. Due to the small sample size for each of the studied impairments, comparisons between countries were not possible. There may be differences that we cannot now report and that need to be studied in future research. Furthermore, the (early) interventional care in the studied countries may explain the possible catching up when people have reached adulthood; such catching up may not occur in other parts of the world. Replication of this study is therefore needed, covering a broader spectrum of the world population.

5. Conclusions

In summary, higher numbers of co-occurrent physical and/or sensory impairments were related to more severe intellectual disability and lower levels of emotional development (ED). Interestingly, movement disorders affected intellectual and ED, while auditory impairment did not affect ED. Epilepsy correlated only with the degree of intellectual disability but not with the level of ED. On the domain level, *Relating to His/Her Own Body* and *Engaging with the Material World* showed associations with visual impairments and movement disorder, the latter disorder also predicting lower levels of ED in the domains *Relating to Significant Others* and *Communicating with Others*. Considering these overall and specific effects of different impairments on the intellectual and emotional functioning of people with multiple disabilities may align early interventions and thereby further improve long-term outcomes.

Author Contributions: M.I. and M.F. conducted the analyses, P.S.S. wrote the introduction and discussion, and T.S. finalized the paper and coordinated the study. All authors have read and agreed to the published version of the manuscript.

Funding: This research was supported by funds of the v. Bodelschwinghsche Stiftungen Bethel (c.f. Board Meeting Protocol from 19.1.2016). PSS was funded by the Bartiméus Fund (reference number P00238).

Institutional Review Board Statement: The study was conducted according to the ethical principles of the 1975 Declaration of Helsinki. All organizations acquired ethical approval separately. For Belgium, the University of Ghent ethics commission of the Faculty of Psychology and Pedagogic Science gave their permission. The ethics board in each Dutch organization gave approval. For Germany, the Charité University Hospital in Berlin (Ethics vote: EA2/193/16) gave their permission; additionally, every hospital received ethical approval from its own ethics commission.

Informed Consent Statement: Informed consent was obtained from all subjects involved in the study.

Data Availability Statement: On request.

Acknowledgments: We thank all the participants, their parents or relatives, and the caregivers who contributed to this study. We thank the caregiving organizations for facilitating the study. Thanks also to Paula Verbon-Dekkers for providing feedback on the manuscript. Great appreciation goes all the members of the Network of Europeans on Emotional Development (NEED) who participated in the data collection.

Conflicts of Interest: T.S. receives royalties from different publishers (esp. Hogrefe, Kohlhammer) for various books and scales and funds of the v. Bodelschwinghsche Stiftungen Bethel.

References

1. Bramston, P.; Bostock, J.; Tehan, G. The Measurement of Stress in People with an Intellectual Disability: A Pilot Study. *Int. J. Disabil. Dev. Educ.* **1993**, *40*, 95–104. [CrossRef]
2. Van Nieuwenhuijzen, M.; De Castro, B.O.; Wijnroks, L.; Vermeer, A.; Matthys, W. The relations between intellectual disabilities, social information processing, and behaviour problems. *Eur. J. Dev. Psychol.* **2004**, *1*, 215–229. [CrossRef]
3. Gardner, W.I.; Sovner, R. *Self-injurious Behaviors, Diagnosis and Treatment: A Multimodal Functional Approach*; VIDA Publishing: Miami, FL, USA, 1994.
4. Janssen, C.G.C.; Schuengel, C.; Stolk, J. Understanding challenging behaviour in people with severe and profound intellectual disability: A stress-attachment model. *J. Intellect. Disabil. Res.* **2002**, *46*, 445–453. [CrossRef]
5. Doodeman, T.W.M.; Schuengel, C.; Sterkenburg, P.S. Expressions of stress of people with severe intellectual disabilities and sensitive caregiving to regulate stress: A qualitative study. *J. Intellect. Dev. Disabil.* **2022**, *47*, 308–317. [CrossRef]
6. Giltaij, H.P.; Sterkenburg, P.S.; Schuengel, C. Adaptive behaviour, comorbid psychiatric symptoms, and attachment disorders. *Adv. Ment. Health Intellect. Disabil.* **2016**, *10*, 82–91. [CrossRef]
7. Sappok, T.; Budczies, J.; Dziobek, I.; Bölte, S.; Dosen, A.; Diefenbacher, A. The Missing Link: Delayed Emotional Development Predicts Challenging Behavior in Adults with Intellectual Disability. *J. Autism Dev. Disord.* **2014**, *44*, 786–800. [CrossRef]
8. Schalock, R.L.; Luckasson, R.; Tassé, M.J. *Intellectual Disability: Definition, Diagnosis, Classification, and Systems of Supports*, 12th ed.; American Association on Intellectual and Developmental Disabilities: Silver Spring, MD, USA, 2021.
9. Sterkenburg, P.; Kempelmann, G.; Hentrich, J.; Vonk, J.; Zaal, S.; Erlewein, R.; Hudson, M. Scale of emotional development–short: Reliability and validity in two samples of children with an intellectual disability. *Res. Dev. Disabil.* **2020**, *108*, 103821. [CrossRef]
10. Sappok, T.; Barrett, B.F.; Vandevelde, S.; Heinrich, M.; Poppe, L.; Sterkenburg, P.; Vonk, J.; Kolb, J.; Claes, C.; Bergmann, T.; et al. Scale of emotional development—Short. *Res. Dev. Disabil.* **2016**, *59*, 166–175. [CrossRef]
11. Sappok, T.; Böhm, J.; Birkner, J.; Roth, G.; Heinrich, M. How is your mind-set? Proof of concept for the measurement of the level of emotional development. *PLoS ONE* **2019**, *14*, e0215474. [CrossRef]
12. Sappok, T.; Došen, A.; Zepperitz, S.; Barrett, B.; Vonk, J.; Schanze, C.; Ilic, M.; Bergmann, T.; De Neve, L.; Birkner, J.; et al. Standardizing the assessment of emotional development in adults with intellectual and developmental disability. *J. Appl. Res. Intellect. Disabil.* **2020**, *33*, 542–551. [CrossRef]
13. Sappok, T.; Heinrich, M.; Böhm, J. The impact of emotional development in people with autism spectrum disorder and intellectual developmental disability. *J. Intellect. Disabil. Res.* **2020**, *64*, 946–955. [CrossRef] [PubMed]
14. Meinecke, T.; Flachsmeyer, M.; Sappok, T. Validation of the Scale of Emotional Development-Short (SED-S) in Mentally Healthy Adults with an Intellectual Disability. (*submitted to peer-reviewed journal*).
15. Flachsmeyer, M.; Sterkenburg, P.; Barrett, B.; Zaal, S.; Vonk, J.; Morisse, F.; Gaese, F.; Heinrich, M.; Sappok, T. Scale of Emotional Development—Short: Reliability and validity in adults with intellectual disability. (*submitted to peer-reviewed journal*).
16. Došen, A. Psychische Stoornissen, Probleemgedrag en Verstandelijke Beperking. In *Een Integratieve Benadering bij Kinderen en Volwassenen*; Koninklijke van Gorcum: Assen, The Netherlands, 2014.
17. Claes, L.; Verduyn, A. (Eds.) *SEO-R: Schaal Voor Emotionele Ontwikkeling Bij Mensen met een Verstandelijke Beperking: Revised. Ser.*; Sen-Publicaties: 5; Garant- Uitgevers N.V.: Antwerp, Belgium, 2012.
18. Morisse, F.; Došen, A. *SEO-R2 Schaal Voor Emotionele Ontwikkeling Bij Mensen met een Verstandelijke Beperking-Revised2: Instrument Voor Assessment*; Garant-Uitgevers N.V.: Antwerp, Belgium, 2016.
19. Jansen, D.E.M.C.; Krol, B.; Groothoff, J.W.; Post, D. People with intellectual disability and their health problems: A review of comparative studies. *J. Intellect. Disabil. Res.* **2004**, *48*, 93–102. [CrossRef] [PubMed]
20. Evenhuis, H.M.; Theunissen, M.; Denkers, I.; Verschuure, H.; Kemme, H. Prevalence of visual and hearing impairment in a Dutch institutionalized population with intellectual disability. *J. Intellect. Disabil. Res.* **2001**, *45*, 457–464. [CrossRef] [PubMed]
21. Van Splunder, J.; Stilma, J.S.; Bernsen, R.M.D.; Evenhuis, H.M. Prevalence of visual impairment in adults with intellectual disabilities in the Netherlands: Cross-sectional study. *Eye* **2005**, *20*, 1004–1010. [CrossRef]
22. Meuwese-Jongejeugd, A.; Van Splunder, J.; Vink, M.; Stilma, J.S.; Van Zanten, B.; Verschuure, H.; Bernsen, R.; Evenhuis, H. Combined sensory impairment (deaf-blindness) in five percent of adults with intellectual disabilities. *Am. J. Ment. Retard.* **2008**, *113*, 254–262. [CrossRef]
23. Arvio, M.; Sillanpää, M. Prevalence, aetiology and comorbidity of severe and profound intellectual disability in Finland. *J. Intellect. Disabil. Res.* **2003**, *47*, 108–112. [CrossRef]
24. Theunissen, S.C.P.M.; Rieffe, C.; Soede, W.; Briaire, J.J.; Ketelaar, L.; Kouwenberg, M.; Frijns, J.H.M. Symptoms of Psychopathology in Hearing-Impaired Children. *Ear Hear.* **2015**, *36*, e190–e198. [CrossRef]
25. Hall, W.C.; Li, D.; Dye, T.D.V. Influence of Hearing Loss on Child Behavioral and Home Experiences. *Am. J. Public Health* **2018**, *108*, 1079–1081. [CrossRef]
26. Eisinger, J.; Dall, M.; Fogler, J.; Holzinger, D.; Fellinger, J. Intellectual Disability Profiles, Quality of Life and Maladaptive Behavior in Deaf Adults: An Exploratory Study. *Int. J. Environ. Res. Public Health* **2022**, *19*, 9769. [CrossRef]
27. Stika, C.J.; Eisenberg, L.S.; Johnson, K.C.; Henning, S.C.; Colson, B.G.; Ganguly, D.H.; DesJardin, J.L. Developmental outcomes of early-identified children who are hard of hearing at 12 to 18 months of age. *Early Hum. Dev.* **2015**, *91*, 47–55. [CrossRef]

28. Lederberg, A.R.; Mobley, C.E. The Effect of Hearing Impairment on the Quality of Attachment and Mother-Toddler Interaction. *Child Dev.* **1990**, *61*, 1596–1604. [CrossRef] [PubMed]
29. Rowley, K.; Snoddon, K.; O'Neill, R. Supporting families and young deaf children with a bimodal bilingual approach. *Int. J. Birth Parent Educ.* **2022**, *9*, 15–20.
30. Dirks, E.; Ketelaar, L.; Van Der Zee, R.; Netten, A.P.; Frijns, J.H.; Rieffe, C. Concern for Others: A Study on Empathy in Toddlers with Moderate Hearing Loss. *J. Deaf Stud. Deaf Educ.* **2016**, *22*, 178–186. [CrossRef]
31. Dale, N.; Salt, A. Early support developmental journal for children with visual impairment: The case for a new developmental framework for early intervention. *Child: Care Health Dev.* **2007**, *33*, 684–690. [CrossRef] [PubMed]
32. Alfaro, A.U.; Meinz, P.; Morash, V.S.; Lei, D.; Kronberg, J.; Lara, S.; Jian, S.; Moore, M. Applicability and attachment findings of the Strange Situation Paradigm in infants with visual impairment. *Infant Ment. Health J.* **2019**, *40*, 835–849. [CrossRef] [PubMed]
33. Fraiberg, S. Blind Infants and Their Mothers: An Examination of the Sign System. In *Before Speech: The Beginning of Interpersonal Communication, Bullowa, M., Ed.*; Cambridge University Press: Cambridge, UK, 1975; pp. 149–169.
34. Sterkenburg, P.S.; Van den Broek, E.; Van Eijden, A. Promoting positive parenting and attachment in families raising a young child with a visual or visual-and-intellectual disability. *Int. J. Birth Parent Educ.* **2022**, *9*, 23–27.
35. Fraiberg, S. *Insights From the Blind*; Souvenir Press: London, UK, 1977.
36. Enkelaar, L.; Smulders, E.; van Schrojenstein, H.; Geurts, A.C.; Weerdesteyn, V. A review of balance and gait capacities in relation to falls in persons with intellectual disability. *Res. Dev. Disabil.* **2012**, *33*, 291–306. [CrossRef]
37. Vandesande, S.; Bosmans, G.; Sterkenburg, P.; Schuengel, C.; Van Keer, I.; Maes, B. Variation in differential reactions to comfort by parents versus strangers in children with severe or profound intellectual disabilities: The role of parental sensitivity and motor competence. *Curr. Psychol.* **2022**, *2022*, 1–14. [CrossRef]
38. Došen, A. *Psychische Störungen und Verhaltensauffälligkeiten bei Menschen mit Intellektueller Beeinträchtigung: Ein Integrativer Ansatz für Kinder und Erwachsene*; Hogrefe: Göttingen, Germany, 2018.
39. Parenti, I.; Rabaneda, L.G.; Schoen, H.; Novarino, G. Neurodevelopmental Disorders: From Genetics to Functional Pathways. *Trends Neurosci.* **2020**, *43*, 608–621. [CrossRef]
40. Sappok, T.; Hassiotis, A.; Bertelli, M.; Dziobek, I.; Sterkenburg, P. Developmental Delays in Socio-Emotional Brain Functions in Persons with an Intellectual Disability: Impact on Treatment and Support. *Int. J. Environ. Res. Public Health* **2022**, *19*, 13109. [CrossRef]
41. Flachsmeyer, M.; Sterkenburg, P.; Barrett, B.; Zaal, S.; Vonk, J.; Morisse, F.; Gaese, F.; Sappok, T. Validation and Extensions of the Scale of Emotional Development—Short. EAMHID Congress 2021 in Berlin. *J. Intellect. Disabil. Res.* **2021**, *65*, 745.
42. Holmes, N.; Shah, A.; Wing, L. The Disability Assessment Schedule: A brief screening device for use with the mentally retarded. *Psychol. Med.* **1982**, *12*, 879–890. [CrossRef] [PubMed]
43. Meins, W.; Süssmann, D. Evaluation of an adaptive behaviour classification for mentally retarded adults. *Soc. Psychiatry* **1993**, *28*, 201–205. [CrossRef] [PubMed]
44. Mccullagh, P. Regression Models for Ordinal Data. *J. R. Stat. Soc. Ser. B Methodol.* **1980**, *42*, 109–142. [CrossRef]
45. Gunther, F. *Diagnostiek en Behandeling van Mensen met een Visuele en Verstandelijke Beperking*; Bartiméus: Doorn, The Netherlands, 2004.
46. Jaiswal, A.; Aldersey, H.; Wittich, W.; Mirza, M.; Finlayson, M. Participation experiences of people with deafblindness or dual sensory loss: A scoping review of global deafblind literature. *PLoS ONE* **2018**, *13*, e0203772. [CrossRef]
47. Dirks, E.; Rieffe, C. Are You There For Me? Joint Engagement and Emotional Availability in Parent–Child Interactions for Toddlers with Moderate Hearing Loss. *Ear Hear.* **2019**, *40*, 18–26. [CrossRef]
48. Hughes, J. Getting it right from the start . . . What makes good support for families of deaf children? *J. Birth Parent Educ.* **2022**, *9*, 14–16.
49. Böhm, J.; Dziobek, I.; Sappok, T. Emotionale Entwicklung, Aggressionsregulation und herausforderndes Verhalten bei Menschen mit Intelligenzminderung [Emotional development, aggression regulation and challenging behavior in individuals with intellectual disbility]. *Fortschr. Der Neurol.-Psychiatr.* **2019**, *87*, 437–443.
50. Hoffman, N.; Sterkenburg, P.S.; Van Rensburg, E. The effect of technology assisted therapy for intellectually and visually impaired adults suffering from separation anxiety: Conquering the fear. *Assist. Technol.* **2017**, *31*, 98–105. [CrossRef]
51. Sterkenburg, P.S. *Developing Attachment: A Workbook for Building up A Secure Relationship with Children or Adults with Severe Intellectual or Multiple Disabilities. Bartiméus Reeks*; Microweb Edu: Doorn, The Netherlands, 2012; ISBN 9789461071477.
52. Lee, M.; MacWilliam, L. *Learning Together: A Creative Approach to Learning for Children with Multiple Disabilities and A Visual Impairment*; Royal National Institute for the Blind: London, UK, 2008; ISBN 13 9781858785318.
53. Nielsen, L. *Space and Self*; Sikon: New York, NY, USA, 1992.
54. Dyzel, V.; Dekkers-Verbon, P.; Toeters, M.; Sterkenburg, P.S. For happy children with a visual or visual-and-intellectual disability: Efficacy research to promote sensitive caregiving with the Barti-mat. *Br. J. Vis. Impair.* **2021**, 1–20. [CrossRef]
55. Enkelaar, L.; Oosterom-Calo, R.; Zhou, D.; Nijhof, N.; Barakova, E.; Sterkenburg, P. The LEDs move pilot study: The Light Curtain and physical activity and well-being among people with visual and intellectual disabilities. *J. Intellect. Disabil. Res.* **2021**, *65*, 971–988. [CrossRef] [PubMed]

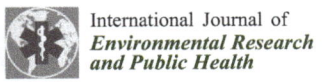

Article

Intellectual Disability Profiles, Quality of Life and Maladaptive Behavior in Deaf Adults: An Exploratory Study

Johanna Eisinger [1], Magdalena Dall [1,*], Jason Fogler [1,2,3], Daniel Holzinger [1,4,5] and Johannes Fellinger [1,4,6]

1 Research Institute for Developmental Medicine, Johannes Kepler University, 4020 Linz, Austria
2 Division of Developmental Medicine, Boston Children's Hospital, Boston, MA 02115, USA
3 Leadership Education in Neurodevelopmental and Related Disabilities/Institute for Community Inclusion (LEND/ICI), Boston Children's Hospital, Boston, MA 02115, USA
4 Institute of Neurology of Senses and Language, Hospital of St. John of God, 4020 Linz, Austria
5 Institute of Linguistics, University of Graz, 8010 Graz, Austria
6 Division of Social Psychiatry, University Clinic for Psychiatry and Psychotherapy, Medical University of Vienna, 1090 Vienna, Austria
* Correspondence: magdalena.dall@jku.at

Citation: Eisinger, J.; Dall, M.; Fogler, J.; Holzinger, D.; Fellinger, J. Intellectual Disability Profiles, Quality of Life and Maladaptive Behavior in Deaf Adults: An Exploratory Study. *Int. J. Environ. Res. Public Health* **2022**, *19*, 9919. https://doi.org/10.3390/ijerph19169919

Academic Editor: Shoumitro Deb

Received: 14 July 2022
Accepted: 7 August 2022
Published: 11 August 2022

Publisher's Note: MDPI stays neutral with regard to jurisdictional claims in published maps and institutional affiliations.

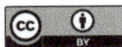

Copyright: © 2022 by the authors. Licensee MDPI, Basel, Switzerland. This article is an open access article distributed under the terms and conditions of the Creative Commons Attribution (CC BY) license (https://creativecommons.org/licenses/by/4.0/).

Abstract: Individuals who are prelingually deaf and have intellectual disabilities experience great challenges in their language, cognitive and social development, leading to heterogeneous profiles of intellectual and adaptive functioning. The present study describes these profiles, paying particular attention to domain discrepancies, and explores their associations with quality of life and maladaptive behavior. Twenty-nine adults with prelingual deafness (31% female) and mild intellectual functioning deficits (mean IQ = 67.3, SD = 6.5) were administered the Vineland Adaptive Behavior Scales-II (VABS-II) and an adapted sign language version of a quality of life scale (EUROHIS-QOL 8). Intellectual disability domain discrepancies were characterized as at least one standard deviation difference between the social domain and IQ and the practical domain and IQ, and a significant difference, according to the VABS-II manual, between the social and practical domains. Domain discrepancies were found between intellectual functioning and both the practical (58.6%) and social domain (65.5%). A discrepancy between intellectual and social functioning was significantly associated with a higher level of internalizing maladaptive behavior (T = 1.89, $p < 0.05$). The heterogeneous profiles highlight the importance of comprehensive assessments for adequate service provision.

Keywords: intellectual disability; deaf; adaptive behavior; intellectual functioning; domain discrepancy; maladaptive behavior; quality of life

1. Introduction

Deafness is a heterogeneous condition that can impact communication, social–emotional development and cognitive development [1]. Around 7 per 10,000 people have severe to profound hearing loss, with onset before language acquisition [2,3].

Approximately one-third to one-half of individuals who are prelingually deaf or hard of hearing have additional disabilities [4,5], most commonly intellectual disability [6]. Additive deprivation of language and communication, stemming from delayed identification, insufficient or late provision of hearing technology and little or no access to sign language, further impedes these individuals' community participation [7–10].

The diagnostic criteria for intellectual disability have been revised in the Diagnostic and Statistical Manual of Mental Disorder-Fifth edition (DSM-5; [11]) to encourage a more comprehensive patient assessment, with greater weight given to adaptive functioning than intellectual functioning for the purpose of ascribing intellectual disability severity [11]. Whereas intellectual functioning generally involves abilities such as reasoning, problem solving, knowledge and experience [12], adaptive functioning refers to the skills that are learned and performed to meet the everyday demands of one's community or society [13], suggesting that adaptive behavior may be the more malleable (and hence important) intervention target to unlock an individual's full potential. Adaptive functioning includes three domains: the conceptual domain, including applied skills in language, reading, writing, math, reasoning, knowledge and memory; the social domain, referring to empathy, social judgment, interpersonal communication skills and the ability to make and retain friendships; and the practical domain, including self-management in areas such as personal care, job responsibilities, money management, recreation and organizing school and work tasks [11].

Intellectual and adaptive functioning, the two aspects of intellectual disability, are related but separate constructs [13]: a large meta-analysis of 148 samples containing a total of 16,468 participants showed a moderate relationship ($r = 0.51$) between intelligence and adaptive behavior, which is stronger in lower IQ groups [14].

With this more nuanced definition of adaptive functioning has come greater interest in intellectual disability domain discrepancy, in which one domain is markedly more deficient than another, as well as inquiry into whether different populations have unique, or at least specific, intellectual disability profiles. Sparrow, Cicchetti and Balla [15], authors of the Vineland Adaptive Behavior Scales-II (VABS-II), provide various adaptive functioning profiles based on pairwise comparison of the four adaptive behavior domains (communication, socialization, daily living skills and motor skills) outlined in the Vineland-II manual. When comparing the specific profile of individuals with hearing impairment with samples matched by age range and controlled for sex, ethnicity and education level, the researchers found that individuals with hearing impairment had lower levels of communication and daily living skills than the IQ-matched sample with typical hearing. The socialization scale appeared as a relative strength, though still lower than the non-clinical group [15].

There is a growing body of research on adaptive profiles in individuals with different neurodevelopmental disorders [16–22]. Tillmann et al. [23] examined how IQ and levels of ASD symptom and autistic trait severity are associated with adaptive functioning and suggested that core ASD-related social communication problems contribute both to adaptive functioning impairments and to the discrepancy between IQ and adaptive functioning. Further supporting this point, a discrepancy between intellectual functioning and adaptive skills was found to be significantly correlated with depression and anxiety in a sample of adults with ASD without intellectual disability, in which socialization was by far the largest weakness [24].

Studies correlating adaptive profiles with such clinically relevant variables as quality of life (QOL) and problem behavior (e.g., [13,25]) show divergent results. Tassé [13] and Simoes et al. [26] found a positive correlation between adaptive behavior and QOL in samples of individuals with mild-to-moderate intellectual disability, whereas Graves et al. [18] did not find significant associations between adaptive functioning and self-reported QOL in a sample of adults with Down syndrome. Jones et al. [27] found higher levels of problem behavior to be associated with more severe degrees of intellectual disability. Curiously, Balboni et al. [25] found that a subgroup of individuals with intellectual disability with the highest levels of problem behavior also had higher levels of adaptive behavior, explaining that a basal level of adaptive skills appears to be necessary for the person to be able to engage in their environment, positively or negatively.

No research to date has investigated the intellectual disability profiles and the relationships between intellectual disability domain discrepancies, QOL and maladaptive behavior in a population with prelingual deafness and intellectual functioning deficits. Hence, the main aim of this study is twofold: (a) to describe the intellectual disability profiles and potential intellectual disability domain discrepancies in a sample of adults who are deaf with borderline and mild cognitive functioning impairment and (b) to explore how these intellectual disability profiles and domain discrepancies are related to maladaptive behavior and self-reported QOL in this population. We explored whether expressed intellectual disability domain discrepancies between cognitive potential and lower social and practical abilities are experienced as stressful barriers to unlock one's potential and therefore may be linked with lower quality of life and increased rates of maladaptive behavior.

2. Materials and Methods

2.1. Participants

This cross-sectional exploratory study was conducted within three therapeutic living communities (Lebenswelt) specifically developed to accommodate the needs of individuals with deafness and additional disabilities, focusing on supporting communication, social relationships, conflict resolution and work satisfaction. They are characterized by the constant use of sign language; one-quarter of the staff members are deaf themselves [7].

We recruited 29 individuals (9 women and 20 men) who met the inclusion criteria of having at least moderate hearing impairment and an IQ score between 50 and 85 (see Table 1). Of these participants, 93% were profoundly deaf and 7% had moderate hearing loss. Nearly all the participants joined their therapeutic communities with lifetime histories of potentially traumatic events—a sadly common finding among members of the deaf community [28,29]—and about 38% had experienced at least one depressive episode [30]; however, no participant was experiencing an active depressive episode during the time of data collection. Their length of enrollment in the therapeutic living communities ranged from 6 months to 20 years. Most of the participants (n = 23; 79.3%) lived and worked in these communities, and the remaining participants (n = 6; 20.7%) only took part in the workshop facilities. Their mean age was 46.89 years (SD = 16.42, range 20–73 years), and their mean IQ score was 67.31 (SD = 6.49, range 57–82). Based on the ICD-10/WHO criteria, the majority (72.4%) were classified as having mild deficits indicated by an IQ score between 50 and 69 [31]. In addition, half (51.7%) of the participants were currently diagnosed with intellectual disability with challenging behavior (F70.1 (ICD-10)), 20.7% with cerebral palsy, 13.8% with epilepsy and 13.8% with autism. Table 1 displays the sample characteristics in detail.

Table 1. Sample characteristics.

Characteristics	N	%	Mean	SD	min	max
Lebenswelt						
Full program (residential and vocational)	23	79.31				
Day program/workshops only	6	20.69				
Sex						
Male/Female	20/9	68.97/31.03				
Age			46.90	16.421	20	73
Hearing status						
Moderate hearing loss (40–69 db)	2	6.90				
Profound hearing loss and deafness (>70 db)	27	93.10				
Co-occurring disorders						
Autism	4	13.79				
Epilepsy	4	13.79				
Cerebral palsy	6	20.69				
Intellectual disability with challenging behavior (F70.1 ICD-10)	15	51.72				
Lifetime depressive episodes	11	37.93				

This study was approved by the ethical committee of the hospital St. John of God in Linz, Austria. Consent was given by the participants themselves and/or by their legal guardians (if applicable).

2.2. Instruments

2.2.1. Intellectual and Adaptive Functioning

The Vineland Adaptive Behavior Scales-II [15] is a comprehensive measure of adaptive behavior. This standardized norm-referenced assessment instrument provides information on an individual's adaptive behavior from birth to 90 years of age across motor, communication, daily living and socialization skills. A standard score (M = 100, SD = 15) for each domain is calculated as well as a summary adaptive behavior composite score. The subscales of the Vineland-II do not perfectly align with the current tripartite model of adaptive behavior described in the DSM-5's definition of intellectual disability. Tassé and Mehling [12] proposed the following alignment or "cross-walking" of the VABS-II domains with the three domains of adaptive functioning identified in DSM-5: communication = conceptual skills; socialization = social skills; and daily living skills = practical skills. Accordingly, the socialization and daily living skills subscales of the Vineland-II were used to address the social and practical domains. However, two of the three sections of the communication subscale relate to the comprehension and production of spoken language. After adapting comprehension items to a visual modality, many items specifically referring to the structure of spoken language (e.g., intonation, verb inflection, prepositions, pronunciation, pronouns) had to be replaced by Austrian sign language items estimated to be functionally equivalent and of a comparable level of complexity. This non-validated adaptation resulted in significant floor effects that strongly weighed against its being considered for measuring the conceptual domain in this group of adults who are deaf with intellectual disability (see Figure 1).

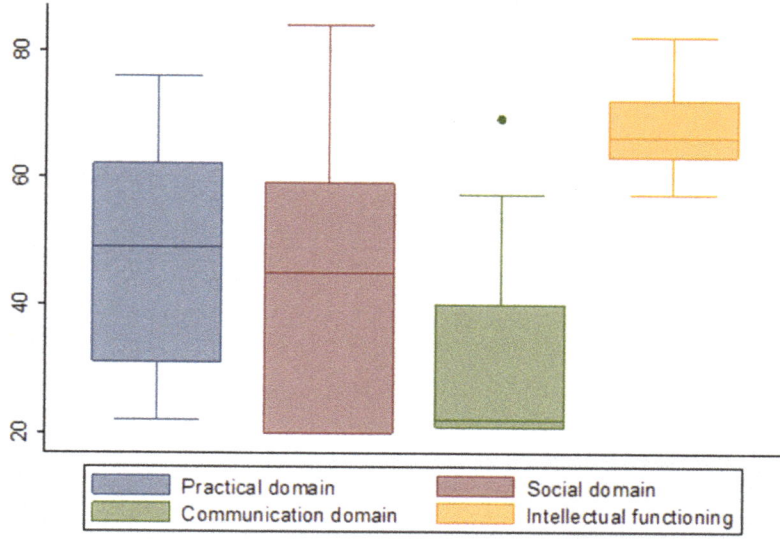

Figure 1. Boxplots of the domains of intellectual disability (standard scores of Vineland-II domains and SON-R 6-40).

To assess participants' intellectual functioning, we administered the Snijders-Oomen Non-verbal Intelligence Scale for individuals (SON-R 6-40; [32]). The SON-R 6-40 assesses the participant's non-verbal cognitive developmental level and provides a standard IQ score (M = 100, SD = 15), making it relatively easy to compare with the standard scores derived from the two VABS-II subscales.

2.2.2. QOL

The EUROHIS-QOL 8-item index (European Health Interview Surveys) is a short version of the WHOQOL-BREF. It consists of 8 questions that are also included in the

26 questions of the WHOQOL-BREF [33]. All four domains (physical, psychological, social and environmental) are represented, each with two questions. A normative study in Germany showed good construct validity and reliability [34]. An adapted, easy-to-understand sign language version of the EUROHIS-QOL 8-item index was administered to assess participants' self-rated QOL [35]. Fellinger et al. (2021) [35] demonstrated that reliable and valid self-reports of QOL can be obtained from adults who are deaf with mild-to-moderate intellectual disability using standard inventories such as the EUROHIS-QOL adapted to the linguistic and cognitive levels of these individuals. The EUROHIS-QOL 8-item index score was computed as the mean score across the eight items, ranging from 1 (worst QOL) to 5 (best QOL). The test–retest reliability was good (0.75), and internal consistency showed a Cronbach's Alpha of 0.78.

2.2.3. Maladaptive Behavior

The VABS-II includes two subscales for internalizing and externalizing maladaptive behavior. The two subscales are reported as v-scale scores. A v-scale score below 18 indicates a non-clinical level of maladaptive behavior; a score between 18 and 20 indicates an elevated level; and a score between 21 and 24 indicates a clinically significant level of maladaptive behavior [15].

2.3. Data Collection

Data collection took place between September 2017 and March 2018. Participants' clinical characteristics (i.e., type and degree of hearing loss; psychiatric, behavioral and neurological diagnoses) were extracted from the medical records of the individuals at the hospital St. John of God. The QOL self-reports were gathered through a structured interview between the resident and a sign language-competent staff member who was not directly involved in the care of the residents (non-involvement in direct care was considered important in order for the participants not to feel pressured to give answers that they thought would be preferred by the interviewer).

VABS-II data were collected for each participant by the staff psychologist in consultation with either a family member or the participant's primary caregiver. Primary caregivers serve the roles of coach, case manager, advocate and personal assistant for residents and were therefore thought to be particularly well-qualified to serve as informants for this study.

2.4. Computing Intellectual Disability Domain Discrepancies

Within the context of this paper, we use the term *intellectual disability domain discrepancy* to indicate that there is a substantial difference between the level of intellectual, social and/or practical adaptive functioning. For the purpose of this study, when comparing intellectual functioning with the social or practical domain, a difference of at least 15 points (=1 SD) between the IQ score (SON-R 6-40) and the socialization and daily living skills (DLS) standard scores indicates an intellectual disability domain discrepancy. When comparing the social and practical domains, a difference between the socialization and the DLS standard scores with a significance level of 0.05 according to the VABS-II manual indicates a domain discrepancy between these two domains.

2.5. Statistical Analysis

First, univariate analysis of the key variables was applied to describe intellectual disability domains, QOL and maladaptive behavior, as well as domain discrepancies. Next, Spearman's correlation was performed to test for a correlation between intellectual disability domains (social, practical and intellectual functioning), QOL and maladaptive behavior. To investigate whether there were significant differences in the means of self-reported QOL and internal and external maladaptive behavior with and without intellectual disability domain discrepancies, an independent samples *t*-test was performed.

3. Results

3.1. Intellectual Disability Domains, QOL and Maladaptive Behavior

Figure 1 shows the distribution of the median standard scores of (a) SON-R 6-40 intellectual functioning and (b) the three domains of Vineland-II adaptive functioning (practical, social and communication). Intellectual functioning emerged as the strongest domain, with a mean standard score of 67.31 (SD = 6.49) and no standard scores lower than 57 (see Table 2). The individuals also demonstrated a low level of practical functioning with a mean score of 48.97 (SD = 17.41), with more than half of the sample classified as having moderate or severe deficits. The social domain was the weakest domain with a mean score of 41.45 (SD = 19.66), indicating a moderate level of impairment according to the classification of the ICD-10 [31], and 12 (41.4%) individuals can be classified as having severe deficits in this domain. The communication domain of the Vineland-II, with a median standard score of 22, emphasizing the floor effect described earlier, was impossible to use as a proxy for the conceptual domain.

Table 2. Descriptive results for intellectual disability domains, QOL and maladaptive behavior.

Intellectual Disability Domains, QOL and Maladaptive Behav	N	%	Mean	SD	min	max
Levels of intellectual functioning impairments (based on SON-R 6-40)	29		67.31	6.492	57	82
Borderline (standard score 70–84 according to ICD-10)	8	27.59				
Mild (50–69)	21	72.4				
Levels of adaptive functioning impairments						
Social domain (based on Vineland-II socialization)	29		41.45	19.66	20	84
Borderline (standard score 70–84 according to ICD-10)	1	3.45				
Mild (50–69)	12	41.38				
Moderate (35–49)	4	13.79				
Severe (20–34)	12	41.38				
Practical domain (based on Vineland-II DLS)	29		48.97	17.41	22	76
Borderline (standard score 70–84 according to ICD-10)	3	10.34				
Mild (50–69)	11	37.93				
Moderate (35–49)	7	24.14				
Severe (20–34)	8	27.59				
Communication domain (based on Vineland-II communication)	29		31.45	14.01	21	69
Borderline (standard score 70–84 according to ICD-10)	0	0.00				
Mild (50–69)	5	17.24				
Moderate (35–49)	5	17.24				
Severe (20–34)	19	65.52				
Self-reported QOL (EUROHIS)	27		4.384	0.59	3	5
Maladaptive behavior (Vineland-II)						
Internalizing maladaptive behavior	29		17.138	2.42	13	21
Externalizing maladaptive behavior	29		18.276	2.3	13	24

3.2. Correlations between the Intellectual Disability Domains and QOL and Maladaptive Behavior

Table 3 shows the Spearman's correlation coefficients between the three domains. The social and practical domains are significantly positively correlated (r = 0.783, p = 0.000), as are the practical domain and intellectual functioning (r = 0.453, p < 0.05). The social domain and intellectual functioning are not significantly correlated (see Table 3). There are neither significant correlations between adaptive behavior and self-reported QOL nor significant relationships between adaptive behavior and maladaptive behavior, although correlations with social functioning approached the trend level of significance (p < 0.1).

Table 3. Zero-order correlation matrix among intellectual, social and practical functioning variables; quality of life; and maladaptive behavior (N = 29).

	Practical Functioning	Social Functioning	Externalizing Maladaptive Behavior	Internalizing Maladaptive Behavior	Quality of Life
Intellectual Functioning	0.453 *	0.151	0.078	−0.075	0.128
Practical Functioning		0.783 **	−0.019	−0.226	0.292
Social Functioning			−0.218	−0.351 †	0.354 †

Spearman's correlation coefficient: † $p < 0.1$; * $p < 0.05$, ** $p < 0.001$.

3.3. Intellectual Disability Domain Discrepancies

Almost two-thirds of the individuals had an intellectual disability domain discrepancy between their intellectual functioning level and the social domain (n = 19, 65.5%), and more than half had an intellectual disability domain discrepancy between their intellectual functioning and the practical domain (n = 17, 58.6%). About one-quarter of the individuals had an intellectual disability domain discrepancy between the social and the practical domains (n = 7, 24.1%), where in all cases the social domain was the weaker domain. Thus, participants' social adaptive skills were often poorer than their intellectual functioning and practical adaptive skills.

3.4. Associations between Intellectual Disability Domain Discrepancies and Self-Reported QOL as Well as Maladaptive Behavior (Independent Samples t-Tests)

When comparing participants with and without intellectual disability domain discrepancies, high mean QOL was endorsed across both groups, and no significant differences were found (see Table 4). Participants with a discrepancy between intellectual functioning and social domain had significantly higher levels of internalizing maladaptive behavior than the other groups (T = 1.889, $p < 0.05$).

Table 4. Mean differences in self-reported QOL and internal and external maladaptive behavior with and without intellectual disability domain discrepancies (independent samples t-test).

	Practical and Social Domains			Intellectual Functioning and Social Domain			Intellectual Functioning and Practical Domain		
	QOL, M (SD)	Internal, M, (SD)	External, M(SD)	QOL, M (SD)	Internal, M(SD)	External, M(SD)	QOL, M(SD)	Internal, M(SD)	External, M(SD)
No Discrepancy	4.381 (0.627)	17.182 (2.462)	18.091 (2.505)	4.597 (0.437)	15.900 (3.071)	17.300 (2.584)	4.506 (0.517)	16.583 (2.999)	18.667 (1.723)
N	21	22	22	9	10	10	11	12	12
Present Discrepancy	4.396 (0.501)	17.000 (2.449)	18.857 (1.464)	4.278 (0.640)	17.789 (1.751)	18.789 (2.016)	4.297 (0.640)	17.529 (1.908)	18.000 (2.646)
N	6	7	7	18	19	19	16	17	17
Mean Difference	−0.015	−0.182	0.766	0.319	1.889 *	1.489	0.209	0.946	−0.667

Self-reported QOL is indicated by a 5-point scale; * = $p < 0.05$; maladaptive behavior is reported as v-scale scores: <18 indicates average level, 18–20 indicates elevated level and 21–24 indicates a clinically significant level.

4. Discussion

The aim of this study was to describe profiles of intellectual disability and domain discrepancies in a sample of adults who are prelingually deaf with mild and borderline cognitive impairment and to explore how these domains of intellectual disability are related with each other and associated with self-reported QOL and maladaptive behavior. Our findings provide a first indication of possible intellectual disability domain discrepancies among individuals with deafness and intellectual disability and highlight the value—as well as potential challenges or limitations—of DSM-5's definition of intellectual disability for the deaf population. Furthermore, we investigated differences between those with and without domain discrepancies with respect to QOL and internalizing and externalizing maladaptive behavior.

Heterogeneous intellectual disability profiles were highly common among our participants, with only 24% showing no discrepancy between intellectual and adaptive functioning. In nearly two-thirds of the sample, intellectual disability domain discrepancies could be observed between intellectual functioning (65.5%) and both the practical (58.6%) and the social domain (65.5%). Domain discrepancy between the practical and social domain occurred in about one-fourth of cases (24.1%). Less than half of the sample had adaptive functioning levels in the practical and social domains that corresponded to their level of mild intellectual impairment, whereas severe levels of impairment were evident in the practical domain in 28% of the sample and in the social domain in 41%.

In our sample, the results of the communication subscales of the VABS-II, which were adapted but not originally designed for use in deaf populations, indicated severe deficits in 65.5% of the sample. Due to pronounced floor effects, the values of this domain were used neither as an equivalent for the conceptual domain nor for further calculations. Language is an important driver of acquiring social and practical skills above a rudimentary basal level [36], and the huge discrepancies seen in our sample with cognitive impairments may be due to the force multiplier effect of communication deprivation on the development of adaptive skills in this vulnerable population. These findings underscore how severe early childhood language deprivation impacts communication skills [10], even in our population where great effort has been taken to optimize access to communication through sign language in adult life. Other research in individuals with intellectual disabilities could show a strong association between communicative competences and QOL [37], which highlights the importance of access to language and communication. In contrast to the findings of Sparrow et al. 2005, in the present study with a sample who is prelingually deaf with mild cognitive deficits, the socialization domain appeared to be the weakest [15].

The relationship between intellectual functioning and the practical domain in our sample was moderately significant ($r = 0.453$, $p < 0.05$) and in line with the results of the meta-analysis of Alexander and Reynolds [14], whereas no significant correlations between intellectual functioning and the social functioning domain could be found in our sample.

Tassé [13] and Simoes et al. [26] both found a positive correlation between adaptive behavior and QOL in samples with mild-to-moderate intellectual disability. A similar effect is hinted at in our sample, with correlations trending toward statistical significance between social functioning and self-reported QOL ($r = 0.354$, $p < 0.1$), as well as a negative correlation between social functioning and internalizing maladaptive behavior ($r = -0.351$, $p < 0.1$). Conversely, neither intellectual functioning nor adaptive functioning in the practical domain were correlated with QOL or maladaptive behavior, a comparable finding to that observed by Graves et al. [18], who found no correlation between adaptive behavior and quality of life in adults with Down syndrome.

Having a statistically significant adaptive domain discrepancy between intellectual and social functioning was significantly correlated with higher levels of internalizing maladaptive behavior, a phenomenon that has also been observed in Autism Spectrum Disorder (e.g., [24,38]). Pending replication, one is tempted to query whether social connection is the critical ingredient in the positive adjustment and emotional well-being of individuals who are deaf (see, e.g., [39,40]), as well as individuals who are deaf and have intellectual disabilities, and we will pursue and welcome further inquiry in this area.

Limitations

We must also note this study's limitations. First and foremost, this is a small sample drawn from a highly enriched therapeutic residential care setting for adults who are deaf and have intellectual disabilities. Since this sample has only borderline-to-mild cognitive impairment, we make no claim to generalizability to the larger population of adults who are deaf with intellectual disability; much larger replication trials are needed.

Second, we must query whether the VABS-II, widely regarded as the "gold standard" adaptive measure in the majority of cases, is the most appropriate measure for this population. We therefore encourage further research in the service of formulating an optimal assessment battery both to gauge and, we hope, discover how to unlock these individuals' full potential. We would emphasize the importance of developing and validating a communication scale that is independent of (or less conflated with) solely spoken and auditory modalities.

5. Conclusions

Clearly, the assessment of intellectual disability transcends IQ, and we hope to inspire efforts toward an even higher level of measure refinement and collaborative research between investigators and participants. Underscoring the DSM-5's incorporation of adaptive functioning into its definition of intellectual disability, our population of participants who were prelingually deaf with mild cognitive impairments had a broad array of strengths and challenges. Intellectual functioning emerged as a relative strength, whereas almost half our participants had severe deficits in the social domain. Critically, a higher level of internalizing maladaptive behavior was observed in those participants with a domain discrepancy between their intellectual and social functioning. We must acknowledge that, even with our best efforts in providing accessible therapeutic communities in adulthood, deficits in the social domain could not be fully compensated after histories marked by severe trauma and deprivation. This finding constitutes a strong case for the early prevention of communicative and social deprivation by providing full access to spoken and/or signed communication. Nevertheless, nuanced measurement of adaptive skills gives us a good opportunity to identify and target malleable factors to improve QOL in individuals who are deaf and have intellectual disability more broadly.

Author Contributions: Conceptualization, J.F. (Johannes Fellinger) and M.D.; methodology, J.E.; validation, J.F. (Johannes Fellinger), D.H., J.F. (Jason Fogler), J.E. and M.D.; formal analysis, J.E.; investigation, M.D. and J.F. (Johannes Fellinger); data curation, M.D.; writing—original draft preparation, J.E., J.F. (Jason Fogler), M.D., D.H. and J.F. (Johannes Fellinger); writing—review and editing, J.E., J.F. (Jason Fogler), M.D., D.H. and J.F. (Johannes Fellinger); supervision, J.F. (Johannes Fellinger); project administration, M.D.; funding acquisition, J.F. (Johannes Fellinger). All authors have read and agreed to the published version of the manuscript.

Funding: Supported by Johannes Kepler Open Access Publishing Fund.

Institutional Review Board Statement: The study was conducted in accordance with the Declaration of Helsinki and approved by the Ethics Committee of the Hospital of St. John of God in Linz (approval number: 14-08).

Informed Consent Statement: Informed consent was obtained from all subjects involved in the study or their legal guardians.

Data Availability Statement: Data are not publicly available due to data protection issues.

Acknowledgments: We would like to thank Johannes Kepler Open Access Publishing Fund.

Conflicts of Interest: The authors declare no conflict of interest.

References

1. World Health Organization. World Report on Hearing. Available online: https://www.who.int/publications/i/item/world-report-on-hearing (accessed on 12 July 2022).
2. Bubbico, L.; Rosano, A.; Spagnolo, A. Prevalence of prelingual deafness in Italy. *Acta Otorhinolaryngol. Ital.* **2007**, *27*, 17–21. [PubMed]
3. Mitchell, R.E. How many deaf people are there in the United States? Estimates from the Survey of Income and Program Participation. *J. Deaf Stud. Deaf Educ.* **2006**, *11*, 112–119. [CrossRef]
4. Mitchell, R.E.; Karchmer, M.A. Demographics of Deaf Education: More Students in More Places. *Am. Ann. Deaf* **2006**, *151*, 95–104. [CrossRef]
5. Gallaudet Research Institute. *Regional and National Summary Report of Data*; GRI Gallaudet University: Washington, DC, USA, 2013.

6. van Naarden Braun, K.; Christensen, D.; Doernberg, N.; Schieve, L.; Rice, C.; Wiggins, L.; Schendel, D.; Yeargin-Allsopp, M. Trends in the prevalence of autism spectrum disorder, cerebral palsy, hearing loss, intellectual disability, and vision impairment, metropolitan atlanta, 1991–2010. *PLoS ONE* **2015**, *10*, e0124120. [CrossRef] [PubMed]
7. Fellinger, J.; Linzner, D.; Holzinger, D.; Dall, M.; Fellinger, M.; Fogler, J. Development of Deaf Adults with Intellectual Disability in a Therapeutic Living Community. *J. Deaf Stud. Deaf Educ.* **2020**, *25*, 261–269. [CrossRef]
8. Hall, W.C.; Levin, L.L.; Anderson, M.L. Language deprivation syndrome: A possible neurodevelopmental disorder with sociocultural origins. *Soc. Psychiatry Psychiatr. Epidemiol.* **2017**, *52*, 761–776. [CrossRef]
9. Kushalnagar, P.; Ryan, C.; Paludneviciene, R.; Spellun, A.; Gulati, S. Adverse Childhood Communication Experiences Associated With an Increased Risk of Chronic Diseases in Adults Who Are Deaf. *Am. J. Prev. Med.* **2020**, *59*, 548–554. [CrossRef]
10. Glickman, N.S.; Hall, W.C. (Eds.) *Language Deprivation and Deaf Mental Health*; Routledge: New York, NY, USA, 2019; ISBN 9781351680837.
11. American Psychiatric Association. *Diagnostic and Statistical Manual of Mental Disorders: DSM-5*, 5th ed.; American Psychiatric Publishing: Washington, DC, USA, 2013; ISBN 9780890425572.
12. Tassé, M.J.; Mehling, M.H. Measuring Intellectual Functioning and Adaptive Behavior in Determining Intellectual Disability. In *Handbook of Research-Based Practices for Educating Students with Intellectual Disability*; Wehmeyer, M.L., Shogren, K.A., Shogren, K.A., Eds.; Routledge Taylor & Francis Group: New York, NY, USA; London, UK, 2017; pp. 71–86, ISBN 9781138832107.
13. Tassé, M.J. Adaptive Behavior and Functional Life Skills Across the Lifespan: Conceptual and Measurement Issues. In *Adaptive Behavior Strategies for Individuals with Intellectual and Developmental Disabilities: Evidence-Based Practices Across the Life Span*, 1st ed.; Lang, R., Sturmey, P., Eds.; Springer International Publishing: Cham, Switzerland, 2021; pp. 1–20, ISBN 978-3-030-66440-4.
14. Alexander, R.M.; Reynolds, M.R. Intelligence and Adaptive Behavior: A Meta-Analysis. *Sch. Psychol. Rev.* **2020**, *49*, 85–110. [CrossRef]
15. Sparrow, S.; Cicchetti, D.; Balla, D. *Vineland-II. Vineland Adaptive Behavior Scales*; AGS Publishing: Circle Pines, MN, USA, 2005.
16. Di Nuovo, S.; Buono, S. Behavioral phenotypes of genetic syndromes with intellectual disability: Comparison of adaptive profiles. *Psychiatry Res.* **2011**, *189*, 440–445. [CrossRef]
17. Mouga, S.; Almeida, J.; Café, C.; Duque, F.; Oliveira, G. Adaptive profiles in autism and other neurodevelopmental disorders. *J. Autism Dev. Disord.* **2015**, *45*, 1001–1012. [CrossRef] [PubMed]
18. Graves, R.J.; Zlomke, K.; Graff, J.C.; Hall, H.R. Adaptive behavior of adults with Down syndrome and their health-related quality of life. *Adv. Neurodev. Disord.* **2020**, *4*, 27–35. [CrossRef]
19. Madduri, N.; Peters, S.U.; Voigt, R.G.; Llorente, A.M.; Lupski, J.R.; Potocki, L. Cognitive and adaptive behavior profiles in Smith-Magenis syndrome. *J. Dev. Behav. Pediatr.* **2006**, *27*, 188–192. [CrossRef]
20. Crocker, N.; Vaurio, L.; Riley, E.P.; Mattson, S.N. Comparison of adaptive behavior in children with heavy prenatal alcohol exposure or attention-deficit/hyperactivity disorder. *Alcohol. Clin. Exp. Res.* **2009**, *33*, 2015–2023. [CrossRef]
21. Peters, S.U.; Goddard-Finegold, J.; Beaudet, A.L.; Madduri, N.; Turcich, M.; Bacino, C.A. Cognitive and adaptive behavior profiles of children with Angelman syndrome. *Am. J. Med. Genet. A* **2004**, *128*, 110–113. [CrossRef]
22. Van Ool, J.S.; Snoeijen-Schouwenaars, F.M.; Tan, I.Y.; Schelhaas, H.J.; Aldenkamp, A.P.; Hendriksen, J.G.M. Classification of intellectual disability according to domains of adaptive functioning and between-domains discrepancy in adults with epilepsy. *J. Intellect. Disabil. Res.* **2019**, *63*, 40–48. [CrossRef] [PubMed]
23. Tillmann, J.; San José Cáceres, A.; Chatham, C.H.; Crawley, D.; Holt, R.; Oakley, B.; Banaschewski, T.; Baron-Cohen, S.; Bölte, S.; Buitelaar, J.K.; et al. Investigating the factors underlying adaptive functioning in autism in the EU-AIMS Longitudinal European Autism Project. *Autism Res.* **2019**, *12*, 645–657. [CrossRef]
24. Kraper, C.K.; Kenworthy, L.; Popal, H.; Martin, A.; Wallace, G.L. The Gap Between Adaptive Behavior and Intelligence in Autism Persists into Young Adulthood and is Linked to Psychiatric Co-morbidities. *J. Autism Dev. Disord.* **2017**, *47*, 3007–3017. [CrossRef] [PubMed]
25. Balboni, G.; Rebecchini, G.; Elisei, S.; Tassé, M.J. Factors affecting the relationship between adaptive behavior and challenging behaviors in individuals with intellectual disability and co-occurring disorders. *Res. Dev. Disabil.* **2020**, *104*, 103718. [CrossRef]
26. Simões, C.; Santos, S.; Biscaia, R.; Thompson, J.R. Understanding the Relationship between Quality of Life, Adaptive Behavior and Support Needs. *J. Dev. Phys. Disabil.* **2016**, *28*, 849–870. [CrossRef]
27. Jones, S.; Cooper, S.-A.; Smiley, E.; Allan, L.; Williamson, A.; Morrison, J. Prevalence of, and factors associated with, problem behaviors in adults with intellectual disabilities. *J. Nerv. Ment. Dis.* **2008**, *196*, 678–686. [CrossRef]
28. Anderson, M.L.; Leigh, I.W.; Samar, V.J. Intimate partner violence against Deaf women: A review. *Aggress. Violent Behav.* **2011**, *16*, 200–206. [CrossRef]
29. Francavillo, G.S.R. *Sexuality Education, Sexual Communication, Rape Myth Acceptance, and Sexual Assault Experience among Deaf and Hard of Hearing College Students*; University of Maryland: College Park, MD, USA, 2009.
30. Kvam, M.H.; Loeb, M.; Tambs, K. Mental health in deaf adults: Symptoms of anxiety and depression among hearing and deaf individuals. *J. Deaf Stud. Deaf Educ.* **2007**, *12*, 1–7. [CrossRef] [PubMed]
31. World Health Organization. *The ICD-10 Classification of Mental and Behavioural Disorders*; World Health Organization: Geneva, Switzerland, 1993.
32. Tellegen, P.J.; Laros, A.J.; Petermann, F. *SON-R 6-40: Non-Verbaler Intelligenztest*; Hogrefe: Göttingen, Germany, 2012.

33. World Health Organization. The World Health Organization Quality of life (WHOQOL)—BREF, 2012 Revision. 2004. Available online: https://apps.who.int/iris/handle/10665/77773 (accessed on 22 November 2021).
34. Brähler, E.; Mühlan, H.; Albani, C.; Schmidt, S. Teststatistische Prüfung und Normierung der deutschen Versionen des EUROHIS-QOL Lebensqualität-Index und des WHO-5 Wohlbefindens-Index. *Diagnostica* **2007**, *53*, 83–96. [CrossRef]
35. Fellinger, J.; Dall, M.; Gerich, J.; Fellinger, M.; Schossleitner, K.; Barbaresi, W.J.; Holzinger, D. Is it feasible to assess self-reported quality of life in individuals who are deaf and have intellectual disabilities? *Soc. Psychiatry Psychiatr. Epidemiol.* **2021**, *56*, 1881–1890. [CrossRef]
36. Liss, M.; Harel, B.; Fein, D.; Allen, D.; Dunn, M.; Feinstein, C.; Morris, R.; Waterhouse, L.; Rapin, I. Predictors and correlates of adaptive functioning in children with developmental disorders. *J. Autism Dev. Disord.* **2001**, *31*, 219–230. [CrossRef] [PubMed]
37. García, J.C.; Díez, E.; Wojcik, D.Z.; Santamaría, M. Communication Support Needs in Adults with Intellectual Disabilities and Its Relation to Quality of Life. *Int. J. Environ. Res. Public Health* **2020**, *17*, 7370. [CrossRef]
38. Day, T.C.; McNaughton, K.A.; Naples, A.J.; McPartland, J.C. Self-reported social impairments predict depressive disorder in adults with autism spectrum disorder. *Autism* **2020**, *24*, 297–306. [CrossRef]
39. Antia, S.D.; Jones, P.; Luckner, J.; Kreimeyer, K.H.; Reed, S. Social Outcomes of Students Who are Deaf and Hard of Hearing in General Education Classrooms. *Except. Child.* **2011**, *77*, 489–504. [CrossRef]
40. Gerich, J.; Fellinger, J. Effects of social networks on the quality of life in an elder and middle-aged deaf community sample. *J. Deaf Stud. Deaf Educ.* **2012**, *17*, 102–115. [CrossRef] [PubMed]

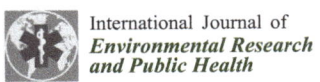

Article

Withdrawing Antipsychotics for Challenging Behaviours in Adults with Intellectual Disabilities: Experiences and Views of Prescribers

Gerda de Kuijper [1,2,*], Joke de Haan [1], Shoumitro Deb [3] and Rohit Shankar [4]

1. GGZ-Drenthe/Centre for ID and Mental Health, Middenweg 19, 9404 LL Assen, The Netherlands
2. Academic Collaboration ID and Mental Health, Department Psychiatry and Department Family Practice, University Medical Centre Groningen, 9713 GZ Hanzeplein, The Netherlands
3. Department of Brain Sciences, Faculty of Medicine, Imperial College London, Du Cane Road, London W12 0NN, UK
4. Peninsula School of Medicine, University of Plymouth and Cornwall Partnership NHS Foundation Trust, Plymouth PL4 8AA, UK
* Correspondence: gerda.de.kuijper@ggzdrenthe.nl; Tel.: +31-6-31623826

Abstract: International current best practice recommends the discontinuation of antipsychotics for challenging behaviours in people with intellectual disabilities (ID), due to lack of evidence of efficacy and risks of harmful side-effects. In clinical practice, discontinuation may be difficult. The aim of this study was to gain insight into prescribers' practice by investigating their experiences with the discontinuation of long-term antipsychotics for challenging behaviour. From professionals' associations thirty-four registered ID physicians, psychiatrists and specialist mental healthcare nurses were recruited who completed an online questionnaire in this survey–study. Almost all participants had attempted to deprescribe antipsychotics for their patients with ID. Sixty-five percent of participants achieved complete discontinuation in 0–25% of their patients, but none in over 50%. Barriers were a lack of non-pharmaceutical treatments for challenging behaviours and caregivers' and/or family concern. Seventy percent of participants indicated that their institutions had encouraged implementing their discontinuation policies in line with the new Dutch Act on Involuntary care and a new Dutch multidisciplinary guideline on problem behaviour in adults with ID. Support and facilitation of clinicians from institutions' managers and political and professional bodies may be helpful in further implementation of best practice in the treatment of challenging behaviour in people with ID.

Keywords: intellectual disabilities; antipsychotics; challenging behaviour; discontinuation; prescribers' policies; survey

1. Introduction

The rates of challenging behaviours displayed by people with intellectual disabilities (ID) vary from 18% in community populations to 85% in people with profound ID who live in institutions [1–3]. The onset and maintenance of challenging behaviours in individuals with ID are associated with biological, psychological and environmental factors [1,2,4–6]. Behaviours include outwardly directed behaviours like aggressive-destructive behaviour, inappropriate (sexual) behaviour and disruptive behaviours. It also includes hyperactivity, irritability, lethargy and self-injurious, stereotypic and withdrawn behaviours [2,7,8]. Challenging behaviours may vary in intensity and be persistent [9–12]. When individuals present with challenging behaviour, this may negatively influence their quality of life [13,14] and social participation [15]. Diagnosis and management require a multidisciplinary and integrative approach as the causes of these behaviours are multi-factorial (physical, genetic, psychiatric, psychological, social, environmental, etc.) [3,6,16].

Psychotropic drugs, especially antipsychotics, are often prescribed for the management of challenging behaviours [17–22]. Significantly higher levels of antipsychotic drug prescribing occur to manage challenging behaviour in people with ID and/or autism [23]. However, the effectiveness of psychotropic drugs for the treatment of challenging behaviours in people with ID has not been proven [24–27]. Moreover, in this population, the risk of side-effects like diabetes, cardio-vascular disorders, sedation and movement disorders is considerable, especially in the case of long-term use of antipsychotics [28–31]. It is recommended by all good practice guidelines that the treatment of challenging behaviours should be, in the first place, non-pharmacological, i.e., psychosocial and behavioural. Practitioners should only prescribe psychotropic drugs after careful weighing of the potential positive and negative effects of this medication and preferably just for the short-term (max. 6–12 weeks). For example, prescription may be beneficial to overcome crisis situations when the person or others are at risk of serious harm, or in conjunction with non-pharmacological interventions [16,32,33].

Although it is recommended that long-term off-label psychotropic drug prescription should be discontinued especially antipsychotics, they are still frequently prescribed for the treatment of challenging behaviours [34–36]. This may, at least partially be, because of failures of successful discontinuation of antipsychotics due to worsening of behaviour upon drug withdrawal [37]. Besides user-related factors, like the occurrence of withdrawal symptoms, symptoms of previously not-recognized mental or physical disorders or other health problems, and staff-related factors, are associated with unsuccessful withdrawal of antipsychotics [38]. For example, staff may experience difficulties in the management of changes in their clients' behaviour, may have negative feelings towards clients' behaviour or lack knowledge or have unrealistic expectations about the effects of psychotropic drugs [39,40]. The involvement of all stakeholders, including the patients and their relatives, seems a key-element in the achievement of successful changes in prescription policies [41].

In some countries, initiatives have been taken to facilitate the deprescribing of antipsychotics for challenging behaviours. For example, in the UK, the "stopping over medication of people with a learning disability, autism or both with psychotropic medicines" (STOMP) is now incorporated within the NHS England long-term plan [42]. The development of a structured pathway with the involvement of all stakeholders led to successful discontinuation in 46% of cases and dose reductions of over 50% in another 11% [43]. A survey among UK psychiatrists about changes in prescription policies as a result of the STOMP initiative showed that the prescriptions practice has changed. The UK psychiatrists are less likely to initiate new prescriptions of antipsychotics. However, complete antipsychotic discontinuation in over 50% of their patients was achieved by only 4.5% of responding psychiatrists [44].

In The Netherlands, Vilans, a knowledge centre on long-term care has conducted a project (2015–2019) to reduce inappropriate psychotropic prescribing in the elderly with dementia and in people with ID and high care needs. In this project, an e-learning on psychotropic drug use in people with ID for support professionals has been developed [45]. Moreover, in The Netherlands, in December 2019, a new multidisciplinary guideline on challenging behaviour [46] and, in January 2020, a new Dutch Act on Involuntary care was published. In both, the prescription of psychotropic drugs for challenging behaviours outside guideline recommendations is regarded as restricted practice. A study among Dutch ID physicians on their experiences with the guideline and new Act showed that they regarded the Act as supportive of reducing the off-label prescriptions of psychotropics. However, because of organisational difficulties, the feasibility of implementing the guideline and new Act is not always possible in practice [47].

In The Netherlands, there are 250 registered ID physicians. Most of them take care of people with ID and complex needs, including people with multiple disabilities and/or behavioural problems.

There are approximately 15–20 ID specialized mental healthcare outpatient clinics spread over The Netherlands. Psychiatrists in mainstream mental healthcare organizations or who have their own private practice may also be consultants at ID institutions. In Dutch mental healthcare, specialist nurses monitor the use of the psychotropic drugs and are authorized to stop or change a prescription in consultation with the psychiatrist who initiated the prescription. In community care, GPs may provide repeat prescriptions and/or the monitoring of psychotropic drug use; however, mostly, they refer to ID physicians or specialized ID mental healthcare when discontinuation or change in medication is necessary. The total number of mental healthcare professionals affiliated with the Dutch ID mental healthcare outpatient clinics, authorized to prescribe psychotropic medication, is unknown. We estimate 100–150 such prescribers based on the number of ID mental healthcare clinics and consultant-psychiatrists specializing in people with ID in The Netherlands.

The present study aimed to gather information about facilitators and barriers to the successful discontinuation of antipsychotic drugs when used for challenging behaviours in people with ID. We conducted a survey, similar to the UK survey [44], about experiences with antipsychotic drug discontinuation among ID physicians, psychiatrists and specialist nurses in The Netherlands who were responsible for the psychotropic drug prescriptions for their patients with ID. We also asked whether their antipsychotic prescribing practice had changed because of the new guideline and new Act.

2. Materials and Methods

2.1. Design

This was a cross-sectional study including a questionnaire survey among Dutch prescribers of psychotropic medications for people with ID.

2.2. Participants and Settings

Participants were registered ID physicians affiliated with ID institutions and institutions' outpatient clinics or having their own practice, and psychiatrists or specialist nurses affiliated with ID-specialized mental healthcare outpatient clinics or having their own practice.

2.3. Materials

The questionnaire items were adapted for the Dutch ID healthcare system from a survey which was developed in a recent study of UK psychiatrists' views on the rationalization of psychotropic use among people with ID [44]. The survey answer options of items were multiple choice with an open field for comments. Supplementary Materials shows the items of the questionnaire and corresponding answer options. The forty-two questionnaire items were grouped under five themes similar to those in the UK survey. These themes included:

(1) Data on working experience and antipsychotic prescription practice in patients with ID;
(2) Experience in deprescribing antipsychotics;
(3) How their antipsychotic prescribing practice including deprescribing, changed over the past five years;
(4) How in the past five years new Dutch Acts and guidelines influenced antipsychotic deprescribing;
(5) Potential facilitators and barriers in achieving the goal of deprescribing.

2.4. Procedures

The participants were recruited from the ID physicians affiliated with the Dutch Intellectual Disabilities physicians' association (NVAVG), psychiatrists affiliated with the Dutch Psychiatrists Association (NVvP) and nurses affiliated with the Dutch specialist nurse care association (VenVNVS). We had to approach all the Dutch psychiatrists and specialist nurses as there is no Register of those who specifically specialize in ID mental healthcare.

The survey was open between 19 February and 1 May 2021. A reminder was sent three weeks before the closing date. A news item with the link to the questionnaire was also placed on the websites of the professionals' associations. Members of the professional organisations/potential responders received an explanatory letter with a link to the program Qualtrics where they could fill in the questionnaire. On average, it took participants 30–45 min to complete the questionnaire.

2.5. Ethics

All responders in the survey participated voluntarily. All data were collected, stored, and safeguarded anonymously, according to the European Act on Protection of Personal Information, in The Netherlands, which was ratified in 2018.

2.6. Analyses

SPSS 26 was used to analyse the survey data. Descriptive statistics were used to calculate frequencies of respondents' characteristics and answer categories as per the multiple-choice questions. Pearson Chi-Square was used to compare characteristics and answer categories between a group consisting of ID physicians on the one hand and psychiatrists and ID specialist mental healthcare nurses on the other.

3. Results

We present the results by the forming of two clusters encompassing the five themes of the questionnaire as described under Methods/Materials (themes 1 and 2, and themes 3, 4 and 5 respectively). The data and analyses of all the 42 questions and corresponding answers (see Supplementary Materials) are available on request.

3.1. Participants and Prescription Patterns (Themes 1 and 2 of the Questionnaire)

Twenty-one of the 250 ID physicians registered in The Netherlands and thirteen of the estimated 100–150 mental healthcare professionals prescribing psychotropics to patients with ID (i.e., psychiatrist or specialist mental healthcare nurse) completed the questionnaire (response rate of 8.5% and estimated response rate 8.6–13%, respectively). The exact response rate of the ID mental healthcare professionals could not be calculated because there are no data on the total number of those in ID mental healthcare in The Netherlands.

Twelve (35%) of the total 34 participants reported that their working experience in the field was for less than 10 years, 10 (30%) had worked in the field for 10–19 years, 11 (32%) 20–29 years, and 1 (3%) for more than 30 years. Five (15%) of the participants stated that 0–25% of their patients, 17 (50%) that 25–50%, 5 (14%) that 50–75% and 4 (12%) that 75–100% of their patients with ID were prescribed antipsychotics. Three participants (9%) could not provide the percentage.

3.2. Participants' Policies and Experiences (Themes 3, 4 and 5 of the Questionnaire)

Table 1 shows the results of participants' practice and experience regarding the deprescribing of antipsychotics in their patients with ID. Participants attempted to deprescribe antipsychotics in a variable part of their patients. In Table 1, the number and percentage of participants is shown who attempted to deprescribe antipsychotics in a certain proportion of their patients.

A considerable number of participants did not attempt to withdraw antipsychotics in their patients with ID and challenging behaviour when there was a clear diagnosis of a psychiatric disorder which justified the prescription. This diagnosis was confirmed recently (i.e., in the two preceding years) in more than half of the total number of respondents (55%). A significantly lesser proportion of ID physicians (38%) compared with ID mental healthcare professionals (ID psychiatrists and nurses) (83%) confirmed the psychiatric diagnosis ($p = 0.01$). Only eight (24%) prescribers confirmed psychiatric diagnosis themselves (ID physicians 10%, ID healthcare professionals 50%, the difference not significant).

In addition, there were differences between these two groups with regard to the mean duration of the discontinuation trajectory, which was, on average, significantly longer in ID physicians (0–6 months, 9% in ID physicians versus 8% in ID mental healthcare professionals, 6–12 months, 24% versus 77%, 12–18 months, 47% versus 0%, and >18 months in 19% versus 15%, respectively, $p = 0.01$)

Table 1. Practice and experience of intellectual disability (ID) physicians and ID mental healthcare professionals [#] who completed the survey (N = 34 participants) in deprescribing antipsychotics for challenging behaviours.

Policies and Experiences of Participants	Percentage of Those Patients with ID on Antipsychotics	Participants Responding to Survey (Number, %)
Attempts to withdraw antipsychotics	0%	0 (0%)
	1–25%	3 (9%)
	26–50%	9 (26%)
	>50%	18 (53%)
	missing	4 (12%)
Achieved complete withdrawal	0%	3 (9%)
	1–25%	22 (65%)
	26–50%	5 (14%)
	>50%	0 (0%)
	missing	4 (12%)
Achieved dose reduction of > 50%	0%	0 (0%)
	1–25%	18 (53%)
	26–50%	9 (26%)
	>50%	3 (9%)
	missing	4 (12%)
Not attempted to withdraw because of licensed indication/clear psychiatric diagnosis	0%	2 (6%)
	1–25%	13 (38%)
	26–50%	9 (26%)
	>50%	6 (18%)
	unknown	4 (12%)

[#] Psychiatrists and specialist mental healthcare nurses affiliated with ID mental healthcare organizations.

Table 2 shows data which complicated the withdrawal process of antipsychotics for challenging behaviour.

Most participants stated that the antipsychotic drug had to be re-instated in some patients. Furthermore, behavioural worsening or other complications like withdrawal dyskinesia or re-emergence of sleep problems or irritability could occur, leading to delay in the discontinuation process. In addition, staff could be unable or need extra time to adapt their guiding style, or to change clients' environment or daily activities when clients became less sedated and more active because of the antipsychotic's withdrawal. These environmental factors could also lead to delay or sometimes failure in the discontinuation process. Nevertheless, complete withdrawal was also achieved in some of the patients, even those whose behaviour deteriorated upon dose reduction.

3.3. Factors Related to Deprescribing Antipsychotics in the Working Field of Participants

Twenty-three (70%) of the thirty-four participants indicated that the institutions they were affiliated with had encouraged their clinicians to reduce antipsychotic drugs because of the new Dutch Act on Involuntary care, which is aimed to reduce restrictive practice and the new Dutch guideline on problem behaviour in adults with ID. They also indicated that they were less likely to initiate antipsychotics for challenging behaviours.

Participants also mentioned some factors that facilitated successful discontinuation and barriers that hindered this process. For example, it was difficult to achieve complete withdrawal among those who received polypharmacy of antipsychotics. On the contrary, the concurrent use of other psychotropics (polypharmacy of psychotropics rather than antipsychotics) facilitated complete withdrawal. Other facilitators were the presence of side effects, first attempt to withdraw, and a positive attitude and involvement of clients' families and support staff. Barriers were resistance against discontinuation from support professionals or family, which was mentioned by 26 (76%) and by 25 (74%) participants, respectively, and unavailability of non-pharmaceutical treatments for clients' challenging behaviours, which was mentioned by 20 (59%) participants. In addition, lack of knowledge about the discontinuation process, e.g., time schedules and steps in dose reductions (20 participants, 59%), and lack of multidisciplinary team involvement (8 participants, 24%) were mentioned.

Table 2. Complications in withdrawing antipsychotics for challenging behaviour in patients with intellectual disabilities as experienced by participants in a survey study (N = 34).

Complications	Proportion of Patients with the Complication	Participants (n, %) Reporting This Complication
Antipsychotic had to be reinstated within - 3 months		14 (41%)
	0%	4
	1–25%	7
	26–50%	1
	>50%	2
Antipsychotic had to be reinstated within - 6 months		17 (50%)
	0%	2
	1–25%	11
	26–50%	4
	>50%	0
Antipsychotic had to be reinstated within - 12 months		25 (74%)
	0%	3
	1–25%	12
	26–50%	6
	>50%	4
	unknown	0
Occurrence of severe behavioural worsening or severe worsening of mental condition	0%	4 (12%)
	1–25%	19 (56%)
	26–50%	6 (18%)
	>50%	1 (3%)
	unknown	4 (12%)
Delay in discontinuation process due to behavioural worsening after complete withdrawal	0%	4 (12%)
	1–25%	13 (38%)
	26–50%	4 (12%)
	>50%	3 (9%)
	unknown	10 (29%)
Delay in discontinuation process due to behavioural worsening after incomplete withdrawal	0%	0 (0%)
	1–25%	8 (24%)
	26–50%	12 (36%)
	>50%	5 (15%)
	unknown	8 (24%)
Complications (multiple answers allowed): Mild behavioural worsening Withdrawal symptoms Re-emergence of psychiatric symptoms Contextual problems		29 (35%) 19 (23%) 24 (29%) 10 (12%)
Delay in discontinuation process due to complications/complete withdrawal	0%	5 (15%)
	1–25%	12 (35%)
	26–50%	8 (24%)
	>50%	1 (3%)
	unknown	8 (24%)
Delay in discontinuation process due to complications/incomplete withdrawal	0%	0 (0%)
	1–25%	11 (32%)
	26–50%	9 (26%)
	>50%	5 (15%)
	unknown	9 (26%)

4. Discussion

In this study, we explored the experiences and views of prescribers regarding withdrawal of long-term antipsychotic drug use for challenging behaviours in people with ID in The Netherlands. Although the long-term prescription of antipsychotics for challenging behaviours in the absence of a psychiatric illness is not recommended [16,46], we found that approximately half of the 21 ID physicians and 13 psychiatrists/specialist mental healthcare nurses who completed the survey questionnaire were still prescribing antipsychotics in the absence of a psychiatric diagnosis in 0–25% of their patients. However, all ID physicians and all but one of psychiatrists/mental healthcare nurses had attempted to deprescribe antipsychotics in the preceding five years. This percentage is higher than in the survey of Deb et al. [44], who found that about half of their 88 respondents had attempted to deprescribe antipsychotics for challenging behaviour in their patients with ID. We found a similar percentage to Deb et al. [44] (65% versus 60% of participants) who succeeded in complete withdrawal in 0–25% of their patients. However, none of the participants in our study was successful in completely discontinuing antipsychotic medications in over 50% of their patients within 12 months compared to 4.5% of participants in the study of Deb et al. [44]. Our participants stated that objections and concerns of family and professional caregivers, and unavailability of non-pharmaceutical treatments and multidisciplinary team input, were barriers in starting or continuing a withdrawal process.

Deb et al. [48] recently completed a qualitative analysis of free text data returned by the UK psychiatrists' during the questionnaire survey [44] and found that the psychiatrists in the UK like the participants in the current Dutch study found that the lack of resources such as multidisciplinary team input and lack of caregiver support for the withdrawal hampered their attempt to deprescribe antipsychotics. As far as we know, there are no studies from other countries reporting prescribers' experiences with antipsychotics discontinuation in patients with ID.

As described above and known from other studies, involvement of all stakeholders in decisions about the withdrawal of long-term used antipsychotics for challenging behaviours is a key factor for success [43,44]. Besides organizational barriers and time-constraints in prescribers' attempts to apply the deprescribing policies [44], staff's attitudes and knowledge around psychotropic drug use are important factors in outcomes of discontinuation trajectories [40]. However, the most important factor may be the involvement of family-caregivers and patients with ID themselves. Studies have shown that family-caregivers, although they have knowledge on the challenging behaviour of their relative and would like to be heard, are often not involved in treatment decisions, e.g., psychotropic drug prescribing [41]. In addition, often individuals with ID themselves lack information and/or their voices are not heard in decisions in prescription of antipsychotics [41,49]. Previous studies of interviews of adults with ID have just touched on the issue of psychotropic medication use [50,51]. To address this knowledge gap, in another study, we also gathered information on the experience of adults with a mild ID who have gone through the experience of psychotropic withdrawal [52]. An important finding was their statement that their own coping style, next to a supportive environment and a good relationship with their doctor, was a key factor for successful discontinuation.

Legal issues may play a role. We found that 70% of the participants in our study indicated that the new Dutch Act on Involuntary care, aimed to reduce restrictive practice, and the new Dutch guideline on problem behaviour in adults with ID had encouraged their service providers to facilitate psychotropic drugs deprescription. However, clinicians are allowed to deviate from this Act and from the Dutch guideline on problem behaviour provided that they can substantiate this decision. Since the present study was the first in The Netherlands on the issue of experiences of prescribers in withdrawing antipsychotics for challenging behaviours of people with ID, it is difficult to know definitely about the possible facilitating effect of these government Act and guidelines, for which future studies are needed.

Other contextual factors also may play a role in our study, since we found differences in antipsychotics discontinuation policies between ID physicians and ID mental healthcare professionals, who have different working settings. ID physicians took significantly more time for the discontinuation process, possibly because their patients' stakeholders' networks are more complex, and it will take more time to coordinate all stakeholders' interests. Another explanation for the longer discontinuation trajectory may be the difference in confirmation of the presence of a psychiatric illness in patients who started the withdrawal process. This was significantly less often confirmed by ID physicians compared with ID mental healthcare professionals. The lack of confirmation will likely lead to uncertainty and fear of family, caregivers and clinicians regarding re-occurrence of maladaptive behaviour or psychiatric symptoms, and delay in the withdrawal process.

Our study has some limitations. First, the response rate of our survey was low. Approximately 10% of ID physicians had completed the survey questionnaire, and we estimated a similar percentage of the ID mental healthcare professionals (psychiatrists and specialist nurses working in ID mental healthcare and/or affiliated with ID institutions). We were not able to calculate the exact response rate of the latter group because there is no data on the number of those professionals. Therefore, the results of our survey may not be representative of all ID physicians, ID psychiatrists and ID specialist nurses in The Netherlands. However, the low response itself raises some interesting observations. A similar survey conducted two years ago in the UK with the same equivalent target audience i.e., psychiatrists who work with people with ID had a response rate of approximately 40%. This raises questions on the differences in attitudes of the prescribers towards this challenging topic. There could be complex confounders, such as time, resource, training, education, knowledge acquisition and cultural attitudes, which might have influenced these response rates. It could be that a different methodology such as face to face interviews might result in better response rates and better understanding of the barriers to the current survey response. However, such projects can be time consuming and resource intensive.

Furthermore, because this study was conducted in Dutch healthcare settings, the results cannot be generalized to other countries. However, it is known that, in many countries, prescribers encounter the same problems in deprescribing antipsychotics in their patients with ID [37]. Therefore, the results of this study may also be applicable to other Western countries.

5. Conclusions

In line with the available international guidelines and a new Dutch Act on Involuntary care, most of the thirty-four participants in our survey of ID physicians, psychiatrists and specialist mental healthcare nurses in The Netherlands had attempted to discontinue their long-term prescriptions of antipsychotics for challenging behaviours in patients with ID. However, complete discontinuation could be achieved in only a small proportion of cases. Concerns of relatives and care and support staff, lack of non-pharmaceutical treatments and lack of multidisciplinary teams' input were perceived as barriers to successful antipsychotic withdrawal attempts.

Besides improvement in the availability of multidisciplinary teams and non-pharmaceutical treatments, education of care-professionals in supporting clients in the management of medication use is recommended.

Facilitation and support from managers at the institutional level, and creating conditions at the political and professional level, seem to be prerequisites in the successful implementation of deprescribing antipsychotic medication for challenging behaviours in patients with ID.

Supplementary Materials: The following supporting information can be downloaded at: https://www.mdpi.com/article/10.3390/ijerph192417095/s1, Supplementary File S1. Survey among prescribers of psychotic drugs to people with intellectual disabilities.

Author Contributions: The study was set up and conducted, and analysis of the results was done by J.d.H. under supervision of G.d.K. The conceptualization of the survey was done by S.D. and R.S. The writing of drafts was done by G.d.K. All authors have read and agreed to the published version of the manuscript.

Funding: This research received no external funding.

Institutional Review Board Statement: Not applicable.

Informed Consent Statement: A written and signed participants' consent was not required because this was not a study involving patients, but volunteers who talked about their experiences.

Data Availability Statement: The data are available on request and with a substantiated explanation at GGZ Drenthe/department research https://ggzdrenthe.nl/research, (accessed on 14 December 2022).

Acknowledgments: We thank the intellectual disability physicians, psychiatrists and specialist nurses who completed the survey for their cooperation.

Conflicts of Interest: The authors declare no conflict of interest.

References

1. Poppes, P.; van der Putten, A.; Vlaskamp, C. Frequency and severity of challenging behaviour in people with profound intellectual and multiple disabilities. *Res. Dev. Disabil.* **2010**, *31*, 1269–1275. [CrossRef] [PubMed]
2. Bowring, D.; Totsika, V.; Hastings, R.; Toogood, S.; Griffith, G. Challenging behaviours in adults with an ID: A total population study and exploration of risk indices. *Br. J. Clin. Psychol.* **2017**, *56*, 16–32. [CrossRef] [PubMed]
3. Deb, S.; Unwin, G.; Cooper, S.; Rojahn, J. Problem behaviours. In *Textbook of Psychiatry for Intellectual Disability and Autism Spectrum Disorder*; Bertelli, M.O., Deb, S., Munir, K., Hassiotis, A., Salvador-Carulla, L., Eds.; Springer Nature: Cham, Switzerland, 2022; Chapter 7; pp. 145–186.
4. Crocker, A.; Prokić, A.; Morin, D.; Reyes, A. ID and co-occurring mental health and physical disorders in aggressive behaviour. *J. ID Res.* **2014**, *58*, 1032–1044.
5. Dworschak, W.; Ratz, C.; Wagner, M. Prevalence and putative risk markers of challenging behavior in students with ID. *Res. Dev. Disabil.* **2016**, *58*, 94–103. [CrossRef]
6. Hemmings, C.; Deb, S.; Chaplin, E.; Hardy, S.; Mukherjee, R. Research for people with intellectual disabilities and mental health problems: A view from the UK. *J. Ment. Health Res. Intellect. Disabil.* **2013**, *6*, 127–158. [CrossRef]
7. Poppes, P.; Putten, A.J.J.; Post, W.J.; Vlaskamp, C. Risk factors associated with challenging behaviour in people with profound intellectual and multiple disabilities. *J. ID Res.* **2016**, *60*, 537–552. [CrossRef]
8. Deb, S. Psychopharmacology. In *Handbook of Evidence-Based Practices in Intellectual and Developmental Disabilities, Evidence-Based Practices in Behavioral Health*; Singh, N.N., Ed.; Springer International Publishing: Cham, Switzerland, 2016; pp. 347–381.
9. Murphy, G.; Beadle-Brown, J.; Wing, L.; Gould, J.; Shah, A.; Holmes, N. Chronicity of Challenging Behaviours in People with Severe ID and/or Autism: A Total Population Sample. *J. Autism Dev. Disord.* **2005**, *35*, 405–418. [CrossRef]
10. Totsika, V.; Toogood, S.; Hastings, R.; Lewis, S. Persistence of challenging behaviours in adults with ID over a period of 11 years. *J. ID Res. JIDR* **2008**, *52*, 446–457.
11. Davies, L.; Oliver, C. The age-related prevalence of aggression and self-injury in persons with an ID: A review. *Res. Dev. Disabil.* **2013**, *34*, 764–775. [CrossRef]
12. Davies, L.; Oliver, C. Self-injury, aggression and destruction in children with severe ID: Incidence, persistence and novel, predictive behavioural risk markers. *Res. Dev. Disabil.* **2016**, *49*, 291–301. [CrossRef]
13. Ramerman, L.; Hoekstra, P.J.; de Kuijper, G. Health-related quality of life in people with ID who use long-term antipsychotic drugs for challenging behaviour. *Res. Dev. Disabil.* **2018**, *75*, 49–58. [CrossRef] [PubMed]
14. Meade, C.; Martin, R.; McCrann, A.; Lyons, J.; Meehan, J.; Hoey, H.; Roche, E. Prader-Willi Syndrome in children: Quality of life and caregiver burden. *Acta Paediatr.* **2021**, *110*, 1665–1670. [CrossRef] [PubMed]
15. Bigby, C. Social inclusion and people with ID and challenging behaviour: A systematic review. *J. Intellect. Dev. Disabil.* **2012**, *37*, 360–374. [CrossRef] [PubMed]
16. NICE. *Challenging Behaviour and Learning Disabilities: Prevention and Interventions for People with Learning Disabilities Whose Behaviour Challenges*; National Collaborating Centre for Mental Health, National Institute for Health and Care Excellence (NICE): London, UK, 2015.
17. de Kuijper, G.; Hoekstra, P.; Visser, F.; Scholte, F.A.; Penning, C.; Evenhuis, H. Use of antipsychotic drugs in individuals with ID (ID) in the Netherlands: Prevalence and reasons for prescription. *J. Intellect. Disabil. Res.* **2010**, *54*, 659–667. [CrossRef] [PubMed]
18. Sheehan, R.; Hassiotis, A.; Walters, K.; Osborn, D.; Strydom, A.; Horsfall, L. Mental illness, challenging behaviour, and psychotropic drug prescribing in people with ID: UK population based cohort study. *BMJ* **2015**, *351*, h4326. [CrossRef]

19. O'Dwyer, M.; Peklar, J.; Mulryan, N.; McCallion, P.; McCarron, M.; Henman, M.C. Prevalence, patterns and factors associated with psychotropic use in older adults with ID in Ireland. *J. Intellect. Disabil. Res.* **2017**, *61*, 969–983. [CrossRef]
20. Lunsky, Y.; Khuu, W.; Tadrous, M.; Vigod, S.; Cobigo, V.; Gomes, T. Antipsychotic Use With and Without Comorbid Psychiatric Diagnosis among Adults with Intellectual and Developmental Disabilities. *Can. J. Psychiatry. Rev. Can. De Psychiatr.* **2018**, *63*, 361–369. [CrossRef]
21. Perry, B.I.; Cooray, S.E.; Mendis, J.; Purandare, K.; Wijeratne, A.; Manjubhashini, S.; Dasari, M.; Esan, F.; Gunaratna, I.; Naseem, R.A.; et al. Problem behaviours and psychotropic medication use in ID: A multinational cross-sectional survey. *J. Intellect. Disabil. Res.* **2018**, *62*, 140–149. [CrossRef]
22. Deb, S.; Bertelli, M.; Rossi, M. Psychopharmacology. In *Textbook of Psychiatry for Intellectual Disability and Autism Spectrum Disorder*; Bertelli, M.O., Deb, S., Munir, K., Hassiotis, A., Salvador-Carulla, L., Eds.; Springer Nature: Cham, Switzerland, 2022; Chapter 11; pp. 247–280.
23. Fusar-Poli, L.; Brondino, N.; Rochetti, M.; Petrosino, B.; Arillotta, D.; Damiani, S.; Provenzani, U.; Petrosino, C.; Aguglia, E.; Politi, P. Prevalence and predictors of psychotropic medication use in adolescents and adults with autism spectrum disorder in Italy: A cross-sectional study. *Psychiatry Res.* **2019**, *276*, 203–209. [CrossRef]
24. Tyrer, P.; Oliver-Africana, P.C.; Ahmed, Z.; Bouras, N.; Cooray, S.; Deb, S.; Murphy, D.; Hare, M.; Meade, M.; Reece, B.; et al. Risperidone, haloperidol, and placebo in the treatment of aggressive challenging behaviour in patients with ID: A randomised controlled trial. *Lancet* **2008**, *371*, 57–63. [CrossRef]
25. McQuire, C.; Hassiotis, A.; Harrison, B.; Pilling, S. Pharmaceutical interventions for challenging behaviour in children with ID: A systematic review and meta-analysis. *BMC Psychiatry* **2015**, *26*, 303. [CrossRef] [PubMed]
26. Deutsch, S.I.; Burket, J.A. Psychotropic medication use for adults and older adults with ID; selective review, recommendations and future directions. *Prog. Neuropsychopharmacol. Biol. Psychiatry* **2021**, *104*, 110017. [CrossRef] [PubMed]
27. Deb, S.; Bethea, T.; Havercamp, S.; Rifkin, A.; Underwood, L. Disruptive, impulse-control, and conduct disorders. In *Diagnostic Manual—Intellectual Disability: A Textbook of Diagnosis of Mental Disorders in Persons with Intellectual Disability*, 2nd ed.; Fletcher, R., Barnhill, J., Cooper, S.-A., Eds.; NADD Press: Kingston, NY, USA, 2016; pp. 521–560.
28. de Kuijper, G.; Mulder, H.; Evenhuis, H.; Scholte, F.; Visser, F.; Hoekstra, P.J. Determinants of physical health parameters in individuals with ID who use long-term antipsychotics. *Res. Dev. Disabil.* **2013**, *34*, 2799–2809. [CrossRef] [PubMed]
29. Matson, J.L.; Mahan, S. Antipsychotic drug side effects for persons with ID. *Res. Dev. Disabil.* **2010**, *31*, 1570–1576. [CrossRef]
30. Scheifes, A.; Walraven, S.; Stolker, J.J.; Nijman, H.L.; Egberts, T.C.; Heerdink, E.R. Adverse events and the relation with quality of life in adults with ID and challenging behaviour using psychotropic drugs. *Res. Dev. Disabil.* **2016**, *49–50*, 13–21. [CrossRef]
31. Sheehan, R.; Horsfall, L.; Strydom, A.; Osborn, D.; Walters, K.; Hassiotis, A. Movement side effects of antipsychotic drugs in adults with and without ID: UK population-based cohort study. *BMJ Open* **2017**, *7*, e017406. [CrossRef]
32. Trollor, J.N.; Salomon, C.; Franklin, C. Prescribing psychotropic drugs to adults with an ID. *Aust. Prescr.* **2016**, *39*, 126–130. [CrossRef]
33. Deb, S.; Kwok, H.; Bertelli, M.; Salvador-Carulla, L.; Bradley, E.; Torr, J.; Barnhill, J. International guide to prescribing psychotropic medication for the management of problem behaviours in adults with intellectual disabilities. *World Psychiatry* **2009**, *8*, 181–186. [CrossRef]
34. de Kuijper, G.M.; Hoekstra, P.J. Physicians' reasons not to discontinue long-term used off-label antipsychotic drugs in people with ID. *J. Intellect. Disabil. Res.* **2017**, *61*, 899–908. [CrossRef]
35. Koch, A.D.; Dobrindt, J.; Schützwohl, M. Prevalence of psychotropic medication and factors associated with antipsychotic treatment in adults with ID: A cross-sectional, epidemiological study in Germany. *J. ID Res.* **2021**, *65*, 186–198.
36. García-Domínguez, L.; Navas, P.; Verdugo, M.Á.; Arias, V.B.; Gómez, L.E. Psychotropic drugs intake in people aging with ID: Prevalence and predictors. *J. Appl. Res. ID (JARID)* **2022**, *35*, 1109–1118. [CrossRef]
37. Sheehan, R.; Hassiotis, A. Reduction or discontinuation of antipsychotics for challenging behaviour in adults with ID: A systematic review. *Lancet Psychiatry* **2017**, *4*, 238–256. [CrossRef] [PubMed]
38. de Kuijper, G.M.; Hoekstra, P.J. An Open-Label Discontinuation Trial of Long-Term, Off-Label Antipsychotic Medication in People With ID: Determinants of Success and Failure. *J. Clin. Pharmacol.* **2018**, *58*, 1418–1426. [CrossRef] [PubMed]
39. de Kuijper, G.M.; Hoekstra, P.J. An open label discontinuation trial of long-term used off-label antipsychotic drugs in people with ID: The influence of staff-related factors. *J. Appl. Res. ID* **2019**, *32*, 313–322.
40. Kleijwegt, B.; Pruijssers, A.; Jong-Bakker, L.; Haan, K.; Os-Medendorp, H.; Meijel, B. Support staff's perceptions of discontinuing antipsychotics in people with ID in residential care: A mixed-method study. *J. Appl. Res. ID* **2019**, *32*, 861–870.
41. Sheehan, R.; Hassiotis, A.; Strydom, A.; Morant, N. Experiences of psychotropic medication use and decision-making for adults with ID: A multistakeholder qualitative study in the UK. *BMJ Open* **2019**, *9*, e032861. [CrossRef] [PubMed]
42. Shankar, R.; Wilcock, M.; Oak, K.; McGowan, P.; Sheehan, R. Stopping, rationalising or optimising antipsychotic drug treatment in people with ID and/or autism. *Drug Ther. Bull.* **2019**, *57*, 10–13. [CrossRef]
43. Shankar, R.; Wilcock, M.; Deb, S.; Goodey, R.; Corson, E.; Pretorius, C.; Praed, G.; Pell, A.; Vujkovic, D.; Wilkinson, E.; et al. A structured programme to withdraw antipsychotics among adults with ID: The Cornwall experience. *J. Appl. Res. Intellect. Disabil.* **2019**, *32*, 1389–1400. [CrossRef]

44. Deb, S.; Nancarrow, T.; Limbu, B.; Sheehan, R.; Wilcock, M.; Branford, D.; Courtenay, K.; Perera, B.; Shankar, R. UK psychiatrists' experience of withdrawal of antipsychotics prescribed for challenging behaviours in adults with ID and/or autism. *BJPsych Open* **2020**, *6*, 112. [CrossRef]
45. Jonker, J. Online learning intervention' Psychotropic drug: Changing views, changing actions. *J. Appl. Res. Intellect. Disabil.* **2018**, *31*, 608. Available online: https://onlinelibrary.wiley.com/doi/epdf/10.1111/jar.12478 (accessed on 14 December 2022).
46. Embregts, P.; Kroezen, M.; Mulder, E.J.; Van Bussel, C.; Van der Nagel, J.; Budding, M.; Busser, G.; De Kuijper, G.; Duinkerken-Van Gelderen, P.; Haasnoot, M.; et al. Multidisciplinaire richtlijn Probleemgedrag bij volwassenen met een verstandelijke beperking. *Ned. Ver. Van Artsen Voor Verstand. Gehandicap. (NVAVG)* **2019**. Available online: https://nvavg.nl/wp-content/uploads/2022/06/Richtlijn-Probleemgedrag_definitief-update-2022.pdf (accessed on 14 December 2022).
47. de Weg, J.C.b.; Honingh, A.K.; Teeuw, M.; Sterkenburg, P.S. An Exploratory Study among ID Physicians on the Care and Coercion Act and the Use of Psychotropic Drugs for Challenging Behaviour. *Int. J. Environ. Res. Public Health* **2021**, *18*, 10240. [CrossRef] [PubMed]
48. Deb, S.; Limbu, B.; Nancarrow, T.; Gerrard, D.; Shankar, R. The effect of the STOMP initiative on the UK psychiatrists' prescribing practice: A qualitative data analysis of free-text questionnaire responses. *J. Appl. Res. Intellect. Disabil.* **2022**, *under review*.
49. Crossley, R.; Withers, P. Antipsychotic Medication and People with ID: Their Knowledge and Experiences. *J. Appl. Res. ID* **2009**, *22*, 77–86.
50. Hall, S.; Deb, S. A qualitative study on the knowledge and views that people with learning disabilities and their carers have of psychotropic medication prescribed for behaviour problems. *Adv. Ment. Health Learn. Disabil.* **2008**, *2*, 29–37. [CrossRef]
51. Hassiotis, A.; Kimona, K.; Moncrieff, J.; Deb, S. A Stakeholder Consultation about Future Research of Psychotropic Medication Use and Behaviour Support for Adults with Intellectual Disabilities Who Present with Behaviours That Challenge: Feasibility of Future Research. *NOCLOR* **2016**. Available online: https://www.ucl.ac.uk/psychiatry/sites/psychiatry/files/stakeholder-consultation-document.pdf (accessed on 14 December 2022).
52. de Kuijper, G.; de Haan, J.; SDeb Shankar, R. Withdrawing antipsychotics for challenging behaviours in adults with intellectual disabilities; experiences and views of prescribers. *Int. J. Environ. Res. Public Health* **2022**, *19*, 15637. [CrossRef]

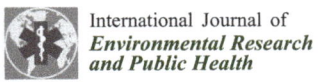

Article

Withdrawing Antipsychotics for Challenging Behaviours in Adults with Intellectual Disabilities: Experiences and Views of Experts by Experience

Gerda de Kuijper [1,2,*], Joke de Haan [1], Shoumitro Deb [3] and Rohit Shankar [4]

1. GGZ-Drenthe/Centre for ID and Mental Health, 9404 LL Assen, The Netherlands
2. Academic Collaboration ID and Mental Health, University Medical Centre Groningen, 9713 GZ Groningen, The Netherlands
3. Faculty of Medicine, Department of Brain Sciences, Imperial College London, London SW7 2BX, UK
4. Peninsula School of Medicine, University of Plymouth, Plymouth PL4 8AA, UK
* Correspondence: gerda.de.kuijper@ggzdrenthe.nl; Tel.: +31-6-3162-3826

Abstract: People with intellectual disabilities (PwID) are frequently prescribed long-term antipsychotics for behaviours that challenge (BtC) despite the lack of proven effectiveness and the increased risks for side effects of these medications in this population. National and international good clinical practice guidelines recommend deprescribing antipsychotics for BtC, which is often not successful due to environmental and other factors. The involvement of all stakeholders, including PwID, is crucial for deprescribing. However, studies showed that PwID and/or their families are often not involved in decision-making regarding the (de)prescribing of antipsychotics despite their desire to get involved. Moreover, studies on the views of PwID regarding their experiences of withdrawing from antipsychotics are lacking. The aim of this study was to gain insight into the views of PwID by investigating their experiences of discontinuation of long-term prescribed antipsychotics for BtC. A qualitative study was set up. Seven experts by experience with mild intellectual disabilities were interviewed. After six interviews, data saturation was achieved. Interviews were transcribed verbatim. Using phenomenological analysis, themes on lived experiences were extracted. Each consecutive interview was analysed. The four main themes extracted from the interviews were the quality of treatment, knowledge and information about psychotropics and the process of withdrawal, support from the participants' environment and the coping style of the interviewees themselves.

Keywords: intellectual disabilities; antipsychotics; challenging behaviour; discontinuation; experts by experience views; qualitative study; interviews

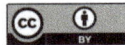

1. Introduction

People with intellectual disabilities (PwID) frequently engage in behaviours that challenge (BtC), especially those with higher care needs and/or who receive residential care [1]. BtC include aggressive behaviour (e.g., verbal abuse, threats and physical violence), destructive behaviour (e.g., breaking or destroying properties and other objects and setting fires), disruptive behaviour (e.g., repetitive screaming, smearing faeces, setting off fire alarms when there is no fire, calling the emergency services when there is no emergency), self-injurious behaviour (e.g., self-biting, head-banging) and sexually harmful behaviour (e.g., sexual assaults, rape and stalking), as described in the National Institute of Care Excellence (NICE, NG11) [2] guidelines.

There are many reasons for BtC, including biological (genetic disorders, physical problems including pain, medication side effects), psychological (psychiatric disorders including anxiety, depression, psychosis and post-traumatic stress disorders) and social factors (inappropriate accommodation and lack of support) [3]. The reported prevalence of psychiatric disorders in PwID varies between 14.4 and 60% depending on the definition of psychiatric diagnosis used (e.g., the inclusion or exclusion of BtC, ADHD and ASD within the psychiatric disorder diagnosis), method of detection using different classification systems (e.g., ICD vs. DSM), use of assessment methods (screening instrument vs. structured interviews), population studied (institutionalised vs. clinic-based vs. community-based), etc. [4–6]. Neurodevelopmental disorders, such as autism spectrum disorder (ASD) and attention deficit hyperactivity disorder (ADHD), are common among PwID [7]. The rate of both psychiatric disorders and BtC increases in PwID with these comorbidities [7,8]. However, both false positive and false negative diagnoses of psychiatric disorders are common in PwID [6].

In the UK, NHS England (NHSE) embarked on a major campaign six years ago called 'STopping Over-Medication of People with learning disabilities, autism or both (STOMP)' [9] to which STAMP (supporting treatment and appropriate medication in paediatrics) was also added recently. The Royal College of Psychiatrists in the UK also published a position paper to support the STOMP STAMP initiative [10]. The National Institute for Health and Care Excellence (NICE) in the UK [2] and the World Psychiatric Association [11] developed guidelines for the use of psychotropics to address BtC among PwID, including recommendations for the initiation, monitoring and potential withdrawal of psychotropic medications.

BtC is best-treated non-pharmacologically, but in some situations, short-term prescriptions of psychotropics may be beneficial [2]. However, BtC is often treated with antipsychotics and prescribed long-term in the absence of a valid psychiatric diagnosis [12,13] despite the lack of evidence for its long-term effectiveness for BtC [14–17]. Moreover, PwID are vulnerable to the side effects of antipsychotics, especially neurological side effects, such as movement disorders; sedation/sleepiness; and metabolic side effects, such as obesity and diabetes [15,18–20]. Therefore, it is important to balance the pros and cons of antipsychotic use carefully and to discontinue them when there is no longer a valid indication, especially in the case of BtC [2].

Furthermore, it is important to involve all the stakeholders. This means that along with staff and healthcare professionals, the PwID themself, their family members and other representatives of PwID showing with BtC should get involved in the decision-making of the (de)prescribing of psychotropic drugs [21]. Indeed, studies showed that PwID and their family members would like to contribute to treatment decisions about BtC and medication use but they are often not involved in decision-making regarding the (ongoing) prescription of medication [22–24].

Although national and international guidelines recommend [2,11,25] that long-term antipsychotics for BtC should be deprescribed, discontinuation often fails [26–29] because of a variety of factors. It is important to involve all stakeholders to increase the proportion of successful discontinuation, as was shown in a study by Shankar and colleagues [28]. In particular, the role of the primary caregivers and other staff should be recognised as the key factors that influence the successful discontinuation of antipsychotics [30–32], as staff may lack knowledge of the effects and side effects of antipsychotics and may have unrealistic expectations of the beneficial effects of psychotropic medications on the psychological functioning of their clients [30,31]. In a recent study of interviews with support staff in the UK, some direct care staff felt that medication is necessary to control BtC in PwID, whereas others felt that these medications were 'chemical restraints' [32].

Furthermore, evaluation of the process of discontinuation is important to identify potential barriers and facilitators for the deprescribing of these agents. A survey among UK psychiatrists showed that family and staff concerns, lack of multidisciplinary input and unavailability of psychosocial interventions were barriers to attempting to discontinue antipsychotics [33]. A Dutch study among direct support professionals about their perceptions of the effect of antipsychotics on BtC and their willingness to cooperate in discontinuing these agents showed that they believed that antipsychotics were effective in the management of BtC [34]. However, they also observed the negative consequences of side effects. Staff were willing to cooperate in reducing the antipsychotic drug use but were not confident about successful complete discontinuation [34].

The current study aimed to add knowledge about facilitators and barriers to the successful discontinuation of antipsychotic drug use for BtC in PwID. Although studies were done on the experiences and views of prescribers and support professionals regarding withdrawing antipsychotics for BtC, as far as we know, studies on users' perspectives are missing. Therefore, in this study, we investigated the views of people with mild ID on the discontinuation of their antipsychotic drugs and their experiences with the withdrawal process.

2. Methods

2.1. Design and Participants

This was a qualitative interview study. Potential participants were selected by their clinicians according to preset eligibility criteria. Eligible participants were adults aged between 18 and 65 years and had mild intellectual disabilities according to the DSM5 classification system (Diagnostic and Statistical Manual of Mental Disorders, 5th revised edition; American Psychiatric Association, 2013). They had to be currently undergoing withdrawal of antipsychotic medications that they had been receiving for more than six months, where either their antipsychotics had already been discontinued recently or they had gone through an attempted withdrawal in the recent past. Potential participants were required to have competency and language skills to take part in the interviews and be able to express their views in the Dutch language. Participants with dementia, bipolar disorder, schizophrenia and chronic psychosis were excluded.

2.2. Procedures

Potential participants were recruited from the responders of a survey that had previously been carried out among Dutch physicians specialising in intellectual disabilities, psychiatrists and mental healthcare specialist nurses [35]. Additionally, the first two authors recruited participants from their networks and by asking their colleagues at the outpatient clinic of the mental healthcare organisations they were affiliated with that provide services for people with intellectual disabilities.

Potential participants were contacted on the phone or visited by the second author (J.d.H.). During these calls or visits, they were informed about the goal and content of the interviews. In these meetings and the interview sessions, the interviewer (J.d.H.) used accessible language, such as short sentences and clear questions. Furthermore, the interviewees could ask a significant other, such as their personal support professional or family member, to accompany them during the interviews.

A topic guide was used for these interviews (see Table 1), the items of which were drawn from the relevant literature on the subject [21–25,36,37].

Table 1. Topic guide with subjects for interviews on users' experiences with the withdrawal of antipsychotics.

Topic Guide
Reasons for antipsychotic drug use
Reason for discontinuation of antipsychotics
Information the participants received about their medication use and the discontinuation process
Mental and physical health problems experienced during the discontinuation process
Opinions of the participants about the decision and process of discontinuation
Tips or advice from the participants for the professionals and other PwID about the discontinuation process

A test interview was done by the second author (J.d.H.) to assess the accessibility of the content and comprehensibility of the interview questions. This test interview took place in the inpatient clinic of the mental healthcare organisation the interviewer was affiliated with. The interviewee was a client who was currently undergoing withdrawal from her antipsychotics. This interview was not recorded and no data from this interview were included in the results section. The test interviewee revealed that there was no need to adapt the topic guide, language use or other subjects.

2.3. Ethics

All participants consented to take part in the interviews and signed an informed consent form before the interview took place. They were informed that the encrypted data would be stored at a safeguarded place and analysed and published anonymously and that they could withdraw from the study at any moment without giving a reason.

The interview study was not a medical, scientific study according to the Dutch Act on Medical Studies with Human Beings, as no personal health-related data were collected, but only the participants' views were captured through these interviews. Therefore, no ethical approval was required for this study. The study was carried out under the responsibility of Mental HealthCare Drenthe (GGZ Drenthe) and was approved by their research committee (declaration is available on request). All data were collected, stored and safeguarded anonymously according to the European Act on Protection of Personal Information, which, in the Netherlands, was ratified in 2018.

2.4. Analyses

The interviews were video-recorded and transcribed verbatim. A phenomenological data analysis method was used to extract themes from the transcriptions by means of (a) thorough reading and re-reading of the transcripts to obtain a general sense of the whole content; (b) extraction of significant statements on the phenomenon under study and formulation and coding of the meaning of these statements; (c) sorting of categories, clusters of themes, and themes of these codes and meanings; and (d) integration of the findings and description of the fundamental structure of the phenomenon that ought to be validated by the interviewees [38].

The sample size was established according to the criteria of data saturation in qualitative studies, which means that qualitative data were collected to the point where a sense of closure was attained because new data yielded redundant information [39]. In the present study, each consecutive interview was analysed. When the last interview yielded no new codes and themes, data saturation was achieved and no new interviews/new participants were needed.

Transferability was maintained (via a thorough reading and re-reading, as well as a rich description of the content of the interviews), along with credibility; confirmability; authenticity via peer-review of the coding of the meanings, categories and themes of the statements; and dependability via the interviewer's log-keeping [40].

Data were analysed by the second author (J.d.H.). A random sample of three interviews (out of seven in total) was independently analysed by the first author (G.d.K.) to assess the agreement with the analyses of J.d.H.

3. Results

Seven experts by experience with mild intellectual disabilities participated in the interview study. These were three men and four women, whose ages ranged from 22 to 62 years. Three used quetiapine; two used aripiprazole; one used olanzapine; and one used a combination of haloperidol, quetiapine and clozapine. All participants were white. The duration of the interviews was 25 min on average. After each interview, the extraction of significant statements and coding and categorising their meanings took place. After the sixth interview, no new categories and themes were extracted; therefore, data saturation was achieved. Four main themes could be extracted from the content of the interviews. These were (a) the quality of the treatment, (b) knowledge and information about the process of withdrawal, (c) the conditions that needed to be met before a discontinuation process could start and (d) the coping style of the person whose medication was discontinued.

(a) The quality of treatment.

All participants indicated that they had used antipsychotics for many years because of various reasons, but none was for a licensed indication. For example, one participant stated:

'Finally, after many years, it was found that I have ADHD, and then quetiapine won't 'work very well, and Concerta will work better, you might say.'

The reasons to discontinue antipsychotics were mainly because participants judged that they no longer had symptoms that needed treatment and/or because of side effects, such as weight gain, tremors, flattened affect and sleepiness. Participants stressed the importance of receiving good treatments from clinicians who take them seriously and provide a clear and understandable explanation about their treatment and the reason for the prescription of their medication, such as (i) What is it for? (ii) How does it work? (iii) What side effects could occur? (iv) When to consult my doctor? However, often they had not been provided explanation and information when the medicine was newly prescribed.

(b) Knowledge and information about the process of withdrawal.

Most participants had some fear of discontinuing because they were afraid that their behavioural problems may re-emerge.

'I was afraid it turned out to go wrong.'

All participants indicated that they and their caregivers were provided with oral information by their doctor or nurse about the discontinuation schedule and dose reductions and the possibility of withdrawal symptoms and changes in behaviour. Four participants experienced withdrawal symptoms, and most of them knew this could happen and what kind of symptoms could be expected.

'I was like, this is just part of it, and then I went reading or doing something else and then it disappeared.'

All participants had informed their caregivers, peers or colleagues that they were discontinuing their drugs and the possibility of withdrawal symptoms.

'They have to know I may react differently.'

(c) Conditions to be met before starting a discontinuation process according to participants' experiences.

Half of the participants found the withdrawal process difficult for various reasons. One participant had problems with providing care for her children, others had physical and emotional problems. In one case, a dose increase of the antipsychotic drug was necessary to relieve these symptoms.

All participants indicated the importance of a good, accessible and trusted relationship with their doctors. This was helpful in continuing their withdrawal process when they had questions or wanted to talk about negative feelings when they experienced difficulties with the withdrawal process.

'All went well in agreement, I could always phone or come for consultation'.

Moreover, others in the participants' environments were important for providing support.

'Support from my parents, brother, sister-in-law, grandmother and grandfather.'

'Good to talk about it with others around you, anyway I think this is important because you won't make it on your own'.

(d) Coping style of the participant.

Most participants indicated that an appropriate mindset and intrinsic motivation are important to start with and continue the discontinuation process.

'Yes, you have to switch and stick to it.'

'Just say to yourself, I can make it.'

'It's also your own mindset, how to deal with yourself when you are afraid to discontinue, then it will be difficult. This was my experience, when you switch your mindset appropriately, then it will be all right.'

Participants also provided tips and advice for their peers. 'Ask help'.

'When you are angry, go to your support professional', *'stick to a structure in your daily activities.'*

4. Discussion

In this study, we explored the experiences and views of adults with mild ID regarding the withdrawal from their long-term-used antipsychotic drugs prescribed for BtC. This process may be difficult because PwID are often dependent on others and/or easily influenced by others and often need support in decision-making around deprescribing and maintaining the process of discontinuation [22,24,41].

Recent studies in the UK and the Netherlands have shown that even after long-term use, it is possible to discontinue antipsychotic medication in 25–61% of adults with intellectual disabilities and have a 50% dose reduction in another 11–19%, although, in up to 20% of cases, antipsychotics were re-instated within 3–4 years of discontinuation, primarily due to the resurgence of BtC [15,26,28]. However, several internal (e.g., comorbid ASD, baseline severity of BtC, an underlying psychiatric disorder) and external (e.g., baseline high dose of antipsychotics, lack of support and contingency plan during the withdrawal process) factors determine the success of any antipsychotic withdrawal [27,42].

The resurgence of BtC may not be related to the withdrawal of medication per se. The withdrawal may unmask a previously undiagnosed psychiatric disorder, such as psychosis, depression or bipolar disorder, or lead to a relapse of them. Discontinuation or dose reduction may lead to withdrawal syndromes, such as insomnia, anxiety and panic. A supersensitivity syndrome consisting of extrapyramidal symptoms, such as akathisia, Parkinsonism and dyskinesia, was associated with antipsychotic withdrawal [43,44]. All these can lead to BtC. In some cases, caregivers' anxiety may exacerbate the BtC or its perception, leading to the enhanced reporting of BtC. Therefore, the clinician will need to make a full assessment of the causes and effects of BtC using standard methodologies [45] (https://spectrom.wixsite.com/project/ (accessed on 1 November 2022).

It is known from other studies that the involvement of all stakeholders in decisions around the withdrawal of long-term-used antipsychotics for BtC is a key factor for success [22–25]. However, the most important factor may be the involvement of family caregivers and patients with ID themselves. Studies have shown that even though family caregivers have the appropriate knowledge of the BtC of their relatives and they would like to participate, they are often not involved in treatment decisions, e.g., psychotropic drug prescribing [21,41]. Furthermore, individuals with ID themselves often lack information and/or are not asked to contribute to decisions in the prescription of antipsychotics [22–25,41]. Although previous studies of interviews of adults with ID have touched on the issue of psychotropic medication use [41], as far as we know, the current study is the first one that specifically targeted the experience of PwID who have gone through the experience of psychotropic withdrawal.

In the current study, a phenomenological analysis of interviews with seven experts by experience extracted four themes that may be of importance in the successful discontinuation of long-term antipsychotic drugs. These themes were (a) the quality of treatment, (b) knowledge and information about the discontinuation process, (c) the conditions that should be met in a withdrawal process according to participants' experiences of taking part in the withdrawal process and (d) the participants' own coping style.

The interviewed participants indicated that a good relationship with their doctor was important. This meant that they were taken seriously and had been provided information about the indications, effects and side-effects of the antipsychotic agents they received, the reason why this medication was no longer indicated/could be discontinued and information about the discontinuation process. Furthermore, their doctor was reliable, had a personal approach and was accessible. The prescribing doctor had to be available when there were problems during the discontinuation process, e.g., withdrawal symptoms or negative feelings. Furthermore, interviewees mentioned that support from their peers, family and support professionals was important. The finding of the fourth theme, namely, the interviewees' own coping style as an important factor in successful discontinuation, was new and surprising. This may suggest that promoting and stimulating patients' feelings of self-confidence and self-efficacy in the management of and decisions around their own medication use may be helpful in the successful discontinuation of inappropriate (long-term) medication. Perhaps, there is a role for support professionals and healthcare workers to support PwID to achieve this. A recently developed training programme for support staff to help with the deprescribing of psychotropics for people with ID, which is called SPECTROM (https://spectrom.wixsite.com/project/ (accessed on 1 November 2022), developed resources that could be used for this purpose [30].

Our study had some limitations. For the interview study, we had to recruit participants from our own networks, which may have influenced the representativeness of participants in the study. For example, all participants were white. Moreover, we did not interview representatives of people with moderate, severe and profound intellectual disabilities who discontinued antipsychotics; therefore, the results of this interview study are not applicable to these populations. Moreover, we only had seven participants in this qualitative interview study. However, we may assume that this sample size was sufficient because data saturation was achieved in the sixth interview. Finally, because this study was carried out among Dutch clients in Dutch healthcare settings, the results might not be generalisable to other countries. Yet, it may be assumed that the occurrence of withdrawal symptoms and the need for support during the process of medication withdrawal are universal among all people with mild intellectual disabilities. Therefore, the results of this study may also be applicable to other countries with comparable service- and care-providing systems for PwID.

5. Conclusions

The experiences and opinions of experts by experience with mild intellectual disabilities who had discontinued their antipsychotic drugs were that the reliability and accessibility of their doctors and being taken seriously; a clear explanation and information about the discontinuation trajectory; support from peers, families and care professionals; and their own coping styles were important factors in successful discontinuation.

In addition to the education of care professionals in supporting their clients with mild intellectual disabilities in the decision-making around their medication use, the clients' own coping style in decisions around the start of and management of difficulties during an antipsychotic discontinuation process may be an important factor for the successful completion of discontinuation.

Author Contributions: Conceptualisation, J.d.H.; data curation, J.d.H.; formal analysis, J.d.H.; investigation, J.d.H.; methodology, J.d.H.; supervision, G.d.K.; writing—original draft, G.d.K.; writing—review and editing, G.d.K., J.d.H., S.D. and R.S. All authors have read and agreed to the published version of the manuscript.

Funding: This research received no external funding.

Institutional Review Board Statement: The study was conducted in accordance with the Declaration of Helsinki, and approved by the Institutional Review Board of Commissie Onderzoek en Zorginnovatie GGZ Drenthe at 28 June 2021.

Informed Consent Statement: Written and signed participants' consent forms were collected.

Data Availability Statement: The data are available on request and with a substantiated explanation at the GGZ Drenthe department research website (https://ggzdrenthe.nl/research, accessed on 1 November 2022).

Acknowledgments: We are very grateful for the cooperation of the experts by experience who consented to be interviewed on their experiences with the topic of this study.

Conflicts of Interest: R.S. received institutional and research support from LivaNova, UCB, Eisai, Veriton Pharma, Bial, Angelini, UnEEG and Jazz/GW pharma outside the submitted work. The other authors declare no conflict of interest.

References

1. Dworschak, W.; Ratz, C.; Wagner, M. Prevalence and putative risk markers of challenging behavior in students with ID. *Res. Dev. Disabil.* **2016**, *58*, 94–103. [CrossRef] [PubMed]
2. National Institute for Health and Care Excellence (NICE) Challenging behaviour and learning disabilities: Prevention and interventions for people with learning disabilities whose behaviour challenges. Available online: https://www.nice.org.uk/guidance/ng11 (accessed on 1 November 2022).
3. Deb, S.; Bethea, T.; Havercamp, S.; Rifkin, A.; Underwood, L. Disruptive, impulse-control, and conduct disorders. In *Diagnostic Manual—Intellectual Disability: A Textbook of Diagnosis of Mental Disorders in Persons with Intellectual Disability*, 2nd ed.; Fletcher, R., Barnhill, J., Cooper, S.-A., Eds.; NADD Press: Kingston, NY, USA, 2016; pp. 521–560.
4. Mazza, M.G.; Rossetti, A.; Crespi, G.; Clerici, M. Prevalence of co-occurring psychiatric disorders in adults and adolescents with intellectual disability: A systematic review and meta-analysis. *J. Appl. Res. Intellect. Disabil.* **2020**, *33*, 126–138. [CrossRef] [PubMed]
5. Peña-Salazar, C.; Arrufat, F.; Santos, J.M.; Fontanet, A.; González-Castro, G.; Más, S.; Valde's-Stauber, J.; Roura-Poch, P. Underdiagnosis of psychiatric disorders in people with intellectual disabilities: Differences between psychiatric disorders and challenging behaviour. *J. Intell. Disabil.* **2020**, *24*, 326–338. [CrossRef] [PubMed]
6. Deb, S.; Perera, B.; Krysta, K.; Ozer, M.; Bertelli, M.; Novell, R.; Wieland, J.; Sappok, T. The European guideline on the assessment and diagnosis of psychiatric disorders in adults with intellectual disabilities. *Eur. J. Psych.* **2022**, *36*, 11–25. [CrossRef]
7. Bertelli, M.O.; Azeem, M.W.; Underwood, L.; Scattoni, M.L.; Persico, A.M.; Ricciardello, A.; Sappok, T.; Bergmann, T.; Keller, R.; Bianco, A.; et al. Autism Spectrum Disorder. In *Textbook of Psychiatry for Intellectual Disability and Autism Spectrum Disorder*; Bertelli, M.O., Deb, S., Munir, K., Hassiotis, A., Salvador-Carulla, L., Eds.; Springer Nature: Cham, Switzerland, 2022; pp. 369–455.
8. Deb, S.; Perera, B.; Bertelli, M.O. Attention Deficit Hyperactivity Disorder. In *Textbook of Psychiatry for Intellectual Disability and Autism Spectrum Disorder*; Bertelli, M.O., Deb, S., Munir, K., Hassiotis, A., Salvador-Carulla, L., Eds.; Springer Nature: Cham, Switzerland, 2022; pp. 457–482. [CrossRef]
9. Branford, D.; Gerrard, D.; Saleem, N.; Shaw, C.; Webster, A. Stopping over-medication of people with intellectual disability, Autism or both (STOMP) in England part 1-history and background of STOMP. *Adv. Ment. Health Intellect. Disabil.* **2019**, *13*, 31–40. [CrossRef]
10. Biswas, A.; Baldwin, D.; Hiremath, A.; Jaydeokar, S.; Lovell, M.; McAlister, H.; Shankar, R.; Deb, S.; Devapriam, J.; Branford, D.; et al. *Stopping the Overmedication of People with Intellectual Disability, Autism or Both (Stomp) and Supporting Treatment and Appropriate Medication in Paediatrics (Stamp)*; Royal College of Psychiatrists: London, UK, 2021; pp. 1–21.
11. Deb, S.; Kwok, H.; Bertelli, M.; Salvador-Carulla, L.; Bradley, E.; Torr, J.; Barnhill, J. International guide to prescribing psychotropic medication for the management of problem behaviours in adults with intellectual disabilities. *World Psychiatry* **2009**, *8*, 181–186. [CrossRef]
12. Bowring, D.L.; Totsika, V.; Hastings, R.P.; Toogood, S.; Griffith, G.M. Challenging behaviours in adults with an ID: A total population study and exploration of risk indices. *Br. J. Clin. Psychol.* **2017**, *56*, 16–32. [CrossRef]
13. Sheehan, R.; Hassiotis, A.; Walters, K.; Osborn, D.; Strydom, A.; Horsfall, L. Mental illness, challenging behaviour, and psychotropic drug prescribing in people with ID: UK population-based cohort study. *Br. Med. J.* **2015**, *351*, h4326. [CrossRef]
14. Unwin, G.L.; Deb, S. Efficacy of atypical antipsychotic medication in the management of behaviour problems in children with intellectual disabilities and borderline intelligence: A systematic review. *Res. Dev. Disabil.* **2011**, *32*, 2121–2133. [CrossRef]
15. Deb, S.; Roy, M.; Limbu, B. Psychopharmacological treatments for psychopathology in people with intellectual disabilities and/or autism spectrum disorder. *Br. J. Psych. Adv.* **2022**, 1–12. [CrossRef]
16. Tyrer, P.; Oliver-Africano, P.C.; Ahmed, Z.; Bouras, N.; Cooray, S.; Deb, S.; Murphy, D.; Hare, M.; Meade, M.; Reece, B.; et al. Risperidone, haloperidol, and placebo in the treatment of aggressive challenging behaviour in patients with intellectual disability: A randomised controlled trial. *Lancet* **2008**, *371*, 57–63. [CrossRef]

17. McQuire, C.; Hassiotis, A.; Harrison, B.; Pilling, S. Pharmacological interventions for challenging behaviour in children with intellectual disabilities: A systematic review and meta-analysis. *BMC Psychiatry* **2015**, *15*, 303. [CrossRef]
18. Sheehan, R.; Horsfall, L.; Strydom, A.; Osborn, D.; Walters, K.; Hassiotis, A. Movement side effects of antipsychotic drugs in adults with and without ID: UK population-based cohort study. *Br. Med. J. Open* **2017**, *7*, e017406.
19. Charlot, L.; Doerfler, L.; McLaren, J. Psychotropic medications use and side effects of individuals with intellectual and developmental disabilities. *J. Intellect. Disabil. Res.* **2020**, *64*, 852–863. [CrossRef]
20. Iasevoli, F.; Barone, A.; Buonaguro, E.; Vellucci, L.; de Bartolomeis, A. Safety and tolerability of antipsychotic agents in neurodevelopmental disorders: A systematic review. *Expert. Opin. Drug. Saf.* **2020**, *19*, 1419–1444. [CrossRef]
21. Sheehan, R.; Hassiotis, A.; Strydom, A.; Morant, N. Experiences of psychotropic medication use and decision-making for adults with ID: A multistakeholder qualitative study in the UK. *Br. Med. J. Open* **2019**, *9*, e032861.
22. Crossley, R.; Withers, P. Antipsychotic Medication and People with ID: Their Knowledge and Experiences. *J. Appl. Res. Intellect. Disabil.* **2009**, *22*, 77–86. [CrossRef]
23. Fish, R.; Hatton, C.; Chauhan, U. "Tell me what they do my body": A survey to find out what information people with learning disabilities want with their medications. *Br. J. Learn. Disabil.* **2017**, *45*, 217–225. [CrossRef]
24. Hall, S.; Deb, S. A qualitative study on the knowledge and views that people with learning disabilities and their carers have of psychotropic medication prescribed for behaviour problems. *Adv. Ment. Health Learn. Disabil.* **2008**, *2*, 29–37. [CrossRef]
25. Embregts, P.; Kroezen, M.; Mulder, E.J.; Van Bussel, C.; Van der Nagel, J.; Budding, M.; Busser, G.; de Kuijper, G.; Duinkerken-Van Gelderen, P.; Haasnoot, M.; et al. Multidisciplinary guideline on Problem behavior in adults with intellectual disabilities. *Ned. Ver. Van Artsen Voor Verstand. Gehandicap. (NVAVG)* **2019**, *2019*, 2–9. (In Dutch)
26. Sheehan, R.; Hassiotis, A. Reduction or discontinuation of antipsychotics for challenging behaviour in adults with ID: A systematic review. *Lancet Psychiatry* **2017**, *4*, 238–256. [CrossRef] [PubMed]
27. De Kuijper, G.M.; Hoekstra, P.J. An Open-Label Discontinuation Trial of Long-Term, Off-Label Antipsychotic Medication in People With ID: Determinants of Success and Failure. *J. Clin. Pharmacol.* **2018**, *58*, 1418–1426. [CrossRef]
28. Shankar, R.; Wilcock, M.; Deb, S.; Goodey, R.; Corson, E.; Pretorius, C.; Praed, G.; Pell, A.; Dee, V.; Wilkinson, E.; et al. A structured programme to withdraw antipsychotics among adults with ID: The Cornwall experience. *J. Appl. Res. Intellect. Disabil.* **2019**, *32*, 1389–1400. [CrossRef] [PubMed]
29. De Kuijper, G.M.; Hoekstra, P.J. An open-label discontinuation trial of long-term used off-label antipsychotic drugs in people with ID: The influence of staff-related factors. *J. Appl. Res. Intellect. Disabil.* **2019**, *32*, 313–322. [CrossRef] [PubMed]
30. Deb, S.; Limbu, B.; Unwin, G.; Woodcock, L.; Cooper, V.; Fullerton, M. Short-term Psycho-Education for Caregivers to Reduce OverMedication of people with intellectual disabilities (SPECTROM): Development and field testing. *Intern. J. Environ. Res. Public Health* **2021**, *18*, 13161. [CrossRef] [PubMed]
31. De Kuijper, G.; van der Putten, A. Knowledge and expectations of direct support professionals towards effects of psychotropic drugs in people with intellectual disabilities. *J. Appl. Res. Intellect. Disabil.* **2017**, *30*, 1–9. [CrossRef] [PubMed]
32. Deb, S.; Limbu, B.; Unwin, G.L.; Weaver, T. Causes of and alternatives to medication for behaviours that challenge in people with intellectual disabilities: Direct care providers' perspectives. *Intern. J. Environ. Res. Public Health* **2022**, *19*, 9988. [CrossRef] [PubMed]
33. Deb, S.; Nancarrow, T.; Limbu, B.; Sheehan, R.; Wilcock, M.; Branford, D.; Courtenay, K.; Perera, B.; Shankar, R. UK psychiatrists' experience of withdrawal of antipsychotics prescribed for challenging behaviours in adults with ID and/or autism. *Br. J. Psych. Open* **2020**, *6*, 112. [CrossRef]
34. Kleijwegt, B.; Pruijssers, A.; Jong-Bakker, L.; Haan, K.; Os-Medendorp, H.; Meijel, B. Support staff's perceptions of discontinuing antipsychotics in people with ID in residential care: A mixed-method study. *J. Appl. Res. Intellect. Disabil.* **2019**, *32*, 861–870. [CrossRef]
35. De Kuijper, G.; de Haan, J. Withdrawing antipsychotics for challenging behaviours in adults with intellectual disabilities; prescribers' experiences and views. *Int. J. Environ. Res. Public Health* **2022**, submitted.
36. De Kuijper, G.; Hoekstra, P.; Visser, F.; Scholte, F.A.; Penning, C.; Evenhuis, H. Use of antipsychotic drugs in individuals with ID (ID) in the Netherlands: Prevalence and reasons for prescription. *J. Intellect. Disabil. Res.* **2010**, *54*, 659–667. [CrossRef]
37. Došen, A. *Psychische Stoornissen, Probleemgedrag en Verstandelijke Beperking*; Chapter 7; Koninklijke van Gorcum: Assen, The Netherlands, 2014; pp. 140–147. (In German)
38. Shosha, G. Employment of Colaizzi's Strategy in Descriptive Phenomenology: A Reflection of a Researcher. 2012. Available online: https://eujournal.org/index.php/esj/article/view/588 (accessed on 1 November 2022).
39. Polit, D.; Beck, C. *Nursing Research. Generating and Assessing Evidence for Nursing Practice*; Wolters Kluwer: Amsterdam, The Netherlands, 2017; Volume 10, p. 744.
40. Mortelmans, D. *Handboek Kwalitatieve Onderzoeksmethoden*; Acco: Leuven, Belgium, 2020; Volume 3.
41. Hassiotis, A.; Kimona, K.; Moncrieff, J.; Deb, S. A stakeholder Consultation about Future Research of Psychotropic Medication Use and Behaviour Support for Adults with Intellectual Disabilities Who Present with Behaviours that Challenge: Feasibility of Future Research. NOCLOR. 2016. Available online: https://www.ucl.ac.uk/psychiatry/sites/psychiatry/files/stakeholder-consultation-document.pdf (accessed on 1 November 2022).

42. Branford, D. Factors associated with successful or unsuccessful withdrawal of antipsychotic drug therapy prescribed for people with learning disabilities. *J. Intellect. Disabil. Res.* **1996**, *40*, 322–329. [CrossRef]
43. Cerovecki, A.; Musil, R.; Klimke, A.; Seemüller, F.; Haen, E.; Schennach, R.; Kühn, K.-U.; Volz, H.-P.; Riedel, M. Withdrawal symptoms and rebound syndromes associated with switching and discontinuing atypical antipsychotics: Theoretical background and practical recommendations. *CNS Drugs* **2013**, *27*, 545–572. [CrossRef]
44. Chouinard, G.; Chouinard, V.-A. Atypical antipsychotics: CATIE study, drug-induced movement disorder and resulting iatrogenic psychiatric-like symptoms, supersensitivity rebound psychosis and withdrawal discontinuation syndromes. *Psychother. Psychosom.* **2008**, *77*, 69–77. [CrossRef] [PubMed]
45. Deb, S.; Unwin, G.L.; Cooper, S.-A.; Rojahn, J. Problem behaviours. In *Textbook of Psychiatry for Intellectual Disability and Autism Spectrum Disorder*; Bertelli, M.O., Deb, S., Munir, K., Hassiotis, A., Salvador-Carulla, L., Eds.; Springer Nature: Cham, Switzerland, 2022; pp. 145–186. [CrossRef]

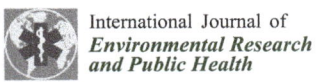

Article

Causes of and Alternatives to Medication for Behaviours That Challenge in People with Intellectual Disabilities: Direct Care Providers' Perspectives

Shoumitro (Shoumi) Deb [1,*], Bharati Limbu [1], Gemma L. Unwin [2] and Tim Weaver [3]

[1] Department of Brain Sciences, Faculty of Medicine, Imperial College London, 2nd Floor Commonwealth Building, Du Cane Road, London W12 0NN, UK
[2] School of Psychology, University of Birmingham, 52 Pritchatts Road, Room 314, Edgbaston, Birmingham B15 2TT, UK
[3] Department of Health & Social Care, School of Health Social Care and Education, Middlesex University, London NW4 4BT, UK
* Correspondence: s.deb@imperial.ac.uk

Abstract: Behaviours that challenge (BtC), such as aggression and self-injury, are manifested by many people with intellectual disabilities (ID). National and international guidelines recommend non-pharmacological psychosocial intervention before considering medication to address BtC. Support staff play a pivotal role in the prescription process. Using coproduction, we developed a training programme for support staff, called SPECTROM, to give them knowledge and empower them to question inappropriate prescriptions and ask for the discontinuation of medication if appropriate and instead look for ways to help people with ID when they are distressed without relying on medication. We have presented data from two focus groups that we conducted during the development of SPECTROM: one that included support staff, and another that had service managers and trainers. In these focus groups, we explored participants' views on the use of medication to address BtC with a particular emphasis on the causes of and alternatives to medication for BtC. Along with the participants' views, we have also presented how we have addressed these issues in the SPECTROM resources.

Keywords: people with intellectual disabilities; the causes of behaviours that challenge; alternatives to medication for behaviours that challenge; social care services; support staff; service/home managers; trainers

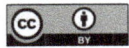

1. Introduction

Behaviours that challenge (BtC), or challenging behaviour, can be defined as "culturally abnormal behaviour of such an intensity, frequency or duration that the physical safety of the person or others is likely to be placed in serious jeopardy, or behaviour which is likely to seriously limit the use of, or result in the person being denied access to, ordinary community facilities" [1]. BtC is common in people with intellectual (learning) disabilities (ID), with up to 60.4% of adults with ID showing at least one form of BtC [2–4]. BtC includes aggression, destructive behaviour, and self-injurious behaviour [5]. BtC can be difficult to manage and may lead to exclusion from community facilities, community placement breakdown and hospitalisation, and the use of restrictive practices such as physical restraint and inappropriate medication use [2,5].

To help a person with BtC, it is crucial to understand the reason behind the BtC rather than to inappropriately use medication [2,6]. BtC can be considered a form of communication whereby a person with ID conveys their distress [7]. For example, if someone is in pain or frustrated because of the demand put on them, they may shout and scream if they cannot communicate their distress to others. According to Matson and colleagues [8], the function of BtC could be categorised under six headings: attention (receive attention), escape (avoid something), non-social (factors internal to the person), physical (physical problems such as relief from pain), and tangible (achieve something). The function of the behaviour is assessed using functional behavioural analysis through Antecedent (situation before the BtC), Behaviour (the description of the actual behaviour), and Consequences (the consequences of the behaviour) ABC charts [9].

Both pharmacological and non-pharmacological psychosocial interventions such as positive behaviour support (PBS) [10] have been used to manage BtC [11,12]. A recent meta-analysis found a significantly long-lasting moderate overall effect of non-pharmacological interventions on BtC (effect size = 0.573) [13]. Interventions combining mindfulness and behavioural techniques, such as a PBS approach, showed greater impact than other interventions. Other PBS-based non-pharmacological interventions have also been shown to be effective in reducing BtC when compared with treatment as usual [14]. Another recent study has shown that a significantly higher number of adults with intellectual disabilities managed to come off their psychotropic medications when PBS was implemented in comparison to the group where no PBS was implemented [15].

Despite the poor evidence for the effectiveness of medications in managing BtC [6], psychotropic medications are used widely among people with ID (49–63%) and often off-license [16], which is a major public health concern [17].

Support (care) staff play a pivotal role in influencing the prescription process, such as by asking doctors to prescribe medication for BtC to begin with, and, given the lack of evidence of the effectiveness of the medications, are overly optimistic about the medication's potential effect [18,19]. Support staff also are most anxious and obstructive to psychiatrists' attempts to withdraw antipsychotic medication when appropriate [20]. Previous surveys of support staff in Australia [21] and the Netherlands [22] showed that most staff felt the use of psychotropic medications for BtC is justified. In our recent focus groups of support staff in the UK, some staff felt the use of medication is appropriate, whereas others felt that it is a 'chemical restraint' [23]. Among other factors, poor staff training and organisational policies are crucial factors in successfully withdrawing psychotropic medications [19–21]. Proper training and support for support staff are thus particularly important for successful programmes concerning the rationalisation of psychotropic medication use in adults with ID.

Training programmes are shown to be useful in many psychiatric disorders, including schizophrenia (30 RCTs) [24] and bipolar disorder [25], in improving patients and their caregivers' quality of life (QoL). They have also been found useful in different neurodevelopmental disorders. For example, our recent meta-analysis has shown a moderate effect size of parental training on improving autism symptoms in children with autism spectrum disorder (ASD) [26]. A review of training programmes directed at parents and teachers included four RCTs and found improvement in attention deficit hyperactivity disorder (ADHD) symptoms with effect sizes of 0.05 to 0.77 [27]. A Cochrane review showed that training support staff helped to reduce antipsychotic prescriptions in people with dementia by 40–50% [28]. This was reflected in a nationwide trend in the reduction of antipsychotic prescriptions by 11% over 10 years (2005–2015) in the UK [29].

We have addressed the aforementioned issues by developing online training resources implemented through face-to-face interactive workshops for support staff caring for adults with ID in community settings. The training programme, SPECTROM (Short-term Psycho-Education for Carers To Reduce Over Medication of people with intellectual disabilities) (https://spectrom.wixsite.com/project accessed on 12 July 2022), was developed using a co-production method [30,31]. This was achieved by putting stakeholders' experiences at the centre of the study and ensuring close and equal collaboration among them from the outset. The ultimate aim of SPECTROM is to empower, inform, and equip support staff with skills to understand the person they support, manage their own psychological responses to their behaviour, negotiate the care pathway, advocate on behalf of the person they care for, and take the views of adults with ID fully into account. The intended goal is to reduce requests from staff for medication and encourage staff to ask the prescribers questions about the necessity of the continued use of psychotropic medication, which should lead to a significant reduction in the use of medication and an increase in psychosocial interventions instead.

As part of the development of SPECTROM training, focus groups were conducted to explore staff perceptions on the use of psychotropic medication to manage BtC in people with ID and gather suggestions regarding the contents and format of SPECTROM. The aim of this paper is to present the findings of the first set of focus groups where support staff, service/home managers, and PBS trainers discussed their perceptions of and views on the use of psychotropic medications to address BtC in adults with ID. In this paper, we have presented two themes related to BtC: participants' views on 'the causes of BtC' and 'the alternatives to medication for BtC'.

2. Materials and Methods

We conducted two focus groups: one involving support staff and another with house/service managers and PBS trainers. These focus groups explored participants' views on the use of psychotropic medication for BtC in adults with ID with a particular emphasis on the potential 'causes of BtC', and 'alternatives to medication for BtC'.

2.1. Participants

We invited nine support staff, seven of whom agreed to attend, but eight ultimately took part. Five service/house managers and three trainers were invited, and all took part in the focus groups. We have not collected any demographic data on the participants.

2.2. Conduct of the Focus Groups

A topic guide (see Supplementary Material S1) was developed based on the literature review findings and the project's aims and objectives. After discussion with the core team (BL, SD, TW, and GU) and other relevant stakeholders, the topic guide was finalised. This was employed flexibly and was open to emergent themes but framed using the Theory of Planned Behaviour model [32], thus examining beliefs and attitudes (e.g., about psychotropic medication and alternative approaches such as PBS) and how these might influence behaviour (e.g., in terms of requesting support from professionals to prescribe medication or provide help with alternative approaches). The interviews started with an exploration of participants' experiences dealing with BtC in adults with ID and the use of medication for BtC. Then, the topic guide moved into issues related to potential causes of BtC, including physical, psychiatric, and environmental causes. From there, the topic guide entered into the issue of participants' views on alternatives to medication, particularly psychosocial interventions such as PBS, for BtC. The sample size was a pragmatic decision. No formal sample size calculation was required for this study. This was a small study with limited resources and included primarily qualitative data collection. The minimum sample size we aimed for was 6–8 participants in each focus group. Participants were purposively sampled for each group to include a range of support staff in terms of their experience and from different organisations.

A researcher (BL) with previous experience in conducting qualitative research ran the focus groups with the help of the chief investigator (SD) under the supervision of an expert in qualitative research (TW). We used the approach utilised in our previous studies of interviewing the carers of people with ID as well as head injury [33–35]. Any paid carers, service/home managers, and trainers working with people with ID who showed BtC were eligible to participate in the study. A research advertisement was sent through the UK Voluntary Organisations Disability Group (VODG), an umbrella organisation of more than 35 social care service providers in the UK (social service, voluntary, and independent sectors). Nine service provider organisations agreed to take part, but, ultimately, only eight got involved. The organisations are Mencap, Challenging Behaviour Foundation, Achieve together, AT-Autism, Avenues Group, Dimensions UK, Milestones Trust, and National Autistic Society. Each organisation identified one available manager and trainer for the focus groups, and each manager identified two support staff. The focus groups were held face-to-face at a venue in London, England in March 2019. Eligible participants were then sent a SPECTROM study summary and information on the study. Once participants agreed, written informed consent was taken. Two separate focus groups were conducted, one with support staff and the other with service managers and trainers. Each lasted for approximately 90 min. The same topic guide was used for both groups, and a semi-structured interview was carried out. The focus groups were recorded using pseudonyms and professionally transcribed. Two authors (BL and SD) independently analysed the data to achieve a consensus. In the focus groups, care staff, service managers, and trainers explored issues around their perception and views on medication use for and causes and assessment of BtC.

2.3. Thematic Analysis

The transcriptions were analysed using thematic analysis. Thematic analysis is the process of identifying patterns and themes within qualitative data and texts. The data are interpreted to examine underlying meaning and ideas. Thematic analysis can be top-down deductive, driven by specific research questions, or bottom-up inductive, driven by data [36]. We used a top-down deductive approach to analyse the gathered data based on the topic guide and research questions we developed. NVivo 12 plus for windows software [37] was used to manage and analyse the data. The authors first familiarised themselves with the data. The transcripts were then read and interpreted for meaning and significance. Then, a code was given to each interpretation, and an initial coding frame was developed to organise the identified codes. This initial frame included main themes under 'physical cause of BtC', 'psychiatric cause of BtC', 'environmental cause for BtC', and 'psychosocial interventions for BtC'. The coding frame developed was continuously reviewed and refined as new codes emerged or as it was searched for patterns. The data and quotes were indexed on identified codes or new emerging codes. The coding framework was then searched for patterns for emerging themes. Similar codes were categorised together to produce patterns and themes. The identified categories were also reviewed to ensure the emerging category was discrete and modified as necessary. The identified themes were then reviewed and revised if needed. Once no new themes emerged, the themes were finalised and defined. The themes and analysis process were also overseen and verified by two authors (GU and TW) who were experienced qualitative researchers.

3. Results

We have presented two themes and six subthemes from the thematic analysis of focus group discussions: (a) causes of BtC, including psychiatric disorders, and (b) alternatives to medication including PBS, person centred approaches, understanding the person, developing relationships, and collaborative working. In the results section, we present the main themes and subthemes followed by relevant quotes directly taken from the transcripts. We have used codes in the parenthesis such as 'SS' for support staff, 'SM' for service/house manager, and 'TR' for trainer to identify the quotes from the different groups of participants.

4. Causes of BtC and How Understanding Them Can Help the Person with ID

Participants discussed the causes of BtC and how understanding them would help address BtC using alternatives to medication. The central emerging theme was 'behaviour is a means of communication'. Triggers for BtC were discussed, including the environmental factors, particularly if the people are not placed in the right environment, and the help they need to accommodate any changes in their life. Participants felt it would be good to have a checklist to recognise the factors that lead to BtC. We have addressed this issue by developing a Checklist for the Assessment of Triggers for the behaviour of concern Scale (CATS) [38]. Staff can use this list to identify the triggers for BtC, which will help complete the Antecedent-Behaviour-Consequence (ABC) chart and functional behaviour analysis.

" ... when she was aggressive, and all she wanted was the curtains tied back. So, what someone else would think of that, you know it's just, it's just knowing." (TR)

"I think it was literally a checklist of going through the whole thing with her. What could it be?" (SM)

"To be considered, the environment, how they feel in the environment, do they feel comfortable there?" (SS)

" ... placement staff comes into it a lot on whether someone who is in the right placement." (SM)

Some participants felt it is not helpful when people come with a label such as being very aggressive. They thought they should thoroughly reassess the person and their behaviour to draw a new person-centred support plan.

"Looking at the support plan. I mean had to rewrite her support plan with in the space of two weeks because she came labelled as being a very difficult person, very challenging. And naturally she was scared so her way of reacting was to fight. And the treatment assessment unit, she was in where I visited her, I was scared, so she must have been absolutely petrified." (SM)

Participants discussed how physical problems, such as pain in the body, can manifest as BtC and be wrongly treated with antipsychotics.

"I know for a fact people have been given anti-psychotic medication and actually it's something physical that's wrong. They've got toothache or they've got tummy ache or they don't like the colour of their room. Something as simple as that, you know." (SM)

"Um, but recently I had someone who was exhibiting behaviour but it was because he had chest infection and he was in pain but he couldn't vocalise or tell someone I'm in pain. So, then staff log it as challenging behaviour, we need to talk to a psychiatrist." (SM)

The issue of communication came up in the discussion. SPECTROM has a module on effective communication and another on effective engagement with people with ID. Both modules encourage staff to learn the best ways to communicate with the person they support so that they can concentrate on their skill-building rather than BtC.

"I think often people are perceived as showing behaviours because of the condition, but actually its external factors and things in the environment or how they're being supported. Um, the communication strategies that they've got." (SM)

"Sometimes when you have challenging behaviours it's not, it's because someone wants something. It's like you said. Yeah, they can't communicate. They're telling you they want something done or to do something. Communication. It's always communication." (TR)

Causes of BtC: Psychiatric Disorder

While discussing the causes of BtC, the role of psychiatric disorders was raised. All participants unanimously agreed that no meaningful training currently exists on the issue of psychiatric disorders in ID, although there is an increasing awareness of Autism Spectrum Disorder (ASD).

" ... we've not really, we've never really given any sort of any specific training on psychosis or um, mine was just basically what I've read from you know carer plans and things like that. Um, but nothing, we've never ever attended any training on it." (SS)

Staff found it difficult to distinguish between psychiatric disorders and BtC. They felt that when the person is trying to communicate their needs through BtC, it is often misinterpreted as a psychiatric illness.

"When is it challenging behaviour and when is it psychosis, like you say? When is it that he's hearing voices that's telling him to do something and when is it when he's doing it because of his own accord that he's trying to communicate something or maybe an expression?" (SS)

" ... how much of what they're displaying is because of their mental illness or how much is that just because they're trying to tell you something and you're not able to understand it? As support staff, something I struggle with personally is knowing the difference." (SS)

Participants felt that when there is a crisis and the person with ID displays BtC, it is often considered part of a psychiatric disorder. As a result, they do not explore other factors, including the environment, to check what is causing the behaviour.

" ... when he attacked staff but he didn't hear voices, was that because of the psychosis or what that because he was having a, he was going through, he was going through that crisis." (SS)

There was significant confusion about the overlap between what may be ASD symptoms (e.g., living within an inner world) and psychiatric symptoms. SPECTROM has comprehensive modules on ASD and ADHD. The ASD module discusses the potential overlap between the ASD phenotype and psychiatric symptoms in detail, but acknowledges that many psychiatric disorders, including psychosis, are common in people with ASD [39].

" ... there was too much stimulation going on and that frustrated him so that he just lashed out. Because he's also diagnosed with autism, there's also that to consider as well. So that was due to the environment why he acted that way rather than it being psychosis because something told him to lash out." (SS)

Participants discussed the difficulty of distinguishing between trauma-related symptoms and psychiatric symptoms. Some participants thought that psychotic symptoms might, in fact, be the memories of past traumatic events spoken aloud rather than genuine psychosis. There is also the possibility of past traumatic experiences inducing real psychotic symptoms [40,41]. This issue has been discussed in the psychiatric disorder module of SPECTROM.

"He believes that he hears people, and he will say that they made me do it and things. .... .is that because he's saying that but actually is that just a past traumatic event that's happened that then he's remembering it?" (SS)

One support staff expressed frustration on the lack of awareness among some general practitioners who take a medical approach to BtC and say that these are often due to a psychiatric disorder.

" ... one of the GP I discussed it. But what do you expect? He's got mental health problems. I'm talking about uh, educating people." (SS)

5. Alternatives to Medication

5.1. Positive Behaviour Support (PBS)

After discussing the possible causes of BtC, the discussion progressed to how to best address BtC without relying on medication. This started with a discussion around PBS and how this framework can be used to reduce inappropriate uses of medication. Some larger service provider organisations seem to have their own PBS support team, which staff found very helpful. However, even in big organisations, the PBS support team resource is not always adequate, and most smaller organisations will not have this kind of support available at all. Most staff in large organisations also only have basic training on PBS.

"She got into crisis, was in crisis for months and regardless of whatever we were doing as a carer, as a care staff, and you know we brought in um, um positive behaviour support team. We were working really closely with them. We've got really, really robust PBS plans." (SS)

"Part of our PBS was to give him space, so we gave him space." (SS)

"So now that he's come .... ..to our company, we said we were going to support him for positive behaviour support plan. .... ..we've seen a different person. He's living a

better life and that's because of the service that he's in that's allowing him to live a better life." (SS)

"You know, staff have PBS training, um, we work with behavioural support analysts that come in and collect data." (SM)

The issue of the cost of providing the service was discussed. One trainer highlighted the fact that using the PBS approach can reduce the frequency of BtC and the use of medication, which will save money in the long run. Therefore, a case could be made for social and health care commissioners to invest the funds needed to implement PBS now in order to save money in the future.

"So that's got big budget implications as well, because certainly similar examples where somebody has come out of long stay and they were on, you know, X amount of medication and all the support plans are saying three to one support in our community. . . . .but two years down the line that three to one support becomes one to one support because somebody's taken a holistic approach to look at what do we need to do to support this person?" (TR)

5.2. Person-Centred Care Approach

Other alternatives to medication based on the PBS approach were discussed, including a person-centred care approach. There seems to be more awareness within the larger social care provider organisations in the UK and their staff about using alternatives to medication to address BtC through a person-centred care approach.

"So our staff are very aware of the, um, other ways to help behaviours rather than prescribing medication." (SM)

"Right now, there has been a lot of awareness that's been created that people are using all those alternatives rather than medication." (SM)

" . . . He's more engaged. He's more willing to communicate, willing to do things. Willing to participate because we are allowing him to do." (SS)

5.3. Understanding the Person

Another person-centred care approach the participants discussed was understanding the person behind the behaviour. Participants felt that, once they got to know the person well, it became easier to help them without using medication when they were distressed. Sometimes people come from a previous placement with a label of being aggressive, but staff felt that this should not deter them from trying to get to know the person and help them with their skill development instead of concentrating on their BtC. One service manager mentioned that, if you do not understand the person and the reason for their BtC, you tend to blame the person for their behaviour which does not help.

"Um she's not written up for anything, PRN at all so her behaviour are managed through um, staff really knowing her well." (SS)

"So, if you don't get to know what they are on about, then they will start to display challenging behaviour." (SS)

"And you find out what they like. Nobody asked them. And show positive interest in what they like and you know to talk to them like they're a real human being." (SS)

"Instead of taking the baggage of their history with them. And it's about stripping all of that out, and almost starting again and saying let's look at this person as a whole now and get the right people involved." (TR)

"And I believe that does have a lot to do with staff attitudes and behaviours. There are still some places where they blame the person and they are behaving because that's the way they are, rather than then behaving in this way because someone has taken something from that person and they don't know how to control it." (SM)

5.4. Developing Relationships

Another vital person-centred care approach that involved developing a positive relationship with the person they support was discussed. One participant said that, even after being scratched by the person with ID on one occasion, she continued to build a relationship with the person, which helped to improve the BtC.

"So, I stayed longer and now we've got a bond that when I'm on annual leave it's a problem because we build that relationship and it got to a point that everything, she wants to do has to be with me." (SS)

" ... where he became heightened and within that he was able to scratch me which left a scar. From that incident, I didn't change my approach towards him but obviously I was cautious because I'm not trying to get injured. But through that, because I hadn't changed the way I was, and no more the next day and even after that, after that incident he saw me at breakfast, I'll still engage with him, still carried on as normal. The relationship that we have now is that you know he, he trusts." (SS)

"But now we got to a point where I can take her to any appointment, we can sit down. So, I, we build a bond." (SS)

5.5. Collaborative Work

Participants felt that multi-disciplinary work was in the best interests of the person with ID. This includes other relevant professionals like doctors and nurses involved in the care of the person and the person with ID themselves and their families.

"With the prescribing, it's also working with families and psychiatrists, because sometimes there's a parent who is going to tell you I know my child and I think they need this, they have been using this." (SM)

"If the families are involved or any other person involved in their circle of support, they will also attend the meeting. And it's a best interest meeting as well." (SM)

" ... um, how you work as a team with those different professionals. We have a pharmacy check." (SM)

One service manager mentioned that they asked key support staff to accompany the person with ID to the clinic for the medication review. She also emphasised the importance of gathering all relevant information before attending the clinic and involving the person with ID and their family, if possible. SPECTROM provides a checklist for staff to go through in preparation for a formal medication review and a set of questions that staff could or should ask the prescribers in the clinic.

" ... before we go to that meeting, let's have a discussion first so there's no surprises. What are we going to say, what are we presenting to the clinical psychiatrist that doesn't know this person as well as what we do. What does the family members got to say about it? So, we go into that meeting with that individual, if they're open to input and they have the capacity to do that, to feed into that meeting so that it's productive for that person." (SM)

6. Discussion

In this paper, we have presented a wealth of data on wide-ranging issues from focus groups, primarily on participants' perception of the causes of BtC and methods to help people with ID without using medication (alternative to medication).

6.1. Causes of BtC Including Physical and Psychiatric Disorders

As for the causes of BtC, the discussion primarily revolved around physical disorders, psychiatric disorders, and environmental factors. There was a consensus among the participants that BtC is often a means of communication and that the causes and effects of BtC need a thorough assessment to draw up an effective person-centred behaviour support plan to reduce overreliance on medication to address BtC. In SPECTROM, we have provided a module on the assessment of behaviour and examples of two assessment schemas: **B.M.P.P.S.** (assessment of the **B**ehaviour itself, **M**edical issues, the **P**erson with ID, **P**sychiatric/psychological issues, and **S**ocial issues) [5] and **H.E.L.P.** (assessment of **H**ealth and medical conditions, **E**nvironment and support, **L**ived experience and emotional well-being, and **P**sychiatric illness) [42].

Physical disorders are more prevalent in people with ID than in the general population [43]. Although it is not uncommon for physical problems that are common in people with ID, such as pain in the body (headache, toothache), constipation, and acid reflux, to lead to BtC, particularly in people who cannot communicate their feelings, it is not always easy to identify these causes. Therefore, a high degree of suspicion and thinking about a physical cause for BtC should help ensure the correct diagnosis. If necessary, a therapeutic trial with a painkiller where pain is suspected may help. We have developed a 'Physical disorder' module in SPECTROM and provided examples of proformas that could be used to detect and rate the severity of pain. Another problem mentioned was the difficulty of carrying out required investigations such as blood tests, X-rays, etc., for many people with ID. SPECTROM provides practical guidelines for addressing these issues, such as using accessible information including pictures of the tests, teaching the person relaxation techniques, etc. SPECTROM also provides videos on 'what happens during a health check', 'what happens during a blood test', 'what happens during an MRI', etc., to familiarise people with ID before they go for any of these investigations.

The issue of the relationship between psychiatric disorders and BtC is a complex one [39]. Most staff did not receive any training or information on this. Participants raised the question of how to distinguish between psychosis and BtC due to environmental factors or when caused by traumatic life events. Therefore, SPECTROM has developed a psychiatric disorder module to provide information to support staff.

The participants discussed the issue of overlap between ASD and BtC. ASD and ID commonly co-occur; 38% of people with ASD have ID, and a similar proportion of people with ID are also known to have ASD. ADHD is equally common in both ASD and ID, although this issue was not discussed in the focus groups. The extensive overlap of symptoms between ID, ASD, and ADHD often makes it difficult to tease apart these diagnoses in people with ID [39,44,45]. As BtC is common in ID (18–60%) [2], ASD (10–15%) [46], and ADHD [44], respectively, the rate of BtC increases when all three conditions co-exist [39]. Therefore, SPECTROM has developed comprehensive modules on ASD and ADHD, with information on strategies to help people with ID and ASD and/or ADHD to reduce BtC. Currently, there is more awareness of the trauma-induced symptoms in people with ID [40], some of which may manifest as psychiatric disorders or BtC [40,41]. Many support staff in large provider organisations seem to be more conscious of this possibility when they draw up a person-centred care plan for the people they support.

6.2. Alternatives to Medicine through the Use of Person-Centred PBS Care Planning

After discussing the causes of BtC, participants progressed to discuss how to address BtC, particularly by using a psychosocial approach and avoiding medication use. The most well-known psychosocial approach is PBS [10], which provides a framework to apply in practice [47]. Most staff from large provider organisations seem familiar with PBS principles, which they use to draw person-centred care plans [48] for people they support. This approach seems to reduce the need to use medication to address BtC. One study found that community team-led implementation of PBS framework did not reduce BtC in community settings [49]. However, others found that PBS and other psychosocial approaches were useful in reducing aggression among people with ID [14].

Participants acknowledged that understanding the person they support is key to understanding BtC and improving them without relying on medication. Service managers and trainers mentioned not focusing on the 'labels' people with ID bring with them but concentrating on the whole person in order to understand their likes and dislikes, strengths and weaknesses, and develop a positive relationship. All participants agreed on a holistic approach to care planning and addressing BtC.

6.3. Shared Decision Making

All participants in the focus group agreed on the need for multidisciplinary work and acknowledged that there is scope to improve shared decision-making by involving the person with ID and their families. In a previous study, we found that adults with ID did not feel sufficiently involved in making the decision about their medication [50]. Some adults with ID who we interviewed were dissatisfied with their medication, mainly due to lack of involvement in the treatment decision, adverse effects, lack of efficacy, and a 'desire to lead a normal life'. In another study, most of the six adults with ID who were interviewed complained about not having enough information on their medication, particularly in an accessible format [51].

A similar sentiment has been echoed by family members, many of whom felt that there is an over-reliance on medication instead of taking a holistic approach to address BtC [52]. In our study, many of the 20 family caregivers interviewed complained about not having enough information about the care of their loved ones and not having enough involvement in the decision-making process [53]. Family caregivers play an essential part in the care of people with ID, even when they do not live in the family home; they are the only constant presence in the life of the person with ID, whereas professionals and care staff come and go. Therefore, the knowledge of their loved ones is of paramount importance in care provisions for people with ID. To address these issues, we have devoted an entire module to 'effective liaison with families' in SPECTROM. This module teaches staff to respect family caregivers' views, acknowledge family caregivers' expertise, communicate with them without jargon, and include family caregivers and the person with ID in care planning, including prescriptions of medication, from the outset in order to promote more shared decision-making.

Although several studies explored care staff views on medication use, they rarely reported on staff perceptions of the causes of BtC, which was at the heart of the discussions within our focus groups. In our previous study, few care staff explicitly reflected that their own behaviour might influence aggressive behaviour in adults with ID [54]. Furthermore, only 16% of staff interviewed in this study mentioned issues around communication despite much of the aggressive behaviour being considered to be communicative [7]. Staff felt that they would benefit from training and information about potential triggers to help them think more about environmental conditions and their own role in precipitating BtC. Many other researchers have highlighted support staff frustration for not having the right training and their desire to gather more knowledge and training on (a) mental health issues, (b) medication prescribing (when to use them and why, and when not to use them and why), (c) medication side effects, (d) and when and how medication could be safely withdrawn [55]. All of these issues are addressed in the SPECTROM programme.

6.4. Strengths of the Study

Previous studies of staff surveys primarily concentrated on staff knowledge of psychotropic medication. They rarely explored their views on the causes of BtC, which our study has addressed. One strength of this study is that it examined not only support staff's opinions, but also service managers' and trainers' opinions. Previous studies have primarily focused on the experiences and perceptions of support staff and family caregivers. Another strength of this study is that support staff, service managers, and trainers were interviewed separately to avoid the influence of service managers on support staff responses. The support staff, managers, and trainers were also from different service provider organisations, allowing us to capture different aspects of the participants' experiences. In addition, the anonymised data analysis allowed support staff to express their opinion freely, thus increasing the face validity of our findings. Another strength was that the data were analysed by two authors.

6.5. Limitations of the Study

All participants were recruited from large service provider organisations. Therefore, the views and experiences of staff working in smaller organisations were not captured, which may have differed significantly. Another weakness is that service managers identified the support staff for the focus groups, thus managers may have chosen support staff that were particularly eager to get their voices heard on this topic.

7. Conclusions

Our exploration of the views of support staff, service managers, and trainers on the causes and management of behaviours that challenge in people with intellectual disabilities used focus groups to reveal that most participants have some knowledge of the physical, psychological, and environmental causes of BtC. Most were also familiar with the concept of positive behaviour support that could be used to support people with intellectual disabilities who display behaviours that challenge without relying on medication. However, it is worth remembering that all participants in our study were employed by large social care service provider organisations in the UK. Most of these organisations are likely to have their own positive behaviour support teams; smaller provider organisations are unlikely to have this in-house support. Participants unanimously expressed concern about their lack of knowledge of psychiatric disorders and their relationship with behaviours that challenge in people with intellectual disabilities. There were no major discrepancies in the views of the support staff and those of the service managers and PBS trainers. All parties have agreed on the need for more information on medication, their indications, and side effects. We have addressed these issues and others raised by the participants in SPECTROM modules.

Supplementary Materials: The following supporting information can be downloaded at: https://www.mdpi.com/article/10.3390/ijerph19169988/s1. S1: Topic Guide for SPECTROM focus groups 1 & 2.

Author Contributions: S.D. is the grant holder. All authors were involved in the conception and design of the study. S.D. conducted the focus groups. B.L. analysed focus group data, and S.D. acted as the second-rater. All authors contributed substantially to the preparation of the manuscript. All authors have read and agreed to the published version of the manuscript.

Funding: This study was funded by the UK's National Institute of Health Research (NIHR) Research for Patient Benefit (RfPB) Programme (grant PBPG-0817-20010). The Imperial Biomedical Research Centre Facility, which is funded by the NIHR, has provided support for the study. The views expressed in this article are those of the authors and not necessarily those of the National Health Service, the NIHR, or the Department of Health, UK.

Institutional Review Board Statement: Not applicable as no new or patient-related data were collected. Also, the participant's views were analysed anonymously, and no personal data were collected from the participants.

Informed Consent Statement: Written informed consent was collected from the participants before the start of the focus groups.

Data Availability Statement: Transcripts of the focus group discussions are available from the authors subject to approval from the study sponsors and the funders.

Acknowledgments: We thank adults with intellectual disabilities, Cornwall Learning Disability Advisory Group, family caregivers and advocates, other stakeholders including service provider organisations, Achieve Together, Dimensions-UK, National Autistic Society, MENCAP, Milestones Trust, Avenues Group, VODG, Challenging Behaviour Foundation, AT-Autism, Mandy Donley and Jeffrey Chan from the Australian National Disability Insurance Scheme Quality and Safeguards Commission, community learning disability team members, Saadia Arshad, Bini Thomas, Sujit

Jaydeokar for taking part in the project. We also acknowledge the help from the co-applicants and project group members, Umesh Chauhan, John Rose, Jean O'Hara, David Branford, Mike Crawford, Rohit Shankar, Caroline Finlayson, Georgina Samuels, Mike Wilcock for helping with the development of SPECTROM.

Conflicts of Interest: The authors declare no conflict of interest.

References

1. Emerson, E.; Bromley, J. The form and function of challenging behaviours. *J. Intellect. Disabil. Res.* **1995**, *39*, 388–398. [CrossRef] [PubMed]
2. Deb, S.; Unwin, G.L.; Cooper, S.-A.; Rojahn, J. Problem behaviours. In *Textbook of Psychiatry for Intellectual Disability and Autism Spectrum Disorder*; Bertelli, M.O., Deb, S., Munir, K., Hassiotis, A., Salvador-Carulla, L., Eds.; Springer Nature: Cham, Switzerland, 2022; pp. 145–186.
3. Deb, S.; Thomas, M.; Bright, C. Mental disorder in adults with intellectual disability. 2: The rate of behaviour disorders among a community-based population aged between 16 and 64 years. *J. Intellect. Disabil. Res.* **2001**, *45*, 506–514. [CrossRef] [PubMed]
4. Hemmings, C.; Deb, S.; Chaplin, E.; Hardy, S.; Mukherjee, R. Research for people with intellectual disabilities and mental health problems: A view from the UK. *J. Ment. Health Res. Intellect. Disabil.* **2013**, *6*, 127–158. [CrossRef]
5. Deb, S.; Bethea, T.; Havercamp, S.; Rifkin, A.; Underwood, L. Disruptive, impulse-control, and conduct disorders. In *Diagnostic Manual-Intellectual Disability: A Textbook of Diagnosis of Mental Disorders in Persons with Intellectual Disability*, 2nd ed.; Fletcher, R., Barnhill, J., Cooper, S.-A., Eds.; NADD Press: Kingston, NY, USA, 2016; pp. 521–560.
6. Deb, S.; Bertelli, M.O.; Rossi, M. Psychopharmacology. In *Textbook of Psychiatry for Intellectual Disability and Autism Spectrum Disorder*; Bertelli, M.O., Deb, S., Munir, K., Hassiotis, A., Salvador-Carulla, L., Eds.; Springer Nature: Cham, Switzerland, 2022; pp. 247–280.
7. Hastings, R.P.; Brown, T. Functional assessment and challenging behaviours: Some future directions. *J. Assoc. Pers. Sev. Handicap.* **2000**, *25*, 229–240.
8. Matson, J.L.; Tureck, K.; Rieske, R. The Questions about Behavioral Function (QABF): Current status as a method of functional assessment. *Res. Dev. Disabil.* **2012**, *33*, 630–634. [CrossRef]
9. Neidert, P.L.; Dozier, C.L.; Iwata, B.A.; Hafen, M. Behavior analysis in intellectual and developmental disabilities. *Psychol. Serv.* **2010**, *7*, 103. [CrossRef]
10. McDonald, A. Positive Behaviour Support. In *Understanding and Responding to Behaviour That Challenges in Intellectual Disabilities*; Baker, P., Osgood, T., Eds.; Pavilion Publishing and Media Limited: West Sussex, UK, 2019; pp. 31–40.
11. Didden, R.; Lindsay, W.; Lang, R.; Sigafoos, J.; Deb, S.; Wiersma, J.; Peters-Scheffer, N.; Marschick, P.B.; O'Rielly, M.F.; Lancioni, G.E. Aggressive behavior. In *Handbook of Evidence-Based Practices in Intellectual and Developmental Disabilities, Evidence-Based Practices in Behavioral Health*; Singh, N.N., Ed.; Springer International Publishing: Cham, Switzerland, 2016; pp. 727–750.
12. Deb, S. Psychopharmacology. In *Handbook of Evidence-Based Practices in Intellectual and Developmental Disabilities, Evidence-Based Practices in Behavioral Health*, 1st ed.; Singh, N.N., Ed.; Springer International Publishing: Cham, Switzerland, 2016; pp. 347–381.
13. Bruinsma, E.; Van Den Hoofdakker, B.J.; Groenman, A.P.; Hoekstra, P.J.; De Kuijper, G.M.; Klaver, M.; De Bildt, A.A. Non-Pharmacological Interventions for Challenging Behaviours of Adults with Intellectual Disabilities: A Meta-Analysis. *J. Intellect. Disabil. Res.* **2020**, *64*, 561–578. [CrossRef] [PubMed]
14. McGill, P.; Vanono, L.; Clover, W.; Smyth, E.; Cooper, V.; Hopkins, L.; Barratt, N.; Joyce, C.; Henderson, K.; Sekasi, S.; et al. Reducing Challenging Behaviour of Adults with Intellectual Disabilities in Supported Accommodation: A Cluster Randomized Controlled Trial of Setting-Wide Positive Behaviour Support. *Res. Dev. Disabil.* **2018**, *81*, 143–154. [CrossRef]
15. Gerrard, D.; Rhodes, J.; Lee, R.; Ling, J. Using positive behavioural support (PBS) for STOMP medication challenge. *Adv. Ment. Health Intellect. Disabil.* **2018**, *13*, 102–112. [CrossRef]
16. Sheehan, R.; Hassiotis, A.; Walters, K.; Osborn, D.; Strydom, A.; Horsfall, L. Mental illness, challenging behaviour, and psychotropic drug prescribing in people with intellectual disability: UK population based cohort study. *BMJ* **2015**, *351*, h4326. [CrossRef]
17. Glover, G.; Williams, R.; Branford, D.; Avery, R.; Chauhan, U.; Hoghton, M.; Bernard, S. *Prescribing of Psychotropic Drugs to People with Learning Disabilities and/or Autism by General Practitioners in England*; Public Health England: London, UK, 2015.
18. de Kuijper, G.; van der Putten, A.A.J. Knowledge and Expectations of Direct Support Professionals towards Effects of Psychotropic Drug Use in People with Intellectual Disabilities. *J. Appl. Res. Intellect. Disabil.* **2017**, *30*, 1–9. [CrossRef] [PubMed]
19. Christian, L.; Snycerski, S.M.; Singh, N.N.; Poling, A. Direct Service Staff and Their Perceptions of Psychotropic Medication in Non-Institutional Settings for People with Intellectual Disability. *J. Intellect. Disabil. Res.* **1999**, *43*, 88–93. [CrossRef] [PubMed]
20. Deb, S.; Limbu, B.; Nancarrow, T.; Gerrard, D.; Shankar, R. The UK psychiatrists' experience of rationalising antipsychotics in adults with intellectual disabilities: A qualitative data analysis of free-text questionnaire responses. *BMC Psychiatry* **2022**. under review.
21. Donley, M.; Chan, J.; Webber, L. Disability Support Workers' Knowledge and Education Needs about Psychotropic Medication. *Br. J. Learn. Disabil.* **2011**, *40*, 286–291. [CrossRef]

22. Kleijwegt, B.; Pruijssers, A.; de Jong-Bakker, L.; de Haan, K.; van Os-Medendorp, H.; van Meijel, B. Support Staff's Perceptions of Discontinuing Antipsychotics in People with Intellectual Disabilities in Residential Care: A Mixed-Method Study. *J. Appl. Res. Intellect. Disabil.* **2019**, *32*, 861–870. [CrossRef] [PubMed]
23. Deb, S.; Limbu, B.; Unwin, G.; Weaver, T. The use of medication for challenging behaviour in people with intellectual disabilities: The direct care providers' perspective. *Psychiatry Int.* **2022**. under review.
24. McFarlane, W.R.; Dixon, L.; Lukens, E. Family psychoeducation and schizophrenia: A review of the literature. *J. Marital. Fam. Ther.* **2003**, *29*, 233–245. [CrossRef]
25. Colom, F.; Vita, E.; Sánchez-Moreno, J.; Palomino-Otiniano, R.; Reinares, M.; Goikolea, J.M.; Benabarre, A.; Martínez-Arán, A. Group psychoeducation for stabilised bipolar disorders: 5-year outcome of a randomised clinical trial *Br. J. Psychiatry* **2009**, *194*, 260–265. [CrossRef]
26. Deb, S.; Retzer, A.; Roy, M.; Acharya, R.; Limbu, B.; Roy, A. The effectiveness of parent training for children with autism spectrum disorders: A systematic review and meta-analyses. *BMC Psychiatry* **2020**, *20*, 583. [CrossRef]
27. Montoya, A.; Colom, F.; Ferrin, M. Is psychoeducation for parents and teachers of children and adolescents with ADHD efficacious? A systematic review. *Eur. Psychiatry* **2011**, *26*, 166–175. [CrossRef]
28. Richter, T.; Meyer, G.; Möhler, R.; Köpke, S. Psychosocial interventions for reducing antipsychotic medication in care home residents. *Cochrane Database Syst. Rev.* **2012**, *12*, CD008634. [CrossRef] [PubMed]
29. Donegan, K.; Fox, N.; Black, N.; Livingston, G.; Banerjee, S.; Burns, A. Trends in diagnosis and treatment for people with dementia in the UK from 2005 to 2015: A longitudinal retrospective cohort study. *Lancet Public Health* **2017**, *2*, e149–e156. [CrossRef]
30. Deb, S.; Limbu, B.; Crawford, M.; Weaver, T. Short-Term PsychoEducation for Carers to Reduce over Medication of people with intellectual disabilities (SPECTROM): Study protocol. *Br. Med. J. Open* **2020**, *10*, e037912. [CrossRef] [PubMed]
31. Deb, S.; Limbu, B.; Unwin, G.; Woodcock, L.; Cooper, V.; Fullerton, M. Short-term Psycho-Education for Caregivers to Reduce over Medication of people with intellectual disabilities (SPECTROM): Development and field testing. *Int. J. Environ. Res. Public Health* **2021**, *18*, 13161. [CrossRef]
32. Breuer, E.; De Silva, M.; Lund, C. Theory of change for complex mental health interventions: 10 lessons from the programme for improving mental healthcare. *Glob. Ment. Health* **2018**, *5*, e24. [CrossRef]
33. Deb, S.; Hare, M.; Prior, L. Symptoms of dementia among adults with Down's syndrome: A qualitative study. *J. Intellect. Disabil. Res.* **2007**, *51*, 726–739. [CrossRef]
34. Morris, P.G.; Prior, L.; Deb, S.; Lewis, G.; Mayle, W.; Burrow, C.; Bryant, E. Patients' views on outcome following head injury: A qualitative study. *BMC Fam. Pract.* **2005**, *6*, 30. [CrossRef]
35. Deb, S.; Aimola, L.; Leeson, V.; Bodani, M.; Li, L.; Weaver, T.; Sharp, D.; Bassett, P.; Crawford, M. Risperidone versus placebo for aggression following traumatic brain injury: A feasibility randomised controlled trial. *BMJ Open* **2020**, *10*, e036300. [CrossRef]
36. Braun, V.; Clarke, V. Using Thematic Analysis in Psychology. *Qual. Res. Psychol.* **2006**, *3*, 77–101. [CrossRef]
37. *NVivo 12 Plus*; QSR international UK LTD: London, UK, 2020.
38. Limbu, B.; Unwin, G.; Deb, S. Comprehensive Assessment of Triggers for Behaviours of Concern Scale (CATS): Initial Development. *Int. J. Environ. Res. Public Health* **2021**, *18*, 10674. [CrossRef]
39. Deb, S.; Perera, B.; Krysta, K.; Ozer, M.; Bertelli, M.; Novell, R.; Wieland, J.; Sappok, T. The European guideline on the assessment and diagnosis of psychiatric disorders in adults with intellectual disabilities. *Eur. J. Psychiatry* **2022**, *36*, 11–25. [CrossRef]
40. McCarthy, J.; Blanco, R.A.; Gaus, V.L.; Razza, N.J.; Tomasulo, D.J. Trauma-and stressor-related disorders. In *Diagnostic Manual-Intellectual Disability: A textbook of Diagnosis of Mental Disorders in Persons with Intellectual Disability*, 2nd ed.; Fletcher, R., Barnhill, J., Cooper, S.-A., Eds.; NADD Press: Kingston, NY, USA, 2016; pp. 353–399.
41. Wieland, J.; Wardenaar, K.J.; Dautovic, E.; Zitman, F.G. Characteristics of post-traumatic stress disorder in patients with an intellectual disability. *Eur. Psychiatry* **2013**, *28*, 1.
42. Bradley, E.; Korossy, M. HELP with behaviours that challenge. *J. Dev. Disabil.* **2016**, *22*, 101–120.
43. Kinnear, D.; Morrison, J.; Allan, L.; Henderson, A.; Smiley, E.; Cooper, S.-A. Prevalence of physical conditions and multimorbidity in a cohort of adults with intellectual disabilities with and without Down syndrome: Cross-sectional study. *Br. Med. J. Open* **2018**, *8*, e018292. [CrossRef]
44. Deb, S.; Perera, B.; Bertelli, M.O. Attention Deficit Hyperactivity Disorder. In *Textbook of Psychiatry for Intellectual Disability and Autism Spectrum Disorder*; Bertelli, M.O., Deb, S., Munir, K., Hassiotis, A., Salvador-Carulla, L., Eds.; Springer Nature: Cham, Switzerland, 2022; pp. 457–482.
45. Bertelli, M.O.; Azeem, M.W.; Underwood, L.; Scattoni, M.L.; Persico, A.M.; Ricciardello, A.; Sappok, T.; Bergmann, T.; Keller, R.; Bianco, A.; et al. Autism Spectrum Disorder. In *Textbook of Psychiatry for Intellectual Disability and Autism Spectrum Disorder*; Bertelli, M.O., Deb, S., Munir, K., Hassiotis, A., Salvador-Carulla, L., Eds.; Springer Nature: Cham, Switzerland, 2022; pp. 369–455.
46. Deb, S.; Roy, M.; Limbu, B. Psychopharmacological treatments for psychopathology in people with intellectual disabilities and/or autism spectrum disorder. *Br. J. Psychiatry Adv.* **2022**, in press.
47. Gore, N.J.; Sapiets, S.J.; Denne, L.D.; Hastings, R.P.; Toogood, S.; MacDonald, A.; Baker, P.; Allen, D.; Apanasionok, M.M.; Austin, D.; et al. Positive Behavioural Support in the UK: A state of the nation report. *Int. J. Posit. Behav. Support* **2022**, *12* (Suppl. 1), 4–39.
48. Ratti, V.; Hassiotis, A.; Crabtree, J.; Deb, S.; Gallagher, P.; Unwin, G. The effectiveness of person-centred planning for people with intellectual disabilities: A systematic review. *Res. Dev. Disabil.* **2016**, *57*, 63–84. [CrossRef]

49. Hassiotis, A.; Poppe, M.; Strydom, A.; Vickerstaff, V.; Hall, I.S.; Crabtree, J.; Omar, R.Z.; King, M.; Hunter, R.; Biswas, A.; et al. Clinical outcomes of staff training in positive behaviour support to reduce challenging behaviour in adults with intellectual disability: Cluster randomised controlled trial. *Br. J. Psychiatry* **2018**, *212*, 161–168. [CrossRef]
50. Hall, S.; Deb, S. A Qualitative Study on the Knowledge and Views That People with Learning Disabilities and Their Carers Have of Psychotropic Medication Prescribed for Behaviour Problems. *Adv. Ment. Health Learn. Disabil.* **2008**, *2*, 29–37. [CrossRef]
51. Hassiotis, A.; Kimona, K.; Moncrieff, J.; Deb, S.; A Stakeholder Consultation about Future Research of Psychotropic Medication Use and Behaviour Support for Adults with Intellectual Disabilities Who Present with Behaviours That Challenge: Feasibility of Future Research. NOCLOR. 2016. Available online: https://www.ucl.ac.uk/psychiatry/sites/psychiatry/files/stakeholder-consultation-document.pdf (accessed on 15 July 2022).
52. Sheehan, R.; Kimona, K.; Giles, A.; Cooper, V.; Hassiotis, A. Findings from an online survey of family carer experience of the management of challenging behaviour in people with intellectual disabilities, with a focus on the use of psychotropic medication. *Br. J. Learn. Disabil.* **2018**, *46*, 82–91. [CrossRef]
53. Deb, S.; Limbu, B. Support staff liaising effectively with family caregivers: Findings from a co-design event and recommendation for a staff training resource. *Front. Psychiatry* **2022**. *under review*.
54. Unwin, G.L. A Longitudinal Observational Study of Aggressive Behaviour in Adults with Intellectual Disabilities. Ph.D. Thesis, University of Birmingham, Birmingham, UK, 2013. Available online: https://etheses.bham.ac.uk/id/eprint/4735/ (accessed on 18 December 2021).
55. Lalor, J.; Poulson, L. Psychotropic medications and adults with intellectual disabilities: Care staff perspectives. *Adv. Ment. Health Intellect. Disabil.* **2013**, *7*, 333–345. [CrossRef]

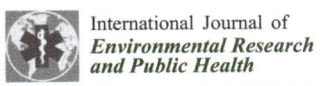

Article

Predictors of Change in Stepping Stones Triple Interventions: The Relationship between Parental Adjustment, Parenting Behaviors and Child Outcomes

Matthew Sanders [1], Nam-Phuong T. Hoang [1,*], Julie Hodges [1], Kate Sofronoff [1], Stewart Einfeld [2], Bruce Tonge [3], Kylie Gray [3,4] and The MHYPEDD Team

[1] Parenting and Family Support Centre, The University of Queensland, Brisbane, QLD 4072, Australia
[2] Brain and Mind Centre, University of Sydney, Camperdown, NSW 2006, Australia
[3] Centre for Developmental Psychiatry and Psychology, Monash University, Clayton, VIC 3800, Australia
[4] Centre for Educational Development, Appraisal, and Research, University of Warwick, Coventry CV4 7AL, UK
* Correspondence: a.phuong@uq.edu.au

Abstract: The current study explored the process of change in Stepping Stones Triple P (SSTP) using a community-based sample of 891 families of children with developmental disabilities (DD) who participated in an SSTP intervention at a community level. A preliminary analysis of outcome data indicated that SSTP intervention was effective in reducing parental adjustment difficulties, coercive parenting, and children's behavioral and emotional difficulties immediately after the intervention. The effects were maintained at 12-month follow-up. The results also indicated that change in parental adjustment over the course of intervention was significantly associated with a change in parenting behaviors. However, change in parenting behaviors but not change in parental adjustment, predicted children's behavioral and emotional problems following the intervention. The results suggest that positive parenting skills are the most salient ingredient driving the change in child behaviors in SSTP interventions.

Keywords: mechanism of change; developmental disability; evidence-based parenting; Triple P

1. Introduction

1.1. Relations between Parental Adjustment, Parenting Behaviors and Children's Outcomes in Families of Children with DD

Research into children with developmental disabilities (DD) has consistently pointed to the elevated risk of the development of behavioral and emotional problems among children of this group [1]. As reported in a recent meta-analysis, the rate of behavioural problems in children with DD is two to three times higher than in typically developing children [2–4]. Different factors can contribute to the development and exacerbation of behavioral and emotional issues within this population. Parental stress has consistently been identified as one of the most prominent contributors. Neece et al. [5] followed two groups of children (144 were typically developing children and 93 were diagnosed with a type of DD) from age three to nine years. Their cross-lagged panel analyses indicated that behavioral problems and parental stress covaried across time, but parental stress consistently arose as a predictor of child behavior problems while the effect of early child behavior problem on parental stress was much less consistent. This finding was supported by Lin et al. [6] study which examined the transactional relations between parenting stress and both internalizing and externalizing behavioral problems in 75 young children with ASD over 1.5 years. The findings also indicated that early parenting stress was significantly associated with later children externalizing problems.

While parental stress directly affects children's emotions and behavior [7], it also influences parenting which may in turn further exacerbate children's behavioral and emotional difficulties. When parents are distressed, they are less likely to be sensitive to their children's behaviors, they might also be more likely to engage in irritable transactions and poor disciplinary practices (inconsistency, coercion) that reinforce undesirable behaviors in children, thus making them more likely to occur again [8,9]. Totsika et al. [10] analyzed data from 555 families of children with DD and found that early parental distress (at nine months) significantly predicted child behavioral and emotional problems at both age seven and age 11 years. This relationship was mediated by adversarial parenting practices between ages 3 and 5 years. Day et al. [11] also surveyed 1392 families of children with a disability aged between 2 and 12 years and found that parental adjustment difficulties (depression, anxiety and stress) were among the strongest predictors of coercive parenting.

Due to the reciprocal transaction between parental stress, parenting behaviors and children's behaviors, it is not uncommon for parents of children with DD who exhibit elevated behavioral problems to also experience a high level of stress and use more coercive parenting. Interventions to reduce behavioral problems in children with DD thus commonly aim to address both parental stress and dysfunctional parenting behaviors [12].

1.2. Stepping Stones Triple P

A number of different parenting programs have been shown to be effective in managing behavioral problems in children with DD. Among those, Stepping Stones Triple P (SSTP) [13]—(a variant of the Triple P Positive Parenting Program) is one of the most extensively studied and widely used. Built on social learning theory, SSTP recognizes the reciprocal nature of parent–child interactions surrounding dysfunctional behaviors [13]. Therefore, the occurrence of child behavioral and emotional problems in children with DD is viewed as both a consequence and an antecedent of dysfunctional parenting and parental adjustment difficulties. In SSTP, the goals are to help parents learn to manage their children's behavior problems without using coercion escalation or harsh discipline and to adopt better strategies to regulate their emotion [13].

Throughout the SSPT program, parents are encouraged to choose their own goals, develop plans and execute their plans which includes the capacity to plan and anticipate, regulate their emotions, solve problems, and collaborate with significant others to provide care for their children. This self-regulatory approach is expected to help reduce parents' use of coercive and punitive disciplining and promote parents' capacity to regulate their emotions and behavior throughout intervention [13]. In addition to the core Triple P strategies, the program incorporates a number of additional disability-related components to reflect the additional challenges faced by parents of children with disabilities as well as a focus on community living and family support movements (such as Being part of the community). These include: (1) Identifying additional factors that are more likely to contribute to the development of behavior problems in persons with disabilities (e.g., the accidental reward for stopping disliked activities). (2) Incorporating other behavior change strategies from the disability literature (such as setting up an activity schedule). (3) Developing additional protocols to deal with self-injurious behavior, repetitive behaviors, and pica that are more prevalent among children with disabilities. (4) Modifying wording and examples in parenting materials to make them more acceptable and sensitive to parents of children with disabilities [13].

Meta-analyses of randomized controlled trials of SSTP have consistently shown that SSTP effectively reduces harsh parenting, child behavioral and emotional problems, and parental distress. For example, Tellegen and Sanders [14] analyzed both controlled and uncontrolled design studies. They found that SSTP had moderate to large effects in reducing coercive parenting behaviors, moderate effects in reducing child behavioral and emotional problems, and moderate effects in reducing parental adjustment problems. In a recent systematic review and meta-analysis of all SSTP levels, Ruane and Carr [15] found that SSTP has small to medium effects on parental adjustment and co-parenting. For parenting behaviors and child behaviors, the effect sizes were medium to large. The growing literature supports the efficacy of SSTP in reducing harsh parenting, child behavioral and emotional problems, and parental adjustment difficulties. Yet, little is known about the process of change explaining the effects of SSTP for families of children with DD. It is not yet understood if a change in parental adjustment over the course of the intervention assists change in parenting behaviors and vice versa. It is also yet to know if changes in parental adjustment or changes in parenting behaviors contribute to the change in children's behaviors and emotional outcomes as proposed by the literature.

1.3. Current Study

The present study examined the process of change in SSTP interventions, explicitly emphasizing the bidirectional association between change in parental adjustment and change in coercive parenting over the course of the SSTP intervention and their association with children's subsequent outcomes. Specifically, we examined (1) how parents' experience of emotional difficulties (parental adjustment) and use of coercive parenting affect one another before, during, and after the intervention and (2) how the change in parental adjustment and use of coercive parenting during the intervention predict subsequently reported a decrease in child behavioral and emotional problems. We hypothesized that: (1) the decrease in parental adjustment difficulties over the course of intervention will be associated with the simultaneous decrease in coercive parenting behaviors and (2) the decrease in parental adjustment difficulties and coercive parenting from pre- to post-intervention will predict a subsequent decrease in child behavioral and emotional problems at follow-up.

2. Materials & Methods

Participants

Participants in this study were 891 parents and caregivers living in the Australian states of Victoria and Queensland and enrolled in the Mental Health of Young People with Developmental Disabilities (MHYPeDD) research study. These were caregivers of a child aged between 2 and 12 years who were recruited via a variety of pathways, e.g., posters, brochures, and newsletters prepared by the project team and disseminated by their current service provider, a project-specific Facebook page, direct contact from the project team or via their child's school. Interested parents then provided evidence of a of diagnosis of DD provided by a suitable professional such as a psychiatrist, psychologist, speech pathologist, neurologist or pediatrician. Although most parents responded to questionnaires online, there was also the option of telephone interviews or hard copies if needed. Most participants (87.65%) were mothers (biological, stepmother, adoptive mother) of at least one child with DD. The majority of target children were male (77.10%) aged between 2 and 12 years old ($M = 4.98$, $SD = 2.65$). At the time of enrolment, 76.77% parents reported their child also had a diagnosis of ASD (Table 1).

Table 1. Demographic characteristics.

Characteristic	Frequency	%
Child gender		
Male	687	77.10
Female	204	22.90
Child age (*Mean* and *SD*)	4.98 (2.65)	
Diagnosis with or without ASD		
With ASD	684	76.77
Without ASD	207	23.23
Caregivers' relationship to the child		
Mother	781	87.65
Father	83	9.32
Grandparents or other relatives	27	3.03

Table 1. Cont.

Characteristic	Frequency	%
Financial hardship		
Financial hardship	115	12.91
No financial hardship	717	80.47
Level of SSTP Intervention		
Level 2	248	27.83
Level 3	57	6.40
Level 4	381	42.76

Note: The accumulate percentage might not equal to 100% due to missing data.

3. Procedure

The study received ethical clearance from the Behavioral and Social Sciences Ethical Review Committee at the University of Queensland. Professionals involved in the MHYPeDD project received training on at least one SSTP program, and they participated in a two-year implementation period to deliver interventions to families of children with DD. Parents were referred by their current service providers, directly via the SSTP project team (including the Facebook page) or their child's school to attend either Primary Care SSTP (3–4 brief individual sessions), SSTP seminars (120-min large-group presentations), Group SSTP (5 group sessions and follow-up telephone calls), Standard SSTP (10 individually delivered sessions); Self-directed Triple P or Triple P Online (self-administered). Parents completed a short package of measures before the intervention, after the intervention and then at six months following their attendance.

To minimize site differences, all practitioners received identical competency- and accreditation-based training and all interventions were delivered with the same practitioners and parent resources. This is a widely used method of Triple P dissemination, ensuring fidelity to the program. Studies of Triple P regular service delivery have shown that there are few differences between training outcomes for practitioners from different disciplines, countries, and levels of programs [16,17].

4. Measures

4.1. Demographics

Demographic variables used for analysis in the present study included the child's age and gender, type of DD (with or without ASD), caregivers' relationship to the child, financial hardship and level of intervention. Responses were mainly based on the primary carer. Financial hardship was assessed using the question: "*Suppose you only had one week to raise $2000 for an emergency. Which of the following best describes how hard it would be for you to get that money?*", with responses ranging from 1 (*I could easily raise the money*) to 4 (*I don't think I could raise the money*). This item has been demonstrated to be a good index of financial hardship [18].

4.2. Parental Adjustment

The parent adjustment subscale of the Parent and Family Adjustment Scale—developmental disability version (PAFAS-DD) was used to measure parental adjustment difficulties. The PAFAS-DD has 30 items measuring parenting and family adjustment [19] on a scale from 0 (None at all) to 3 (Very much/most of the time) with higher scores indicating a higher level of dysfunction within families. The Parental Adjustment subscale has five items that assess parents' emotional adjustment at the time of the survey. Examples of questions include: "*I feel satisfied with my life*" or "*I cope with the demands of being a parent*". PAFAS-DD Parental Adjustment subscale has been shown to be a reliable measure to assess parental adjustment difficulties with internal consistency found in previous studies ranging from $\alpha = 0.81$; [11] to $\alpha = 0.82$ [19]. PAFAS-DD has also been shown to have satisfactory construct and convergent validity [19].

4.3. Coercive Parenting

The Coercive Parenting subscale of the PAFAS-DD was used to measure participants' levels of coercive parenting. The Coercive Parenting subscale is comprised of five items that describe parenting behaviors such as: "*I shout or get angry at my child when they misbehave*" or "*I get annoyed with my child*". Parents indicated how true the statement is to their parenting practice on a scale from 0 (None at all) to 3 (Very much/most of the time). A higher score indicates more use of coercive parenting. This scale has been demonstrated to be a valid and reliable measure of coercive parenting in families of children with DD. Composite internal consistency found for this subscale was 0.75, [19] and internal consistency was $\alpha = 0.73$ [11].

4.4. Child Behavioral and Emotional Problems

Parents reported child behavioral and emotional problems using the Child Adjustment and Parenting Efficacy Scale—Developmental Disability (CAPES-DD) [20]. CAPES-DD has 30 items that describe different behavioral and emotional problems in children. Examples of items are: '*breaks or destroys things*' (Behavioral problems) and '*seems fearful and scared*' (Emotional problems). Parents indicate how accurately the problems describe their children by rating on a scale from 0 ('*Not true of my child at all*') to 3 ('*True of my child very much, or most of the time*'). The CAPES-DD yields three scores. The Behavioral Problems score, Emotional Problems Score and Total Problems score. CAPES-DD has consistently been found to have good internal consistency with Cronbach's alpha ranging between ($\alpha = [0.80–0.90]$) for both the subscales and the total score [11,21]. CAPES-DD total problems scale also correlates strongly with the total behavior problems scale of the Developmental Behavior Checklist for both Primary Carer and Under-4 versions [21].

4.5. Analytic Strategies

Repeated measures ANOVA was adopted to calculate the change of scores across three time points. The relationship between parental adjustment and coercive parenting was explored using latent growth modelling (LGM) in which intercepts represent baseline score and slopes represent latent change over time. LGM allows researchers to explore the growth of individual constructs while simultaneously examining the relationship between several constructs. Bi-directional relationships were estimated with the error covariances, and the unidirectional relationships were estimated with path coefficients. A comparative fit index (*CFI*) value ≥ 0.95 and the root means square error approximation (*RMSEA*) value ≤ 0.08 indicates a good fit.

To estimate the contribution of change in parental adjustment and change in coercive parenting to subsequent child behavioral and emotional problems, hierarchical multiple regression was conducted. Demographic variables of families and child behavioral/emotional problems at baseline were controlled at Step 1 and Step 2 before changes in parental adjustment and coercive parenting (Time 1–Time 2) were entered at Step 3 to predict Time 3 child's emotional and behavioral problems. The analyses were undertaken using AMOS and R software for statistic computing.

5. Results

5.1. Missing Data Analysis

The analysis of missing data indicated there was 18.7% missingness in total. Little's MCAR test was not significant ($X^2 = 175,818.70$, $df = 190,183$, $p > 0.05$). The maximum likelihood estimation method was used to handle missing data.

5.2. Change in Parental Adjustment, Parenting Behaviors, and Child Behaviors

Table 2 shows the mean score of PAFAS- Adjustment, PAFAS—Coercive, CAPES-DD-Behaviors and CAPES-DD Emotion at Time 1, Time 2, and Time 3. The PAFAS- Adjustment score of 5.75 ($SD = 3.00$) pre-intervention, decreased significantly ($F(1,890) = 80.37$, $p < 0.05$)

to 5.11 (SD = 2.61) post-intervention, and was maintained at the 12-month follow-up period ending at 5.02 (SD = 2.56). A significant reduction in the Coercive parenting score was also observed from Time 1 to Time 2. At Time 1, PAFAS- Coercive score was $M = 9.66$ ($SD = 2.61$) which reduced significantly to $M = 8.73$ ($SD = 2.27$) at Time 2 ($F(1,890) = 230.31, p < 0.05$). This effect was maintained at Time 3 at $M = 8.85$, $SD = 2.09$ ($F(1,890) = 157.20, p < 0.05$).

Table 2. Mean, SD of Variables.

	Time 1 M (SD)	Time 2 M (SD)	Time 3 M (SD)	Main Effect of Time	
				Time 1–Time 2	Time 1–Time 3
Parental adjustment	5.75 (3.00)	5.11 (2.61)	5.02 (2.56)	$F(1,890) = 80.37, p < 0.05$	$F(1,890) = 97.72, p < 0.05$
Coercive parenting	9.66 (2.61)	8.73 (2.27)	8.85 (2.09)	$F(1,890) = 230.31, p < 0.05$	$F(1,890) = 157.20, p < 0.05$
Child Behavior	23.04 (6.65)	21.61 (6.15)	21.22 (5.78)	$F(1,890) = 116.274\ p < 0.05$	$F(1,890) = 153.74, p < 0.05$
Child Emotion	5.04 (1.80)	4.73 (1.57)	4.84 (1.50)	$F(1,890) = 42.95, p < 0.05$	$F(1,890) = 14.75, p < 0.05$

To examine whether the change scores are different across different levels of intervention, analysis was conducted controlling for the level of intervention. Results showed no interaction effect between time and level of intervention for any of the variables either short-term or long-term.

Child behavior problems estimated with the CAPES-DD Behavior started at Time 1 at $M = 23.04$ ($SD = 6.65$) then significantly reduced to $M = 21.61$ ($SD = 6.15$) at Time 2 ($F(1,890) = 116.27, p < 0.05$). The comparison between Time 3 and Time 1 was also significant ($F(1,890) = 153.74, p < 0.05$) indicating that the effect was maintained at Time 3.

Child emotional problems measured by CAPES-DD Emotion was 5.04 ($SD = 1.80$) at Time 1 and reduced significantly to $M = 4.73$ ($SD = 1.57$) ($F(1,890) = 42.95, p < 0.05$). This change was maintained at Time 3 ($F(1,890) = 14.75, p < 0.05$).

5.3. The Association between Change in Parental Adjustment and Change in Coercive Parenting

The LGM model to test the correlation of changes between parental adjustment and coercive parenting is presented in Figure 1 and Table 3. The model fits the data well ($X^2 = 29.508$, $df = 7$, $p < 0.05$; $CFI = 0.993$, $RSMEA = 0.060$). At Time 1, parental adjustment was significantly and positively associated with coercive parenting (*covariance coefficient* = 0.40, $p < 0.05$), indicating that those who experienced more adjustment difficulties at Time 1 were more likely to use coercive parenting strategies and vice versa. The examination of the change scores showed that changes in parental adjustment throughout intervention were significantly and positively associated with the change in coercive parenting (*covariance coefficient* = 0.16, $p < 0.05$). This finding suggests that a reduction in parental adjustment difficulties was associated with a reduction in coercive parenting.

Table 3. Estimate, Standard error of Coefficient and *p*-values of slopes and intercepts association.

	Estimate	Standard Error	*p*-Value
Parental Adjustment Intercept -> Coercive Parenting Slope	−0.210	0.22	<001
Coercive Parenting Intercept -> Parental Adjustment Slope	−0.299	0.31	<0.001
Parental Adjustment Intercept <-> Coercive Parenting Intercept	0.396	0.088	<0.05
Parental Adjustment Slope <-> Coercive Parenting Slope	0.161	0.276	<0.001

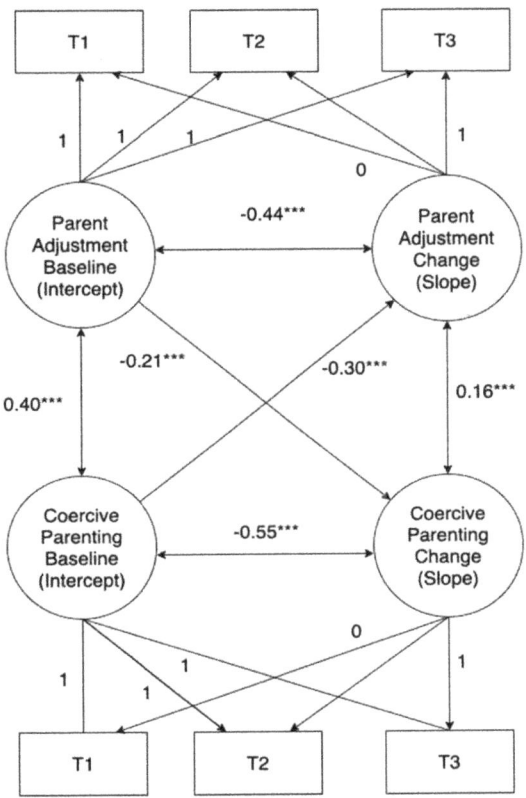

Figure 1. Latent growth Model of Intervention Outcomes. Note: *** $p < 0.001$.

5.4. The Association between Changes in Parental Adjustment and Coercive Parenting to Change in Child Behavioral and Emotional Problems

The association between variables are presented in Table 4.

Table 4. Cross-correlation between variables.

		(1)	(2)	(3)	(4)	(5)	(6)	(7)
1	T1 Child Behavior	1						
2	T3 Child Behavior	0.77 **						
3	T1 Child Emotion	0.559 **	0.431 **					
4	T3 Child Emotion	0.440 **	0.581 **	0.634 **				
5	T1 Coercive Parenting	0.328 **	0.182 **	0.172 **	0.094 **			
6	T2 Coercive Parenting	0.286 **	0.234 **	0.156 **	0.177 **	0.731 **		
7	T1 Parental Adjustment	0.321 **	0.298 **	0.261 **	0.257 **	0.346 **	0.306 **	
8	T2 Parental Adjustment	0.292 **	0.306 **	0.238**	0.305 **	0.278 **	0.390 **	0.760 **

Note: ** $p < 0.01$.

Prior to conducting the regression analysis, all assumptions for multiple regression including linearity, multivariate normality, multicollinearity, and homoscedasticity were conducted. Data met the assumptions required for multiple regression.

After accounting for demographics and child behavioral/emotional problems at Time 1, the change in coercive parenting throughout Intervention (Time 1–Time 2) significantly predicts the behavioral problems ($\beta = 0.10$, $p < 0.01$) and child's emotional problems ($\beta = 0.11$, $p < 0.01$) at Time 3. However, changes in parental adjustment did not significantly predict either child emotional or behavioral problems at Time 3 (Table 5).

Table 5. Hierarchical multiple regression to predict child Behavior and Emotion problems at Time 3.

	Time 3 Behavior Problems			Time 3 Emotion Problems		
	B	SE	β	B	SE	β
Step 3						
Child gender	0.06	0.34	0.00	0.07	0.11	0.02
Child age	−0.24	0.05	−0.11 ***	−0.04	0.02	−0.08 *
With or without ASD	0.85	0.35	0.06 **	0.42	0.11	0.12 ***
Level of intervention	0.10	0.15	0.02	−0.02	0.05	−0.01
Parent education	0.19	0.08	0.06 *	0.00	0.03	0.01
Marital status	0.16	0.32	0.01	0.11	0.10	0.03
Financial hardship	0.60	0.38	0.04	0.33	0.12	0.09 *
Time 1 Behavior/Emotion	0.65	0.02	0.75 ***	0.45	0.03	0.57 ***
T1–T2 Change in Parental Adjustment	−0.03	0.07	−0.01	0.00	0.02	0.00
T1–T2 Change in Coercive Parenting	0.32	0.08	0.10 ***	0.09	0.03	0.11 ***
R^2			0.61 ***			0.38 ***

* $p < 0.05$; ** $p < 0.01$; *** $p < 0.001$. ASD: Autism Spectrum Disorder.

6. Discussion

This study sought to extend the literature by examining how changes in parental adjustment and parenting skills at key timepoints throughout SSTP intervention affect each other and subsequently influence children's outcomes. To our knowledge, this is the first mechanism of change analysis of the SSTP intervention. Results of this study suggested two main findings: First, the changes in parental adjustment over the course of intervention were associated with the changes in coercive parenting such that a decrease in parental emotional adjustment was correlated with a decrease in coercive strategies used. These change processes appear to co-occur such that when there is a reduction in parental emotional adjustment, there is also a reduction in coercive parenting. Second, the decrease in coercive parenting but not parental emotional adjustment achieved via intervention significantly contributed to children's behavioral and emotional performance at follow-up.

When examining the relationship between baseline performance and the trajectory of changes, we found that parents who used more coercive parenting and reported more emotional difficulties at baseline demonstrated greater changes over the course of intervention. Such findings were consistent with and supported previous studies of a behavioral parenting intervention, suggesting that families with more problems at baseline respond better to intervention [22,23]. Families with more problems at baseline may have greater scope for growth thus demonstrating better progress than families with fewer initial concerns of which little improvement was needed.

Research conducted on families of children with DD in the past two decades has highlighted that an effective intervention for children with DD needs to address parental distress in order to bring about change in children. This argument is based on evidence to the link between parental adjustment difficulties and children's outcomes [8,12]. In this study, we hypothesized that as parent's emotional difficulties decrease, children's behavioral and emotional problems will mutually deescalate. In contrast to our hypothesis, we found that change in parental adjustment throughout intervention was significantly associated with the change in coercive parenting, but its increase or decrease over the course of intervention did not contribute directly to the increase or decrease of subsequent child behavioral and emotional problems.

To explain this finding, we need to understand the SSTP program's model of change. SSTPs and Triple P programs are built on the foundation of self-regulation principles.

According to Sanders [24], self-regulation refers to the ability to change one's own behavior and become an independent problem-solver by gaining the skills necessary to achieve one's personal goals. In social cognitive theory, self-regulation is viewed as an essential process through which individuals can guide their behavior through changing circumstances over time. It involves modulating thought, affect, behavior, or attention with specific mechanisms and supportive meta-skills. As a result, SSTP training encourages parents to identify their goals, plan and self-select the most appropriate strategies to manage their emotions, and conduct self-evaluations addressing changes if needed [25]. The parents are thus able to attribute changes to their own behavior and effort rather than the child's difficulties. Furthermore, self-evaluation might help parents become more aware of their own behavior and better able to assess situations before responding to them. By self-regulating, parents may have been able to distinguish their own emotions from their children's difficulties and avoid passing on emotional disturbances to their children [26].

The findings of this study have implications for the development of parenting programs that support families of children with developmental disabilities; suggesting that parenting skills are key to influencing children's behavior. Meanwhile, it is also important to highlight that although parental adjustment was not directly correlated with change in children's behaviors, change in parental adjustment throughout the intervention, actually fostering healthy functioning parenting. As parents experience less emotional distress, they might be able to focus on building a positive, nurturing relationship with their children, resulting in a decrease in child behavioral and emotional problems

The finding of a non-significant relationship between change in parental adjustment and subsequent child outcomes nevertheless needs to be interpreted with care. It is possible too that some aspects of parental adjustment, such as the presence of parental mental health problems (anxiety and depression) might take longer to recover and change in response to reductions in problematic child behavior. There might also be a floor effect for problems, as most parents in our sample did not experience elevated adjustment difficulties hence a relatively small effect size was observed. Future studies with multiple data collection points and with clinically elevated samples might be useful to understand the cumulative and interactionally dependent between parental adjustment and child behavior change over time.

Finally, the mechanism for testing relationships between variables was restricted to three-time point data and was based on single parent reports which might require further validation. As Rutter [27] has suggested, to answer causal questions about development, there is a need for integrating longitudinal data in experimental intervention. More data points would allow a more accurate trajectory of change across individuals using LGM. Additional assessment time points would also allow a more definitive conclusion of the causal relationships which would enhance our understanding of the mechanisms by which changes in parent-related variables produce changes in child outcomes.

This study suggests that positive parenting skills are the most salient intervention ingredient driving the change in child behaviors, and the continued focus on building parenting capacities and parenting skills is justified. Although conducting a moderator analysis was not the primary focus of this study, our findings of baseline effect on family changes over the course of intervention are valuable in pointing to subgroups that might benefit the most from SSTP intervention. Our regression model findings also indicate several potential moderators (baseline status of families, DD with or without ASD, parental education, and family financial hardship) that can impact families' capacity to change through intervention. Future studies with adequate sample sizes and more advanced analytic techniques could conduct moderator-mediator analysis to explore how mechanisms of change might vary by moderator groups.

7. Conclusions

Using a community-based sample of SSTP roll-out, this study emphasizes the significant role of parenting behaviors in improving children's outcomes and suggests that developing warm, positive relationships between parents and their children should continue to be a priority in evidence-based parenting programmes for parents of children with DD. Additionally, this study also highlights the importance of promoting parental emotional well-being throughout intervention in order to mitigate the tendency to engage in coercive or negative parenting practices that are detrimental to children's development.

Author Contributions: Conceptualization, M.S. and N.-P.T.H.; Methodology, N.-P.T.H.; Software, N.-P.T.H.; Validation, N.-P.T.H. Formal Analysis N.-P.T.H.; Investigation, M.S. and N.-P.T.H.; Resources M.S. and J.H.; Data Curation M.S. and N.-P.T.H.; Writing—Original Draft Preparation, N.-P.T.H. and M.S.; Writing—Review and Editing M.S., J.H., K.S., S.E., B.T. and K.G.; Visualization, N.-P.T.H.; Supervision, M.S.; Project Administration, J.H., K.S. and The MHYPEDD team; Funding Acquisition, M.S., J.H., K.S., S.E., B.T. and K.G. All authors have read and agreed to the published version of the manuscript.

Funding: This study was supported by a grant from the Australian Government's National Health and Medical Research Council (NHMRC programme grant APP1016919) for the Mental Health of Young People with Developmental Disabilities (MHYPeDD) project.

Institutional Review Board Statement: The study was conducted according to the guidelines of the Declaration of Helsinki, and approved by the Institutional Review Board (or Ethics Committee) of The University of Queensland (protocol code 2012001065, Date of approval: 20 September 2012).

Informed Consent Statement: Informed consent was obtained from all subjects involved in the study.

Data Availability Statement: The data presented in this study are available on request from the corresponding author. The data are not publicly available due to ethics commitment of data security.

Conflicts of Interest: The Parenting and Family Support Centre is partly funded by royalties stemming from published resources of the Triple P—Positive Parenting Program, which is developed and owned by The University of Queensland (UQ). Royalties are also distributed to the Faculty of Health and Behavioral Sciences at UQ and contributory authors of published Triple P resources. Triple P International (TPI) Pty Ltd. is a private company licensed by Uniquest Pty Ltd. on behalf of UQ, to publish and disseminate Triple P worldwide. The authors of this report have no share or ownership of TPI. Authors Sanders, Hoang and Hodges receive or may in future receive royalties and/or consultancy fees from TPI. TPI had no involvement in the study design, collection, analysis or interpretation of data, or writing of this report. Authors Sanders, Hoang and Hodges are employed by UQ; author Sofronoff holds an honourary appointment with UQ. Other authors have no conflict to declare.

References

1. Baker, E.; Stavropoulos, K.K.; Baker, B.L.; Blacher, J. Daily Living Skills in Adolescents with Autism Spectrum Disorder: Implications for Intervention and Independence. *Res. Autism Spectr. Disord.* **2021**, *83*, 101761. [CrossRef] [PubMed]
2. Buckley, N.; Glasson, E.J.; Chen, W.; Epstein, A.; Leonard, H.; Skoss, R.; Jacoby, P.; Blackmore, A.M.; Srinivasjois, R.; Bourke, J.; et al. Prevalence Estimates of Mental Health Problems in Children and Adolescents with Intellectual Disability: A Systematic Review and Meta-Analysis. *Aust. N. Z. J. Psychiatry* **2020**, *54*, 970–984. [CrossRef] [PubMed]
3. Baker, B.L.; Blacher, J. Disruptive Behavior Disorders in Adolescents with Asd: Comparisons to Youth with Intellectual Disability or Typical Cognitive Development. *J. Ment. Health Res. Intellect. Disabil.* **2015**, *8*, 98–116. [CrossRef]
4. Dekker, M.C.; Koot, H.M.; Ende JV, D.; Verhulst, F.C. Emotional and Behavioral Problems in Children and Adolescents with and without Intellectual Disability. *J. Child Psychol. Psychiatry* **2002**, *43*, 1087–1098. [CrossRef]
5. Neece, C.L.; Green, S.A.; Baker, B.L. Parenting Stress and Child Behavior Problems: A Transactional Relationship across Time. *Am. J. Intellect. Dev. Disabil.* **2012**, *117*, 48–66. [CrossRef]
6. Lin, Y.-N.; Iao, L.-S.; Lee, Y.-H.; Wu, C.-C. Parenting Stress and Child Behavior Problems in Young Children with Autism Spectrum Disorder: Transactional Relations across Time. *J. Autism Dev. Disord.* **2021**, *51*, 2381–2391. [CrossRef]
7. Ben-Sasson, A.; Carter, A.S. The Application of the First Year Inventory for Asd Screening in Israel. *J. Autism Dev. Disord.* **2012**, *42*, 1906–1916. [CrossRef]
8. Hastings, R.P.; Beck, A. Practitioner Review: Stress Intervention for Parents of Children with Intellectual Disabilities. *J. Child Psychol. Psychiatry Allied Discip.* **2004**, *45*, 1338–1349. [CrossRef]
9. Lunkenheimer, E.; Lichtwarck-Aschoff, A.; Hollenstein, T.; Kemp, C.J.; Granic, I. Breaking Down the Coercive Cycle: How Parent and Child Risk Factors Influence Real-Time Variability in Parental Responses to Child Misbehavior. *Parenting* **2016**, *16*, 237–256. [CrossRef]

10. Totsika, V.; Hastings, R.P.; Emerson, E.; Hatton, C. Early Years Parenting Mediates Early Adversity Effects on Problem Behaviors in Intellectual Disability. *Child Dev.* **2020**, *91*, e649–e664. [CrossRef]
11. Day, J.J.; Hodges, J.; Mazzucchelli, T.G.; Sofronoff, K.; Sanders, M.R.; Einfeld, S.; Tonge, B.; Gray, K.M.; MHYPeDD Project Team. Coercive Parenting: Modifiable and Nonmodifiable Risk Factors in Parents of Children with Developmental Disabilities. *J. Intellect. Disabil. Res.* **2021**, *65*, 306–319. [CrossRef] [PubMed]
12. Neece, C.L.; Chan, N. The Stress of Parenting Children with Developmental Disabilities. In *Parental Stress and Early Child Development*; Springer: Berlin/Heidelberg, Germany, 2017; pp. 107–124.
13. Sanders, M.R.; Mazzucchelli, T.G.; Studman, L.J. Stepping Stones Triple P: The Theoretical Basis and Development of an Evidence-Based Positive Parenting Program for Families with a Child Who Has a Disability. *J. Intellect. Dev. Disabil.* **2004**, *29*, 265–283. [CrossRef]
14. Tellegen, C.L.; Sanders, M.R. Stepping Stones Triple P-Positive Parenting Program for Children with Disability: A Systematic Review and Meta-Analysis. *Res. Dev. Disabil.* **2013**, *34*, 1556–1571. [CrossRef] [PubMed]
15. Ruane, A.; Carr, A. Systematic Review and Meta-Analysis of Stepping Stones Triple P for Parents of Children with Disabilities. *Fam. Process* **2019**, *58*, 232–246. [CrossRef] [PubMed]
16. Sethi, S.; Kerns, S.E.U.; Sanders, M.R.; Ralph, A. The International Dissemination of Evidence-Based Parenting Interventions: Impact on Practitioner Content and Process Self-Efficacy. *Int. J. Ment. Health Promot.* **2014**, *16*, 126–137. [CrossRef]
17. Morawska, A.; Sanders, M.; Goadby, E.; Headley, C.; Hodge, L.; McAuliffe, C.; Pope, S.; Anderson, E. Is the Triple P-Positive Parenting Program Acceptable to Parents from Culturally Diverse Backgrounds? *J. Child Fam. Stud.* **2011**, *20*, 614–622. [CrossRef]
18. Emerson, E. Mothers of Children and Adolescents with Intellectual Disability: Social and Economic Situation, Mental Health Status, and the Self-Assessed Social and Psychological Impact of the Child's Difficulties. *J. Intellect. Disabil. Res.* **2003**, *47*, 385–399. [CrossRef]
19. Mazzucchelli, T.G.; Hodges, J.; Kane, R.T.; Sofronoff, K.; Sanders, M.R.; Einfeld, S.; Tonge, B.; Gray, K.M.; MHYPEDD Project Team. Parenting and Family Adjustment Scales (Pafas): Validation of a Brief Parent-Report Measure for Use with Families Who Have a Child with a Developmental Disability. *Res. Dev. Disabil.* **2018**, *72*, 140–151. [CrossRef]
20. Mazzucchelli, T.G.; Sanders, M.R.; Morawska, A. *Child Adjustment and Parent Efficacy Scale-Developmental Disability (Capes-Dd)*; Parenting and Family Support Centre, University of Queensland: Brisbane, Australia, 2011.
21. Emser, T.S.; Mazzucchelli, T.G.; Christiansen, H.; Sanders, M.R. Child Adjustment and Parent Efficacy Scale-Developmental Disability (Capes-Dd): First Psychometric Evaluation of a New Child and Parenting Assessment Tool for Children with a Developmental Disability. *Res. Dev. Disabil.* **2016**, *53*, 158–177. [CrossRef]
22. Gardner, F.; Hutchings, J.; Bywater, T.; Whitaker, C. Who Benefits and How Does It Work? Moderators and Mediators of Outcome in an Effectiveness Trial of a Parenting Intervention. *J. Clin. Child Adolesc. Psychol.* **2010**, *39*, 568–580. [CrossRef]
23. Sanders, M.R.; Kirby, J.N.; Tellegen, C.L.; Day, J.J. The Triple P-Positive Parenting Program: A Systematic Review and Meta-Analysis of a Multi-Level System of Parenting Support. *Clin. Psychol. Rev.* **2014**, *34*, 337–357. [CrossRef] [PubMed]
24. Sanders, M.R. Triple P-Positive Parenting Program as a Public Health Approach to Strengthening Parenting. *J. Fam. Psychol.* **2008**, *22*, 506. [CrossRef] [PubMed]
25. Sanders, M.R.; Mazzucchelli, T.G. The Promotion of Self-Regulation through Parenting Interventions. *Clin. Child Fam. Psychol. Rev.* **2013**, *16*, 1–17. [CrossRef] [PubMed]
26. Koole, S.L.; Rothermund, K. "I Feel Better but I Don't Know Why": The Psychology of Implicit Emotion Regulation. *Cogn. Emot.* **2011**, *25*, 389–399. [CrossRef] [PubMed]
27. Rutter, M. Aetiology of Autism: Findings and Questions. *J. Intellect. Disabil. Res.* **2005**, *49*, 231–238. [CrossRef] [PubMed]

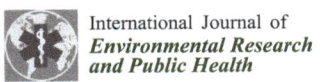

Article

The Global Deterioration Scale for Down Syndrome Population (GDS-DS): A Rating Scale to Assess the Progression of Alzheimer's Disease

Emili Rodríguez-Hidalgo [1,2], Javier García-Alba [3], Ramon Novell [1,2] and Susanna Esteba-Castillo [1,2,*]

1. Specialized Service in Mental Health and Intellectual Disability, Institute of Health Assistance (IAS), Parc Hospitalari Martí i Julià, 17190 Girona, Spain
2. Neurodevelopmental Group [Girona Biomedical Research Institute]-IDIBGI, Institute of Health Assistance (IAS), Parc Hospitalari Martí i Julià, 17190 Girona, Spain
3. Research and Psychology in Education Department, Complutense University of Madrid, 28040 Madrid, Spain
* Correspondence: susanna.esteba@ias.cat; Tel.: +34-972-18-26-00

Abstract: The aim of this study is to adapt and validate the global deterioration scale (GDS) for the systematic tracking of Alzheimer's disease (AD) progression in a population with Down syndrome (DS). A retrospective dual-center cohort study was conducted with 83 participants with DS (46.65 ± 5.08 years) who formed the primary diagnosis (PD) group: cognitive stability (n = 48), mild cognitive impairment (n = 24), and Alzheimer's disease (n = 11). The proposed scale for adults with DS (GDS-DS) comprises six stages, from cognitive and/or behavioral stability to advanced AD. Two neuropsychologists placed the participants of the PD group in each stage of the GDS-DS according to cognitive, behavioral and daily living skills data. Inter-rater reliability in staging with the GDS-DS was excellent (ICC = 0.86; CI: 0.80–0.93), and the agreement with the diagnosis categories of the PD group ranged from substantial to excellent with κ values of 0.82 (95% CI: 0.73–0.92) and 0.85 (95% CI: 0.72, 0.99). Performance with regard to the CAMCOG-DS total score and orientation subtest of the Barcelona test for intellectual disability showed a slight progressive decline across all the GDS-DS stages. The GDS-DS scale is a sensitive tool for staging the progression of AD in the DS population, with special relevance in daily clinical practice.

Keywords: global deterioration scale; rating scale; cognitive decline; cognitive testing; Alzheimer's disease; dementia; down syndrome; intellectual disability

1. Introduction

Life expectancy in people with Down syndrome (DS) has increased considerably, to up to sixty years on average [1], evidencing an accelerated aging phenotype [2]. The risk of developing Alzheimer's disease in people with DS (AD-DS) is greatly elevated due to the gene overexpression produced by the chromosome 21 trisomy, in which amyloid precursor protein and other gene modulations involve an accumulation of extracellular amyloid beta and neurofibrillary tangles [3,4]. AD neuropathology is present in more than 60% of people with DS by the age of 40 to 50 years [5]. Therefore, people with DS are considered at absolute risk of developing AD [6] and become a genetic paradigm for translational research with regard to the general population [7]. Despite these conceptual advances, AD-DS is usually diagnosed around the age of 50 years [8,9], later than expected [10], and these individuals are usually excluded from the clinical trials of typically developing individuals with AD [11].

Some major stages of the natural course of AD-DS have been suggested. Diagnostic categories in some studies are as follows: asymptomatic, cognitively stable, preclinical, prodromal AD, AD dementia, and uncertain [12–14]. Recently, under the biological definition and diagnosis relying on biomarkers, five stages have been proposed for AD-DS [15]:

cognitively stable (CS), preclinical AD, mild cognitive impairment (MCI), prodromal AD and dementia. Bearing these data in mind, it seems self-evident that there is a lack of consensus on the proposed stages to capture the entire clinical continuum of AD-DS which, on the contrary, are based primarily on biological criteria. Furthermore, recent studies in the general population suggest different initial stages on the dementia continuum. In this sense, a subjective cognitive decline (SCD) stage has been proposed as a risk condition announcing possible dementia [16,17], but it must be supported by objective cognitive impairment to be considered part of the AD continuum [18]. Additionally, mild behavioral impairment (MBI) [19,20] has been proposed as a prodromal neuropsychiatric stage of emergent dementia. Due to the high risk of developing AD in subjects with DS, and considering that AD-DS pharmacological interventions are not efficient enough [21,22], it is necessary to arrange a grading scale that captures the whole clinical spectrum of the AD-DS with the inclusion of these recently proposed diagnostic categories to detect early therapeutic windows.

Although the biological perspective research framework has meant a forward leap in the prediction of MCI and AD, cognitive markers continue to be essential. There are several cases in daily clinical practice in which neuroimaging and biomarker findings suggest a certain diagnosis but without being supported by a neuropsychological examination, as in cases of biomarker positivity for AD without associated or progressive cognitive impairment [18]. Because biomarkers may fail in the diagnosis of AD, a neuropsychological examination can provide crucial cognitive information in the diagnostic and follow-up processes of the ID population [23]. In this sense, the aspects that should be explored in any longitudinal assessment for the entire continuum of AD-DS are dysexecutive cognitive or behavioral features, episodic memory, orientation, and general global cognitive decline [24–27].

The high prevalence of MCI and AD in individuals with DS has resulted in much research concerning the detection of both diagnoses. In a recent paper, the diagnostic criteria to delimit MCI in people with DS (MCI-DS) have been proposed [28], a stage that can be considered as prodromal of AD [29]. These authors showed that scores in the behavior rating inventory of the executive function parent form (BRIEF-P) [30] combined with scores on abstract thinking and verbal memory are useful values for detecting MCI-DS. Furthermore, the memory, language, and communication sections of the National Task Group-Early Detection Screen for Dementia (NTG-EDSD) seem to be sensitive to MCI-DS [31]. The Cambridge Cognitive Examination for Older Adults with Down's syndrome—Spanish version (CAMCOG-DS) [32], with different cut-offs points, has been provided to detect prodromal AD or MCI and AD in people with DS and mild or moderate ID [13,32]. Furthermore, visuospatial-paired associate memory, hand–eye coordination, and semantic verbal fluency may be relatively sensitive events in the prodromal stage of AD-DS [10]. Finally, the performance of episodic memory using a modified cued recall test discriminates between individuals with preclinical, prodromal, and clinically manifest AD, albeit of mild degree [33]. Compared with the aforementioned major phases, the later stages of the AD-DS spectrum have not received special attention nor an international official definition.

The progression of the disease in the clinical setting is assessed through cognitive, behavioral, psychiatric, and clinical tests. Additionally, rating scales provide a common language to diagnose, monitor, and evaluate therapeutic interventions. A good rating scale would be practical and properly validated in the target population, embracing different domains beyond cognition, and be sensitive to change in all stages to measure therapeutic effects [34], both pharmacological and non-pharmacological. In the general population, there are two reference scales for grading dementia. One of them is the clinical dementia rating scale (CDR) [35], a semi-structured interview with a patient and a close caregiver, covering six domains (memory, orientation, judgment and problem solving, work in the community, performance at home and in hobbies, and personal care). The results are distributed on a five-point scale from cognitive normality to severe dementia. Interestingly, an adaptation of the CDR, the CDR for frontotemporal lobar degeneration (CDR-FTDL) [36], was developed with the inclusion of language and behavior domains not contemplated in the original CDR, and has been shown to be sensitive in distinguishing disease progression between FTLD and AD in the general population [37]. Additionally, a modified CDR for adults with DS based on questionnaires and patient/caregiver interviews is available [38], capturing the progressive deterioration of AD in this population.

The second grading dementia scale is the global deterioration scale (GDS [39], which determines the degree of functional loss based on the severity of the cognitive impairment. It consists of descriptions of the clinically differentiated stages of the AD continuum, from stage 1 (normal) to 7 (severe AD). Subsequently, the functional assessment staging (FAST) [40] provides the GDS with a division of phases 6 and 7, involving the progressive inability to maintain basic activities of daily living. The GDS is easier to apply than the CDR as it correlates with neuropathological, functional, global, and cognitive changes in the progression of MCI to AD [41] and with the hippocampal volume [42]. Furthermore, in our context, the GDS is the instrument of choice that determines the introduction and withdrawal of pharmacological and non-pharmacological treatment in patients with AD [43,44]. Therefore, it would be desirable to arrange a global deterioration rating scale which contemplates the amnesic [45,46] and the behavioral [47,48] forms of onset classically described in AD-DS. Consequently, such a scale would improve both the response to health needs according to the time point of disease progression and provide researchers in this field with a common language in our context.

The main objective of the present study is to examine the feasibility of an adapted GDS for its use in people with DS on the continuum of AD. We expect to find that the stages proposed for GDS-DS are anchored to the performance of cognitive and behavioral instruments that are well established in people with DS and a mild or moderate level of ID.

2. Materials and Methods

2.1. Study Design and Description of the Sample

This is a retrospective, dual-center cohort study of Caucasian adults with DS. A total of 87 participants were identified from the Servicio Especializado en Salud Mental y Discapacidad Intelectual (Specialized Mental Health ID Unit, Institute of Health Assistance, Girona) and the Unidad de Adultos con Síndrome de Down (Adult Down Syndrome Unit, La Princesa University Hospital, Madrid, Spain).

A neurological, psychiatric, and laboratory examination was applied to all the participants. The neurological examination consisted of taking the participant's history (e.g., previous central nervous system alterations, relevant drug treatment, substance abuse, sleep disorders) and a physical examination. Psychiatric data were collected using the psychiatric assessment schedule for adults with a developmental disability (PAS-ADD) [49]. Blood samples were obtained in order to detect hypothyroidism, vitamin B12 deficiency, and anemia.

The inclusion and exclusion criteria of the study are displayed in Table 1. Going into detail, the age cut-off was chosen based on previous studies which reported that being above 39 years of age represents a high risk of developing cognitive decline from a previous level of efficiency in people with DS [50]. The level of ID was determined according to the DSM-5 criteria [51]. All participants were required to have a reliable informant available to report on the present and past adaptive skills and behavior of the participants.

Those with sensory impairments that prevented the completion of the research protocol, those with a history of alterations of the central nervous system (e.g., brain tumors, head injury, stroke), those with uncontrolled sleep disorders (e.g., obstructive sleep apnoea), and individuals suffering from substance abuse were excluded. Patients were also excluded if they had untreated anemia, vitamin B12 deficiency, or uncontrolled hypothyroidism because of their potential risks of influencing behavior.

Table 1. Inclusion and exclusion criteria.

Inclusion Criteria	Exclusion Criteria
≥39 years old	Severe sensory impairments
Both sexes	No reliable informant
Mild or moderate intellectual disability	Untreated anemia
DS confirmed karyotype	Vitamin B12 deficiency
	Uncontrolled hypothyroidism
	Behavior disorder (comorbid, affecting normal functioning)
	Uncontrolled sleep disorders
	Substance abuse
	Previous central nervous system alterations
	Relevant drug treatment

It should be noted that cases of conduct disorder, depression, and anxiety were not automatically ruled out. Those cases caused by a stressful event in the past six months, were excluded but those (un)treated cases related to normal daily functioning were not, according to clinical judgment.

Finally, participants exposed to a high anticholinergic burden through polypharmacy from psychotropics, gastrointestinal and cardiovascular medications were excluded if the treatment was considered ineffective, according to clinical judgment.

Our study was conducted in accordance with The Code of Ethics of the World Medical Association (Declaration of Helsinki). The study protocol was approved by the Clinical Research Ethical Committee of the Parc Hospitalari Santa Caterina (Girona). Written informed consent was obtained from parents and written and pictorial assent were additionally obtained.

2.2. Clinical Assessment

The protocol consisted of a cognitive test and behavioral and daily living skills questionnaires that have been shown to be most sensitive to cognitive impairment in Spanish-speaking subjects with DS.

2.2.1. Cognitive Assessment

The protocol with the following test was applied to all the participants:

- The level of ID was based on the results from the Kaufman brief intelligence test, second edition (KBIT-II) [52] and Vineland adaptive behavior scales–second Edition (Vineland II) [53].
- The *KBIT-II* is a test designed for the measurement of verbal and non-verbal intelligence. It consists of two sub-tests that assess crystallized intelligence and fluid intelligence and allow the establishment of the level of ID.
- The *Vineland II* scale measures adaptive behaviors, including communication, daily living skills, socialization, and motor skills.
- General cognitive abilities were assessed using the following scales: the Cambridge cognitive examination for older adults with Down's syndrome and other intellectual disabilities—Spanish version (CAMCOG-DS) [32], and the Barcelona test for intellectual disability (BT-ID) [54].
- The CAMCOG-DS comprises seven cognitive domains (orientation, language, memory, attention, praxis, abstract thinking, and perception). The maximum score is 109 points. The psychometrical properties are good: test–retest reliability = 0.92, ICC = 0.91, internal consistency = 0.70 − 0.93, and κ values of 0.95 and 0.97 versus DSM-IV [51] and ICD-10 [55] criteria, respectively. It is a reliable tool for the assessment of cognitive impairment in people with ID with and without DS with mild and moderate levels of ID.

- The *BT-ID* consists of 67 subtests grouped into eight cognitive domains (language, working memory, orientation, praxis, attention, executive function, visuoconstruction, and memory). It shows good psychometric properties: test–retest reliability = 0.91, ICC = 0.95, internal consistency = 0.70 − 0.93. It provides normative data for five groups based on intellectual disability level, age, and curricular competence.
- Planning and problem solving were assessed with the Tower of London—Drexel University: 2nd edition ID version [56]. Its psychometric properties are reliable for differentiation between subjects with mild and moderate ID, and are associated with other measures of executive functions. Additionally, it demonstrated sufficient evidence of reliability and validity in adults with Down syndrome.

2.2.2. Informants' Questionnaires

- The behavior rating inventory of executive function, parents' form (*BRIEF-P*) [30] measures executive functions or self-regulation in their everyday environments. It consists of two indexes: (1) Behavioral regulation index (BRI), composed of inhibit, shift, and emotional control scales; and (2) the metacognitive index (MI), composed of initiate, working memory, planning, organization, and monitor scales.
- The informant interview of the Cambridge examination for older adults with Down's syndrome and other intellectual disabilities—Spanish version (CAMDEX-DS) [32]. It consists of (1) a structured interview with the informant/family member to collect information to detect a decline in the individual's best level of functioning, their cognitive and functional impairment, and the mental and physical health of the participant, including depression, anxiety, paranoid symptoms, delirium, substance abuse, physical disability, hypothyroidism, cerebrovascular problems, and pharmacological treatment; (2) the CAMCOG-DS (see the cognitive test scale section in this article); (3) a guide for the clinical diagnosis of AD, capturing changes in daily adaptive skills (section A), memory (section B), other cognitive domains (section C1), personality/behavior (section C2) and confusional acute syndrome (section D); and (4) suggestions for the correct intervention in people with ID and dementia. In this study, the CAMDEX-DS was used only for clinical diagnostic purposes to avoid the risk of circularity.

The participants of the PD group were classified according to three diagnostic categories: cognitive stability, MCI and AD. The diagnosis of cognitive stability was made when participants had no cognitive impairment or decline in adaptive skills, according to the CAMDEX-DS informant section. As there is currently no internationally accepted official definition for MCI-DS [57], the diagnosis of MCI or AD was based on expert multidisciplinary clinical judgment according to recent publications, as is recommended in standard practice for DS [26,28,58–61]. In detail, a participant fulfilled the diagnosis of MCI when presented with a single or multiple cognitive decline and/or loss of functionality according to the CAMDEX-DS informant section [26]. The diagnosis of AD was obtained if participants had memory decline or another cognitive impairment, such as aphasia, apraxia, agnosia, or dysexecutive syndrome, or loss of functionality [62]. In both conditions, the information about changes from previous levels of performance must be supported by a close caregiver [26,58,60]. It should be noted that the CAMDEX-DS was used only for diagnostic purposes, whereas performance on the neuropsychological tests confirmed the diagnosis through a longitudinal clinical study [26].

2.2.3. Global Deterioration Scale for Down Syndrome (GDS-DS)

The GDS-DS began at stage 1 (cognitive and behavioral stability), in which subjects were placed if they had neither subjective complaints nor cognitive or behavioral impairments identified by the instruments of the study protocol. Stage 2 (subjective cognitive and/or behavioral impairment) included those subjects with changes in cognition, behavior or adaptive skills, as self-reported or reported by caregivers but not supported by objective data. Stage 3 (mild cognitive and/or behavioral impairment) corresponded to those cases with reports of cognitive or behavioral impairment by the patient or confirmed by a reliable informant, supported by objective data, with no or very mild loss of adaptive skills. Stages 4 (mild Alzheimer's disease), 5 (moderate Alzheimer's disease) and 6 (advanced Alzheimer's disease) were reserved for those subjects presenting mild to severe deterioration in cognitive and behavioral domains, as reported by an informant, supported by objective data and demonstrating affected adaptive skills (Table 2).

Table 2. Stages and diagnostic criteria for each stage of the GDS-DS.

	Stages
1	Cognitive and behavioral stability All must be present I. BRIEF-P BRI index: ≥ 33 II. CAMCOG-DS total: ≥ 83 (mild ID); ≥ 65 (moderate ID) III. Any CAMDEX-DS diagnostic criteria (no A, B, C1 or C2)
2	Subjective cognitive and/or behavioral impairment All must be present I. BRIEF-P BRI index: ≤ 33 II. CAMCOG-DS total: ≥ 83 (mild ID); ≥ 65 (moderate ID) III. CAMDEX-DS diagnostic criteria: B or C1 or C2
3	Mild cognitive and/or behavioral impairment (I and/or II) + III must be present I. BRIEF-P BRI index: ≤ 32 II. CAMCOG-DS total: $\leq 82 - 69$ (mild ID), $\leq 64 - 57$ (moderate ID) III. CAMDEX-DS diagnostic criteria: B or C1 or C2 ≤ 2 supporting criteria
4	Mild Alzheimer's disease (I and/or II) + III must be present I. BRIEF-P BRI index: ≤ 32 II. CAMCOG-DS total: ≤ 68 (mild ID), ≤ 56 (moderate ID) III. CAMDEX-DS diagnostic criteria: A, B, C1 or C2, no D ≥ 2 supporting criteria
5	Moderate Alzheimer's disease (I and/or II) + III must be present I. BRIEF-P BRI index: ≤ 32 II. CAMCOG-DS total: ≤ 68 (mild ID), ≤ 56 (moderate ID) III. CAMDEX-DS diagnostic criteria: A, B, C or C2, no D ≥ 3 supporting criteria
6	Advanced Alzheimer's disease (I and/or II) + III must be present, or III and V I. BRIEF-P BRI index: ≤ 32 II. CAMCOG-DS total: ≤ 68 (mild ID), ≤ 56 (moderate ID) III. CAMDEX-DS diagnostic criteria: A, B, C1 or C2, no D ≥ 3 supporting criteria Incomplete or no administered neuropsychological examination

GDS-DS, global deterioration scale for people with Down's syndrome; BRIEF-P BRI, behavior rating inventory of executive function, parents' form behavioral regulation index; CAMCOG-DS, Cambridge cognitive examination for older adults with Down's syndrome and other intellectual disabilities; ID, intellectual disability; CAMDEX-DS, Cambridge examination for older adults with Down's syndrome and other intellectual disabilities.

- GDS-DS adaptation

The GDS-DS was constructed on the basis of the global deterioration scale (GDS) [39]. Some modifications were introduced to adapt this scale to the study population. First, the original GDS scale consists of seven stages (1–7), whereas the GDS-DS consists of six stages (1–6). Secondly, because growing evidence suggests that subjective cognitive decline [16,17] and mild behavioral impairment [19,20] could predict AD, subjective cognitive and behavioral aspects were considered. Therefore, stage 2 was labeled as subjective cognitive and/or behavioral impairment and stage 3 as mild cognitive and/or behavioral impairment.

In general, for the delimitation of the GDS-DS stages, the performance of the participants in the cognitive instruments and the information of the behavioral questionnaire and caregivers gathered from the study protocol were classified as mandatory or supporting criteria, according to the recent literature about AD and DS (Table 2).

- Mandatory criteria

The mandatory criteria were established based on those cognitive and behavioral instruments that had obtained sufficient quantitative data to differentiate MCI and AD, in addition to adaptive skills. The purpose was to establish criteria that were as inclusive as possible; thus, the following instruments and scores were considered:

1. Behavioral Regulation Index—BRIEF-P [30]. This questionnaire demonstrates that, in people with DS, a cut-off point of ≥ 55 allows the classification of stable subjects at the cognitive and behavioral levels (sensitivity = 90), while a cut-off point of <32 allows the classification of subjects with MCI (specificity = 0.90). For scores between 32 and 55, the diagnosis is more doubtful [28]. According to these data, the following cut-off points were assigned for our study: ≥ 33 would be a criterion for cognitive and behavioral stability (stage 1) and subjective cognitive and/or behavioral impairment (stage 2), and ≤ 32 would be a criterion for mild cognitive or behavioral impairment (stage 3) and mild, moderate and advanced AD (stages 4, 5 and 6, respectively).
2. Regarding the total score of the *CAMCOG-DS* [32], it has become clear that a cut-off point of the total score = 68 allows the detection of AD in subjects with DS and mild ID (sensitivity: 80%; specificity: 81%), and a cut-off point of 52 (sensitivity: 85%; specificity: 81%) in those with moderate ID [32]. Additionally, in another study of subjects with DS and mild ID, a cut-off point of 82 (sensitivity: 80%, specificity 80.5%) differentiated between asymptomatic and prodromal AD, and a cut-off point of 80 (sensitivity: 75%, specificity 87.8%) differentiated asymptomatic and dementia AD. In the same study, for those with moderate ID, a cut-off point of 64 (sensitivity: 66.7%, specificity 72.3%) differentiated between asymptomatic and prodromal AD, and a cut-off point of 56 (sensitivity: 84%, specificity 84.3%) between asymptomatic and dementia AD [13]. The data of these two previous studies were incorporated for all the stages of the GDS-DS, according to the ID level and the CAMCOG-DS total score.
3. The Guide to clinical diagnosis of the CAMDEX-DS—Spanish version [32]. The decline of daily life skills is decisive in the diagnostic process of AD, since in the MCI, these are preserved or only very mildly affected. Therefore, in our study, positive scores in sections B (memory), section C1 (other cognitive domains) or section C2 (personality/behavioral) were considered indicative of mild cognitive and/or behavioral impairment (stage 3). Furthermore, positive scores in section A (daily living skills), section B and sections C1 or C2 and negative scores in section D (acute confusional syndrome) are indicative of AD (stages 4, 5 and 6).

It should be noted that the BRIEF-P (BRI index) and the CAMCOG-DS, in addition to providing a quantitative basis for each stage of the GDS-DS, also cover the symptoms of the two most frequent forms of AD onset in the DS population, either the amnestic [45,46] or the behavioral variants [47,48].

- Supporting criteria

The supporting criteria were established based on those cognitive and behavioral instruments of the protocol study that demonstrated a decrease associated with an increase in the clinical intensity of AD-DS from the MCI-DS phase. These criteria might not be mandatory, but their presence helped determine the stage of the GDS-DS that would be assigned to each participant. The instruments considered for this purpose were:

1. BT-ID: the orientation, semantic fluency (eating and drinking), formal fluency, delay verbal memory (stories) and visual discrimination subtests.

2. CAMCOG-DS: abstract thinking subtest.

Recent studies claim that significantly lower scores on the above subtests can be indicative of MCI-DS and the early phase of AD [10,13,26,28]. Therefore, these were added as supporting criteria for AD-DS from stage 3 (mild cognitive and/or behavioral impairment) upward (stages 4, 5 and 6).

It should be emphasized that in order to identify the stages of AD (4, 5 and 6), in addition to the mandatory and supporting criteria established, the degree of deterioration (mild, 4; moderate, 5; and advanced, 6) would have to be determined by the judgment and clinical experience of specialists, who play a decisive role in this regard.

For stage 6 (advanced Alzheimer's disease), an additional criterion was established. Based on our clinical experience and other studies of populations with DS, it has been suggested that some tests cannot be administered to those with advanced stages of AD or in populations with severe intellectual disabilities [57] because they do not provide enough information due to the "floor effect" [22]. Therefore, the criterion of not being able to administer all or any cognitive tests from the screening protocol to participants would, on its own, be an indicator of advanced AD, supported by affected adaptive skills.

2.3. Procedures

Cognitive, behavioral and adaptive skills data from the PD group were used retrospectively to place each participant in a stage of the GDS-DS and thus form the GDS-DS group. Two neuropsychologist specialists in DS blinded to the diagnosis of the PD group (SEC, JGA) placed each subject into one of the six levels of the proposed GDS-DS rating scale, according to the level of ID of each participant and the mandatory and supporting criteria established (Table 1). It should be highlighted that in order to avoid circularity, the two specialists were different to those who made the diagnoses for the PD group. The degree of agreement between the examiners in placing the subjects in the stages of the GDS-DS was checked. The inter-rater reliability test was applied to the two raters' first GDS-DS classifications. Then, the classifications of the two raters was transformed into single values as follows: if they matched the GDS-DS assignment, the same value was maintained, and when the two raters did not agree on the classification using the GDS-DS, the case was discussed until a consensus was reached. Additionally, the demographic and the diagnostic categories of the PD and the GDS-DS groups were analyzed in order to observe possible similarities.

The agreement between the two raters classifying the participants using the GDS-DS compared with the PD group was analyzed. For this purpose, the stages 1 (cognitive and behavioral stability) and 2 (subjective cognitive and/or behavioral impairment) of the GDS-DS were associated with the cognitive stability diagnosis of the PD group; stage 3 (mild cognitive and/or behavioral impairment) of the GDS-DS was associated with the diagnosis of mild cognitive impairment of the PD group; and stages 4, 5 and 6 (Mild, Moderate and Advanced Alzheimer's disease) of the GDS-DS were associated with the Alzheimer's disease of the PD group. Codes associated with each category of the PD group are displayed in Table 3.

Table 3. Recode numeric values.

GDS-DS Stages	Primary Diagnosis
1. Cognitive and behavioral stability 2. Subjective cognitive and/or behavioral impairment	0. Cognitive stability
3. Mild cognitive and/or behavioral impairment	1. Mild cognitive impairment
4. Mild Alzheimer's disease 5. Moderate Alzheimer's disease 6. Advanced Alzheimer's disease	2. Alzheimer's disease

GDS-DS, global deterioration scale for people with Down's syndrome.

Finally, as the progressive deterioration of adaptive skills was an immovable criterion and an analysis with this variable could lead to a circularity problem, the authors checked for a possible association of the GDS-DS stages with a selection of the cognitive and behavioral instruments included as mandatory and supporting criteria for each stage.

2.4. Statistical Analysis

We performed all statistical analyses using the software program SPSS (version 27.0; SPSS Inc., Chicago, IL, USA). Bilateral significance levels were set at a p-value of less than 0.05. The normality of data was assessed using the Kolmogorov–Smirnov test, and subsequently, non-parametric analyses were carried out. For the GDS-DS group, demographic characteristics, level of ID, and performance on selected neuropsychological tests were analyzed by a non-parametric Kruskal–Wallis test followed by the Bonferroni correction for post hoc pairwise comparisons or Pearson's chi-square test for category data. Spearman's correlation analysis was used to determine the associations between the stages of the GDS-DS with the cognitive and behavioral data selected. A Mann–Whitney U test was performed with pairs of the GDS-DS groups because the effect size between the cognitive and behavioral performance across the GDS-DS stages was computed using the non-parametric probability of superiority estimation (PSest), interpreted as small ($\geq$56), medium ($\geq$0.64), and large ($\geq$0.71) [63]. Inter-rater agreement and concordance between the stages issued by rater 1 and rater 2 with the primary diagnosis of the study were analyzed by using Cohen's weighted kappa values.

3. Results

3.1. Sample and Demographics

Of the subjects selected, four ultimately did not agree to participate in the study. The final sample formed the primary diagnosis (PD) group and consisted of 83 subjects (46.65 ± 5.08 years; male = 46 (55.4%), female = 37 (44.6%)) and was divided into three groups: (1) cognitively stable group, with 48 subjects (45.10 ± 3.83 years; male = 24 (50%), female = 24 (50%)); (2) mild cognitive impairment group, with 24 subjects (47.46 ± 5.35 years; male = 16 (66.7%), female = 8 (33.3%)); and (3) Alzheimer's disease group, with 11 subjects (51.64 ± 6.05 years; male = 6 (54.5%), female = 5 (45.6%)). Seven of the initial candidates had to be excluded because they could not undergo the neuropsychological assessment.

The demographic details of the PD group are reported in Table 4. Of the total 83 participants, about half were diagnosed as being cognitively stable, one third as having mild cognitive impairment and a smaller number as having Alzheimer's disease. The mean age of the subjects with AD was significantly higher than the stable subjects but not than the MCI group. No statistical differences were observed in the gender and level of ID across the groups.

Table 4. Demographics of the primary diagnosis sample.

	Total	Cognitive Stability	Mild Cognitive Impairment	Alzheimer's Disease	p
n	83	48	24	11	
Age	46.65 (39–63)	45.10 (39–43)	47.46 (39–61)	51.64 (43–63)	0.01 * a
Gender					0.41
Male	46 (55.4%)	24 (50%)	16 (66.7%)	6 (54.5%)	
Female	37 (44.6%)	24 (50%)	8 (33.3%)	5 (45.6%)	
ID level					0.61
Mild	49 (59.1%)	29 (60.4%)	15 (62.5%)	5 (45.6%)	
Moderate	34 (40.9%)	19 (39.6%)	9 (37.5%)	6 (54.6%)	

Age values are shown as means and range. For the sex and ID level, percentages regarding the group are shown. ID, intellectual disability. * $p < 0.05$, according to Kruskal–Wallis test with Bonferroni correction for age, or χ^2-test for gender and ID level. a, between cognitive stability and Alzheimer's disease.

Within the GDS-DS group (Table 5), 27 participants were diagnosed as having cognitive stability (stage 1) and with subjective cognitive and/or behavioral impairment (stage 2), 25 with mild cognitive and/or behavioral impairment (stage 3) and 31 participants with any degree of AD (stages 4, 5 or 6). Interestingly, comparing these two groups, a similar number of participants were classified as MCI with both methods and 20 more subjects as AD. There were more participants diagnosed as more cognitively stable in the PD group than those placed in stage 1 of GDS-DS (48 and 9, respectively). As expected, subjects diagnosed with AD in the PD group and those placed on the stage 6 of the GDS-DS (advanced Alzheimer's disease) were the oldest.

Table 5. Demographics for each stage of the global deterioration scale for people with Down's syndrome.

	Total	GDS-DS Stages						p
		1	2	3	4	5	6	
		Cognitive/ Behavioral Stability	Subjective Cognitive/ Behavioral Impairment	Mild Cognitive/ Behavioral Impairment	Mild Alzheimer's Disease	Moderate Alzheimer's Disease	Advanced Alzheimer's Disease	
n	83	9	18	25	10	14	7	
Age	46.65 (39–63)	46.44 (40–61)	44.72 (39–54)	45.60 (39–54)	46.60 (42–52)	47.43 (41–54)	54.14 (49–63)	0.02 * a, * b
Gender								0.15
Male	46 (55.4%)	8 (88.9%)	11 (61.1%)	10 (40.0%)	4 (40.0%)	9 (64.3%)	4 (57.1%)	
Female	37 (44.6%)	1 (11.1%)	7 (38.9%)	15 (60.0%)	6 (60.0%)	5 (35.7%)	3 (42.9%)	
ID level								0.08
Mild	49 (59.1%)	4 (44.4%)	15 (83.3%)	17 (68.0%)	4 (40.0%)	6 (42.9%)	3 (42.9%)	
Moderate	34 (40.9%)	5 (55.6%)	3 (16.7%)	8 (32.0%)	6 (60.0%)	8 (57.1%)	4 (57.1%)	

Age values are shown as means and range. For the sex and ID level, percentages regarding the group are shown. ID, intellectual disability. * $p < 0.05$, according to Kruskal–Wallis test with Bonferroni correction for age, or χ^2-test for gender and intellectual disability level. a, between subjective cognitive/behavior impairment and advanced Alzheimer's disease; b, between mild cognitive/behavior impairment and advanced Alzheimer's disease.

3.2. Cognitive and Behavioral Data across the GDS-DS Stages

These analyses were conducted without the data from the stage 6 subjects, who were excluded because they could not complete the study protocol.

The analysis of the correlations revealed negative significant correlations between performance on the tests and the GDS-DS, except for the BRIEF-P and the visual discrimination BT-ID subtest. The correlations were moderate between the GDS-DS and the CAMCOG-DS Total score, orientation subtest and formal fluency, but weak with abstract thinking subtest of the CAMCOG-DS, free memory delay (stories) and semantic fluency of the BT-ID (Table 6).

The performance on the cognitive and behavioral tools across the GDS-DS stages is displayed in Table 7. Overall, the performance on the CAMCOG-DS total score and the orientation subtest (BT-ID) decreased significantly across stage 1 (cognitive and/or behavioral stability) to 5 (moderate Alzheimer's disease).

Table 6. Correlations between GDS-DS stages and cognitive/behavioral assessment.

Cognitive and Behavioral Assessment	Rho
BRIEF-P	
BRI index	−0.17
CAMCOG-DS	
Total score	−0.70 **
Abstract thinking	−0.39 **
BT-ID	
Orientation	−0.78 **
Free delay memory (stories)	−0.37 **
Semantic fluency (eat/drink)	−0.38 **
Formal fluency	−0.54 **
Visual discrimination	−0.11

GDS-DS, global deterioration scale for people with Down's syndrome; BRIEF-P, behavior rating inventory of executive function parents' form; BRI, behavioral regulation index; CAMCOG-DS, Cambridge cognitive examination for older adults with Down's syndrome and other intellectual disabilities; BT-ID, Barcelona test for intellectual disability. ** $p < 0.01$, (two-tailed test), using Spearman's correlation coefficient.

Table 7. Cognitive and behavioral performance across the GDS-DS stages.

		GDS-DS Stages					p
	Total	1 Cognitive/ Behavioral Stability	2 Subjective Cognitive/ Behavioral Impairment	3 Mild Cognitive/ Behavioral Impairment	4 Mild Alzheimer's Disease	5 Moderate Alzheimer's Disease	
BRIEF-P BRI index	40.99 (35–47)	47.00 (39–49)	40.00 (36–47)	36.00 (30–42)	40.00 (36–45)	37.00 (36–51)	
CAMCOG-DS							
Total score	72.00 (55–88)	**84.00 (76–87)**	**82.50 (76–87)**	71.00 (60–78)	61.50 (50–71)	49.5 (44–55)	** a, ** b, ** c, ** c, e **
Abstract thinking	2.00 (0–4.5)	4.00 (1–5)	**4.50 (0–5)**	2.00 (0–4)	1.00 (0–4)	0.00 (0–1)	* b
BT-ID							
Orientation	91.00 (48–109)	**103.00 (97–113)**	**109.00 (102–114)**	91.00 (73–108)	46.00 (35–49)	28.50 (21–40)	** a, ** b, ** c, ** d, ** e, ** f
Delay stories	2.00 (0–4)	3.00 (2–6)	**3.00 (2–5)**	3.00 (1–4)	1.50 (0–4)	**0.00 (0–2)**	* d, * e
Semantic fluency (eat/drink)	9.00 (6.5–12)	10.00 (9–12)	10.5 (8–13)	10.00 (8–11)	9.00 (5–13)	**6.00 (5–8)**	* d
Formal fluency	2.00 (0–4)	**3.00 (2–4)**	4.00 (2–6)	2.00 (1–4)	0.00 (0–3)	**0.00 (0–1)**	** b, ** c, *** d
Visual discrimination	18.00 (16–19)	18.00 (16–19)	18.00 (17–20)	18.00 (16–19)	16.00 (16–19)	18.00 (16–19)	

Values are given as median and range: GDS-DS, global deterioration scale for people with Down's syndrome; BRIEF-P, behavior rating inventory of executive function parents' form; BRI, behavioral regulation index; CAMCOG-DS, Cambridge cognitive examination for older adults with Down's syndrome and other intellectual disabilities; BT-ID, Barcelona test for intellectual disability. * $p < 0.05$, ** $p < 0.01$, *** $p < 0.001$, according to Kruskal–Wallis test with Bonferroni correction. a, between cognitive/behavioral stability and mild Alzheimer's disease; b, between cognitive/behavioral stability and moderate Alzheimer's disease; c, between subjective cognitive/behavioral impairment and mild Alzheimer's disease; d, between subjective cognitive/behavioral impairment and moderate Alzheimer's disease; e, between mild cognitive/behavioral impairment and moderate Alzheimer's disease; f, between mild cognitive/behavioral impairment and mild Alzheimer's disease. Significant differences in bold.

In terms of sectors, performance significantly decreased regarding:

- Delay stories (BT-ID) between stage 2 (subjective cognitive and/or behavioral impairment) and 5 (moderate Alzheimer's disease) and stages 3 (mild cognitive and/or behavioral impairment) and 5 (moderate Alzheimer's disease).
- Formal fluency (TB-ID) between stage 1 (cognitive and/or behavioral stability) and 5 (moderate Alzheimer's disease), stage 2 (subjective cognitive and/or behavioral impairment), stage 3 (mild Alzheimer's disease) and stage 4 (moderate Alzheimer's disease).

- Semantic fluency (BT-ID) between stages 2 (subjective cognitive and/or behavioral impairment) and 5 (moderate Alzheimer's disease).

Note that (i) the performance on abstract thinking, orientation, delay stories, and formal fluency subtest (BT-ID) did not decrease between stage 1 (cognitive and behavioral stability) and 2 (subjective cognitive and/or behavioral impairment); (ii) the performance on the BRI index (BRIEF-P) decreased between 1 (cognitive and behavioral stability) and 3 (mild cognitive impairment), but was heterogeneous from stage 3 (mild cognitive and/or behavioral impairment) to stage 5 (moderate Alzheimer's disease); (iii) the performance on delay stories subtest (BT-ID) did not show significant oscillations between stage 2 (subjective cognitive and/or behavioral impairment) and 3 (mild cognitive and/or behavioral impairment); and the performance on the visual discrimination subtest (BT-ID) was similar across all the stages. These data had an impact on the posterior analysis of the effect sizes values.

The raw differences that showed a progressive decrease between performances on the selected tests across the GDS-DS stages are displayed in Table 8 and Table S1 of the online Supplementary Materials.

Table 8. Effect sizes between the GDS-DS stages.

	GDS-DS Stages							
	1–2		2–3		3–4		4–5	
	P	PS$_{est}$	P	PS$_{est}$	P	PS$_{est}$	P	PS$_{est}$
BRIEF-P								
BRI index	0.395	0.60 [a]	0.061	0.67 [b]	0.183	0.61	0.567	0.51
CAMCOG-DS								
Total score	0.938	0.51	0.010 *	0.80 [c]	0.027 *	0.69 [b]	0.088	0.68 [b]
Abstract thinking	0.595	0.56	0.139	0.63 [a]	0.549	0.51	0.129	0.65
BT-ID								
Orientation	0.314	0.62	0.002 **	0.78 [c]	0.000 ***	0.94 [c]	0.057	0.71 [c]
Free delay memory (stories)	0.775	0.53	0.663	0.54	0.331	0.55	0.467	0.56 [a]
Semantic fluency (eat/drink)	0.856	0.52	0.265	0.60	0.906	0.49	0.114	0.63 [a]
Formal fluency	0.364	0.61	0.011 *	0.73 [c]	0.118	0.66 [b]	0.716	0.44
Visual discrimination	0.733	0.54	0.367	0.58	0.363	0.56 [a]	0.305	0.58

GDS-DS, global deterioration scale for people with Down's syndrome; BRIEF-P, behavior rating inventory of executive function parents' form; BRI, behavioral regulation index; CAMCOG-DS, Cambridge cognitive examination for older adults with Down's syndrome and other intellectual disabilities; BT-ID, Barcelona test for intellectual disability. P, p value; PS$_{est}$, probability of superiority effect size; * $p < 0.05$, ** $p < 0.01$, *** $p < 0.001$; [a] PS$_{est} \geq 56$, [b] PS$_{est} \geq 0.64$, [c] PS$_{est} \geq 0.71$. Significant effect sizes and p values with progressive decrease on the performance across the stages (Table 7) in bold.

Overall, small to large effect sizes were observed between stage 2 (subjective cognitive and/or behavioral impairment) and 5 (moderate Alzheimer's disease) for the CAMCOG-DS total score and orientation subtest (BT-ID).

The effect sizes ranged from small to medium between stages 1 (cognitive and behavioral stability) and 3 (mild cognitive and/or behavioral impairment) for the BRI index (BRIEF-P). Medium to large effect sizes were observed for the formal fluency subtest (BT-ID) between stage 2 (subjective cognitive and/or behavioral impairment) and stage 4 (mild Alzheimer's disease).

The effect sizes ranged from small to medium for free delay memory and semantic fluency subtest (BT-ID) between stage 4 (mild Alzheimer's disease) and 5 (moderate Alzheimer's disease).

A small effect size was observed between stage 3 (mild cognitive and/or behavioral impairment) and 4 (mild Alzheimer's disease) on the *visual discrimination* subtest (BT-ID).

3.3. Reliability

The inter-rater reliability for staging using GDS-DS was excellent, with a mean Cohen weighted κ value of 0.86 (CI: 0.80–0.93). The agreement between the two raters classifying the PD group using the GDS-DS was excellent, as determined by specialists, with κ values of 0.82 (CI: 0.73–0.92) and 0.85 (CI: 0.77–0.94).

4. Discussion

The main goal of the present study was to devise a global rating scale for AD in people with DS based on the GDS scale [39]. The resulting GDS-DS amplifies the classical phases of the AD-DS (stability, prodromal AD and AD). Our purpose was to provide a scale that captures progressive decline in the entire AD-DS continuum. The GDS-DS meets this requirement from the cognitive stability to AD stages, especially in relation to performance on the CAMCOG-DS *total score* and *orientation* subtests of the BT-ID and dementia.

The GDS-DS ranges through six stages from cognitive and behavioral stability (stage 1) to advanced Alzheimer's disease (stage 6), contrasting with the seven stages of the global deterioration scale (GDS) [39] for the general population. In view of the results obtained in the present work, in which an overall decrease in deterioration is detected by the CAMCOG-DS total score, six stages capture the entire continuum of AD in people with DS and, in addition, they are consistent with the stages of AD proposed in research of the National Institute on Aging and the Alzheimer's Association (NIA-AA) [6].

The six stages of the GDS-DS differ from the five stages of the clinical dementia rating scale (CDR) [35] and the modified clinical dementia rating scale for people with Down syndrome questionnaire (CDR-QDS) and interview (CDR-IDS) forms [38]. These two rating scales (CDR and CDR-IDS/CQR-IDS), as opposed to our GDS-DS, do not include stage 2 (subjective cognitive and/or behavioral impairment). This can lead to misdiagnosis because subjective cognitive impairment is increasingly seen as an early symptom of dementia risk in the general population [16,17] and although it is not a sensitive aspect by itself [18], it must be considered with complementary clinical data as a different entity from MCI. In addition, behavioral aspects are also not considered in these scales, although they are important factors for detecting possible changes associated with prodromal AD in subjects with DS [47]. Furthermore, in our clinical dementia contexts, the global deterioration scale (GDS) [39] is used to monitor, design and modify appropriate pharmacological treatment in patients with AD in the general population [43,44]. Thus, the authors consider the GDS-DS a closer instrument for daily clinical practice and recommend its use for clinical trials in subjects with AD-DS.

Seven participants were placed in the stage 6 (advanced Alzheimer's disease) category of the GDS-DS in our study. The criterion to be placed in this stage was that the subject did not endure the neuropsychological examination proposed in the protocol and this was, in turn, an exclusion criterion for the PD group on which the present work is based. Some DS adults in the symptomatic stages of AD are not able to complete a neuropsychological examination [22]. The authors of the present study agree, as routine follow-up visits have encountered this setback. As a result, despite progress in terms of instruments adapted for people with ID, the neuropsychological tests used in the aforementioned studies and in daily clinical practice are not sufficiently valid to capture the deterioration in advanced stages of AD-DS nor for severe/profound intellectual disability [57,64,65]. Therefore, in terms of daily clinical practice, for people placed in stage 6 in our study, the authors recommend the use of adapted tools, such as the cognitive exploration scale for people with intellectual disability and extended support (ECDI-SE) or the modified ordinal scales of psychological development for people with intellectual disability (M-OSPD-ID). However, at the same time, this also means that using these instruments in the early stages of AD can lead to a ceiling effect on the scores. Future studies should focus on valid instruments for all phases of AD, avoiding ceiling and floor effects, regardless of the severity of symptoms.

Performance in the orientation subtest of BT-ID decreased significantly throughout the GDS-DS stages. Although not pathognomonic of AD, temporal disorientation is frequently observed in daily clinical practice in subjects with cognitive impairment. This requires semantic and episodic information activation [66] and has been linked to atrophy in the posterior hippocampus [67] and the disconnection between the posterior part of the right medial temporal gyrus and the posterior cingulate cortex [68]. The progressive loss of orientation has already been described in the transition from MCI to AD in people with DS [26]. In view of these facts, this subtest should be present in longitudinal follow-ups in individuals with ID.

Performance on executive functions (abstract thinking, free delay memory (stories), semantic and formal fluency) shows a slight decline with modest sustained effect sizes in some stages of the AD continuum. The anatomical substrate of these functions is linked with the temporoparietal, precuneus-posterior cingulate and occipital areas [24], which show a decreased volume [41,60] and loss of integrity in white matter tracts [58,69] in individuals with AD-DS. In addition, an increase in alpha band synchronization using magnetoencephalography has been found in the functional connectivity in the AD continuum in the general and in the DS population and is associated with cognitive decline in executive function, language and working memory [62]. Additionally, MCI-DS individuals with confirmed amyloid positivity who progress to AD have shown a pattern of increased delta activity in frontal regions [70]. The clinical relevance of these findings suggests that all these cognitive functions also should be examined in longitudinal clinical follow-ups

Declines in the CAMCOG-DS total score have been shown to be related to changes in all of the stages of the GDS-DS. A decline in performance on CAMCOG-DS has been found in the entire AD-DS continuum [13,26,28,62], regardless of whether the level of ID is mild or moderate [22]. Interestingly, performance on CAMCOG-DS is linked to amyloid deposition [71], and it is recommended that longitudinal studies assess cognitive changes related to ID and dementia [72]. Therefore, CAMCOG-DS could be a suitable instrument for anchoring the GDS-DS stages of our context, in a similar way that the mini examen cognoscitivo (MEC) [73] is anchored to the global deterioration scale [39] in the general population.

The *BRI* index of BRIEF-P [30] does not change significantly across the GDS-DS stages, but it drops slightly from the cognitive/behavioral stability to mild cognitive and/or behavioral impairment, stages 1 to 3, respectively. The authors selected the *BRI* index because worse scores on this index could differentiate between healthy and MCI-DS subjects [28], and our results partially replicate this. In light of these results, the inclusion of behavioral impairment in the GDS-DS seems appropriate. In addition, in the general population, mild behavioral impairment [19] improves the specificity of MCI as an at-risk state for incident dementia [74] and has been associated with higher AD polygenic risk scores [75]. Considering that behavioral changes are able to herald AD in the DS population [47], the authors recommend the use of the *BRI* index scores to detect behavioral impairment in the DS population in the earlier stages.

The main strength of the present study is that the GDS-DS, with the inclusion of behavioral aspects, allows the capture of subjects in the initial stages of AD-DS either due to memory or behavioral difficulties, in addition to being associated with performance in cognitive and behavioral tests that have been shown to be reliable in the DS population.

Additionally, the GDS-DS could be the first step in unifying the criteria for classifying the continuum of Alzheimer's disease in people with DS. It allows a common language for communication between clinicians and researchers and could be a basic instrument for the selection of samples in clinical trials in people with DS.

Furthermore, the GDS-DS, can also be used to inform families about the stages of Alzheimer's disease, when sufficient data from future studies have been collected to construct specific clinical profiles in combination with functional assessment staging. Knowing the continuum can complement the neurological diagnosis and facilitate family members' understanding of the expected prognosis.

However, some limitations have to be acknowledged. In this study, we used cross-sectional information that relied on the longitudinal data of a three-year follow-up study. We first wanted to verify that the GDS-DS was applicable to people with DS. As this has been proven to be feasible, future studies could investigate the application of the scale in longitudinal follow-ups to minimize possible cohort effects.

Additionally, our study was based on data collected from neuropsychological tests, behavioral questionnaires and informant interviews. Today, neuroimaging or neurophysiological techniques provide rich complementary data that correlate brain changes with cognitive features in aging and AD. Thus, future studies must include the linking of neuroimaging and neurophysiological data with the stages of GDS-DS.

5. Conclusions

In summary, GDS-DS is not designed as a diagnostic tool but as a quantitative measure of disability. The insights delivered in this paper show that the proposed GDS-DS rating scale represents an important attempt at staging people with DS throughout the continuum of AD, providing a unique method of classification that can be useful in clinical trials and in daily clinical practice. As noted in the development of the original GDS [39], the limits of each of the GDS-DS stages are not axiomatic, but they do allow graduation as a guideline that facilitates the monitoring of the AD-DS continuum.

Supplementary Materials: The following supporting information can be downloaded at: https://www.mdpi.com/article/10.3390/ijerph20065096/s1, Table S1: Effect sizes between groups of the GDS-DS stages.

Author Contributions: Conceptualization, E.R.-H. and S.E.-C.; methodology, E.R.-H. and S.E.-C.; software, E.R.-H.; validation, S.E.-C., R.N. and J.G.-A.; formal analysis, E.R.-H.; investigation, E.R.-H. and S.E.-C.; data curation, E.R.-H.; writing—original draft preparation, E.R.-H.; writing—review and editing, S.E.-C., R.N. and J.G.-A.; supervision, S.E.-C. and R.N.; project administration, S.E.-C., J.G.-A. and E.R.-H.; funding acquisition, S.E.-C., R.N. and J.G.-A. All authors have read and agreed to the published version of the manuscript.

Funding: This research was funded by the Spanish Government, grant number PI12/02019, PSI-2014-53524-P. The APC was funded by S.E.-C,'s SESMDI research start-up funds.

Institutional Review Board Statement: The study was conducted in accordance with the Declaration of Helsinki and approved by the Institutional Review Board and Research Ethics Committee of the Parc Hospitalari Martí i Julià (Approval Code: S041-775; Approval Date: 4 July 2012).

Informed Consent Statement: Informed consent was obtained from all subjects involved in the study.

Data Availability Statement: The data presented in this study are available on request from the corresponding author.

Acknowledgments: The authors would like to thank the participants and their families enrolled in this study.

Conflicts of Interest: The authors declare no conflict of interest. The funders had no role in the design of the study; in the collection, analyses, or interpretation of data; in the writing of the manuscript; or in the decision to publish the results.

References

1. Englund, A.; Jonsson, B.; Zander, C.S.; Gustafsson, J.; Annerén, G. Changes in Mortality and Causes of Death in the Swedish Down Syndrome Population. *Am. J. Med. Genet. Part A* **2013**, *161*, 642–649. [CrossRef] [PubMed]
2. Zeilinger, E.L.; Gärtner, C.; Janicki, M.P.; Esralew, L.; Weber, G. Practical Applications of the NTG-EDSD for Screening Adults with Intellectual Disability for Dementia: A German-Language Version Feasibility Study. *J. Intellect. Dev. Disabil.* **2016**, *41*, 42–49. [CrossRef]
3. Tosh, J.L.; Rhymes, E.R.; Mumford, P.; Whittaker, H.T.; Pulford, L.J.; Noy, S.J.; Cleverley, K.; Strydom, A.; Fisher, E.; Wiseman, F.; et al. Genetic Dissection of down Syndrome-Associated Alterations in APP/Amyloid-β Biology Using Mouse Models. *Sci. Rep.* **2021**, *11*, 5736. [CrossRef] [PubMed]

4. Wiseman, F.K.; Pulford, L.J.; Barkus, C.; Liao, F.; Portelius, E.; Webb, R.; Chávez-Gutiérrez, L.; Cleverley, K.; Noy, S.; Sheppard, O.; et al. Trisomy of Human Chromosome 21 Enhances Amyloid-b Deposition Independently of an Extra Copy of APP. *Brain* **2018**, *141*, 2457–2474. [CrossRef]
5. Hithersay, R.; Startin, C.M.; Hamburg, S.; Mok, K.Y.; Hardy, J.; Fisher, E.M.C.C.; Tybulewicz, V.L.J.; Nizetic, D.; Strydom, A.; Mok, K.Y.; et al. Association of Dementia with Mortality among Adults with Down Syndrome Older Than 35 Years. *JAMA Neurol.* **2019**, *76*, 152–160. [CrossRef] [PubMed]
6. Jack, C.R.; Bennett, D.A.; Blennow, K.; Carrillo, M.C.; Dunn, B.; Haeberlein, S.B.; Holtzman, D.M.; Jagust, W.; Jessen, F.; Karlawish, J.; et al. NIA-AA Research Framework: Toward a Biological Definition of Alzheimer's Disease. *Alzheimers Dement.* **2018**, *14*, 535–562. [CrossRef]
7. Head, E.; Lott, I.T.; Wilcock, D.M.; Lemere, C.A. Aging in Down Syndrome and the Development of Alzheimer's Disease Neuropathology. *Curr. Alzheimer Res.* **2015**, *13*, 18–29. [CrossRef] [PubMed]
8. Hithersay, R.; Baksh, R.A.; Startin, C.M.; Wijeratne, P.; Hamburg, S.; Carter, B.; Strydom, A.; Strydom, A.; Fisher, E.; Nizetic, D.; et al. Optimal Age and Outcome Measures for Alzheimer's Disease Prevention Trials in People with Down Syndrome. *Alzheimers Dement.* **2021**, *17*, 595–604. [CrossRef]
9. Sinai, A.; Mokrysz, C.; Bernal, J.; Bohnen, I.; Bonell, S.; Courtenay, K.; Dodd, K.; Gazizova, D.; Hassiotis, A.; Hillier, R.; et al. Predictors of Age of Diagnosis and Survival of Alzheimer's Disease in Down Syndrome. *J. Alzheimers Dis.* **2018**, *61*, 717–728. [CrossRef] [PubMed]
10. Firth, N.C.; Startin, C.M.; Hithersay, R.; Hamburg, S.; Wijeratne, P.A.; Mok, K.Y.; Hardy, J.; Alexander, D.C.; Strydom, A. Aging Related Cognitive Changes Associated with Alzheimer's Disease in Down Syndrome. *Ann. Clin. Transl. Neurol.* **2018**, *5*, 741–751. [CrossRef]
11. Strydom, A.; Coppus, A.; Blesa, R.; Danek, A.; Fortea, J.; Hardy, J.; Levin, J.; Nuebling, G.; Rebillat, A.; Ritchie, C.; et al. Alzheimer's Disease in Down Syndrome: An Overlooked Population for Prevention Trials. *Alzheimers Dement. Transl. Res. Clin. Interv.* **2018**, *4*, 703–713. [CrossRef] [PubMed]
12. Lott, I.T.; Head, E. Dementia in Down Syndrome: Unique Insights for Alzheimer Disease Research. *Nat. Rev. Neurol.* **2019**, *15*, 135–147. [CrossRef]
13. Benejam, B.; Videla, L.; Vilaplana, E.; Barroeta, I.; Carmona-Iragui, M.; Altuna, M.; Valldeneu, S.; Fernandez, S.; Giménez, S.; Iulita, F.; et al. Diagnosis of Prodromal and Alzheimer's Disease Dementia in Adults with Down Syndrome Using Neuropsychological Tests. *Alzheimers Dement. Diagnosis, Assess. Dis. Monit.* **2020**, *12*, e12047. [CrossRef]
14. Startin, C.M.; D'Souza, H.; Ball, G.; Hamburg, S.; Hithersay, R.; Hughes, K.M.O.; Massand, E.; Karmiloff-Smith, A.; Thomas, M.S.C.; Strydom, A.; et al. Health Comorbidities and Cognitive Abilities across the Lifespan in down Syndrome. *J. Neurodev. Disord.* **2020**, *12*, 4. [CrossRef] [PubMed]
15. Rafii, M.S.; Ances, B.M.; Schupf, N.; Krinsky-McHale, S.J.; Mapstone, M.; Silverman, W.; Lott, I.; Klunk, W.; Head, E.; Christian, B.; et al. The AT(N) Framework for Alzheimer's Disease in Adults with Down Syndrome. *Alzheimers Dement. Diagnosis, Assess. Dis. Monit.* **2020**, *12*, e12062. [CrossRef]
16. Jessen, F.; Kleineidam, L.; Wolfsgruber, S.; Bickel, H.; Brettschneider, C.; Fuchs, A.; Kaduszkiewicz, H.; König, H.H.; Mallon, T.; Mamone, S.; et al. Prediction of Dementia of Alzheimer Type by Different Types of Subjective Cognitive Decline. *Alzheimers Dement.* **2020**, *16*, 1745–1749. [CrossRef]
17. Rostamzadeh, A.; Bohr, L.; Wagner, M.; Baethge, C.; Jessen, F. Progression of Subjective Cognitive Decline to MCI or Dementia in Relation to Biomarkers for Alzheimer Disease: A Meta-Analysis. *Neurology* **2022**, *99*, e1866–e1874. [CrossRef] [PubMed]
18. Dubois, B.; Villain, N.; Frisoni, G.B.; Rabinovici, G.D.; Sabbagh, M.; Cappa, S.; Bejanin, A.; Bombois, S.; Epelbaum, S.; Teichmann, M.; et al. Clinical Diagnosis of Alzheimer's Disease: Recommendations of the International Working Group. *Lancet Neurol.* **2021**, *20*, 484–496. [CrossRef] [PubMed]
19. Ismail, Z.; Smith, E.E.; Geda, Y.; Sultzer, D.; Brodaty, H.; Smith, G.; Agüera-Ortiz, L.; Sweet, R.; Miller, D.; Lyketsos, C.G. Neuropsychiatric Symptoms as Early Manifestations of Emergent Dementia: Provisional Diagnostic Criteria for Mild Behavioral Impairment. *Alzheimers Dement.* **2016**, *12*, 195–202. [CrossRef] [PubMed]
20. Jiang, F.; Cheng, C.; Huang, J.; Chen, Q.; Le, W. Mild Behavioral Impairment: An Early Sign and Predictor of Alzheimer's Disease Dementia. *Curr. Alzheimer Res.* **2022**, *19*, 407–419. [CrossRef]
21. de Oliveira, L.C.; de Paula Faria, D. Pharmacological Approaches to the Treatment of Dementia in Down Syndrome: A Systematic Review of Randomized Clinical Studies. *Molecules* **2022**, *27*, 3244. [CrossRef] [PubMed]
22. Videla, L.; Benejam, B.; Pegueroles, J.; Carmona-Iragui, M.; Padilla, C.; Fernández, S.; Barroeta, I.; Altuna, M.; Valldeneu, S.; Garzón, D.; et al. Longitudinal Clinical and Cognitive Changes Along the Alzheimer Disease Continuum in Down Syndrome + Supplemental Content. *JAMA Netw. Open* **2022**, *5*, 2225573. [CrossRef]
23. Rösner, P.; Berger, J.; Tarasova, D.; Birkner, J.; Kaiser, H.; Diefenbacher, A.; Sappok, T. Assessment of Dementia in a Clinical Sample of Persons with Intellectual Disability. *J. Appl. Res. Intellect. Disabil.* **2021**, *34*, 1618–1629. [CrossRef]
24. Benejam, B.; Aranha, M.R.; Videla, L.; Padilla, C.; Valldeneu, S.; Fernández, S.; Altuna, M.; Carmona-Iragui, M.; Barroeta, I.; Iulita, M.F.; et al. Neural Correlates of Episodic Memory in Adults with Down Syndrome and Alzheimer's Disease. *Alzheimers. Res. Ther.* **2022**, *14*, 123. [CrossRef]

25. Fonseca, L.M.; Padilla, C.; Jones, E.; Neale, N.; Haddad, G.G.; Mattar, G.P.; Barros, E.; Clare, I.C.H.; Busatto, G.F.; Bottino, C.M.C.; et al. Amnestic and Non-Amnestic Symptoms of Dementia: An International Study of Alzheimer´s Disease in People with Down's Syndrome. *Int. J. Geriatr. Psychiatry* **2020**, *35*, 650–661. [CrossRef]
26. García-Alba, J.; Ramírez-Toraño, F.; Esteba-Castillo, S.; Bruña, R.; Moldenhauer, F.; Novell, R.; Romero-Medina, V.; Maestú, F.; Fernández, A. Neuropsychological and Neurophysiological Characterization of Mild Cognitive Impairment and Alzheimer's Disease in Down Syndrome. *Neurobiol. Aging* **2019**, *84*, 70–79. [CrossRef]
27. Startin, C.M.; Hamburg, S.; Hithersay, R.; Al-Janabi, T.; Mok, K.Y.; Hardy, J.; Strydom, A.; Fisher, E.; Nizetic, D.; Tybulewicz, V.; et al. Cognitive Markers of Preclinical and Prodromal Alzheimer's Disease in Down Syndrome. *Alzheimers Dement.* **2019**, *15*, 245–257. [CrossRef]
28. Esteba-Castillo, S.; Garcia-Alba, J.; Rodríguez-Hildago, E.; Vaquero, L.; Novell, R.; Moldenhauer, F.; Castellanos, M.Á. Proposed Diagnostic Criteria for Mild Cognitive Impairment in Down Syndrome Population. *J. Appl. Res. Intellect. Disabil.* **2022**, *35*, 495–505. [CrossRef]
29. Dubois, B.; Feldman, H.H.; Jacova, C.; Hampel, H.; Molinuevo, J.L.; Blennow, K.; DeKosky, S.T.; Gauthier, S.; Selkoe, D.; Bateman, R.; et al. Advancing Research Diagnostic Criteria for Alzheimer's Disease: The IWG-2 Criteria. *Lancet Neurol.* **2014**, *13*, 614–629. [CrossRef]
30. Gioia, G.A.; Isquith, P.K.; Guy, S.C.; Kenworthy, L.; Baron, I.S. Behavior Rating Inventory of Executive Function. *Child Neuropsychol.* **2000**, *6*, 235–238. [CrossRef]
31. Silverman, W.; Krinsky-McHale, S.J.; Lai, F.; Diana Rosas, H.; Hom, C.; Doran, E.; Pulsifer, M.; Lott, I.; Schupf, N.; Andrews, H.; et al. Evaluation of the National Task Group-Early Detection Screen for Dementia: Sensitivity to 'Mild Cognitive Impairment' in Adults with Down Syndrome. *J. Appl. Res. Intellect. Disabil.* **2021**, *34*, 905–915. [CrossRef]
32. Esteba-castillo, S.; Dalmau-bueno, A.; Ribas-vidal, N.; Vilà-alsina, M.; Novell-alsina, R.; García-alba, J. Adaptación y Validación Del Cambridge Examination for Mental Disorders of Older People with Down's Syndrome and Others with Intellectual Disabilities (CAMDEX-DS) En Población Española Con Discapacidad Intelectual. *Rev. Neurol.* **2013**, *57*, 337–346. [CrossRef]
33. Krinsky-McHale, S.J.; Hartley, S.; Hom, C.; Pulsifer, M.; Clare, I.C.H.; Handen, B.L.; Lott, I.T.; Schupf, N.; Silverman, W. A Modified Cued Recall Test for Detecting Prodromal AD in Adults with Down Syndrome. *Alzheimers Dement. Diagn. Assess. Dis. Monit.* **2022**, *14*, e12361. [CrossRef]
34. Robert, P.; Ferris, S.; Gauthier, S.; Ihl, R.; Winblad, B.; Tennigkeit, F. Review of Alzheimer's Disease Scales: Is There a Need for a New Multi-Domain Scale for Therapy Evaluation in Medical Practice? *Alzheimers. Res. Ther.* **2010**, *2*, 24. [CrossRef]
35. Morris, J.C. The Clinical Dementia Rating (CDR). *Neurology* **1993**, *43*, 2412.2-a. [CrossRef]
36. Knopman, D.S.; Kramer, J.H.; Boeve, B.F.; Caselli, R.J.; Graff-Radford, N.R.; Mendez, M.F.; Miller, B.L.; Mercaldo, N. Development of Methodology for Conducting Clinical Trials in Frontotemporal Lobar Degeneration. *Brain* **2008**, *131*, 2957–2968. [CrossRef]
37. Mioshi, E.; Flanagan, E.; Knopman, D. Detecting Clinical Change with the CDR-FTLD: Differences between FTLD and AD Dementia. *Int. J. Geriatr. Psychiatry* **2017**, *32*, 977–982. [CrossRef]
38. Lessov-Schlaggar, C.N.; Del Rosario, O.L.; Morris, J.C.; Ances, B.M.; Schlaggar, B.L.; Constantino, J.N. Adaptation of the Clinical Dementia Rating Scale for Adults with down Syndrome. *J. Neurodev. Disord.* **2019**, *11*, 39. [CrossRef]
39. Reisberg, B.; Ferris, S.H.; de León, M.J.; Crook, T. The Global Deterioration Scale for Assessment of Primary Degenerative Dementia. *Am. J. Psychiatry* **1982**, *139*, 1136–1139. [CrossRef]
40. Reisberg, B. Functional Assessment Staging (FAST). *Psychopharmacol. Bull.* **1988**, *24*, 653–659.
41. Sabbagh, M.N.; Cooper, K.; DeLange, J.; Stoehr, J.D.; Thind, K.; Lahti, T.; Reisberg, B.; Sue, L.; Vedders, L.; Fleming, S.R.; et al. Functional, Global and Cognitive Decline Correlates to Accumulation of Alzheimers Pathology in MCI and AD. *Curr. Alzheimer Res.* **2010**, *7*, 280–286. [CrossRef] [PubMed]
42. Bobinski, M.; Wegiel, J.; Wisniewski, H.M.; Tarnawski, M.; Mlodzik, B.; Reisberg, B.; de Leon, M.J.; Miller, D.C. Atrophy of Hippocampal Formation Subdivisions Correlates with Stage and Duration of Alzheimer Disease. *Dement. Geriatr. Cogn. Disord.* **1995**, *6*, 205–210. [CrossRef]
43. Bello López, J.; Piñol Ripoll, G.; Lleó Bisa, A.; Lladó Plarrumaní, A. Protocol de Diagnòstic i Tractament de La Malaltia d'Alzheimer. Available online: https://www.scneurologia.cat/wp-content/uploads/2019/01/Actualitzaci%C3%B3-Guia-M%C3%A8dicad%E2%80%99Alzheimer-de-la-Societat-Catalana-de-Neurologia-%E2%80%93-2015.pdf (accessed on 26 December 2022).
44. Lladó Plarrumaní, A.; Santaeugènia González, S.J.; Melendo Azuela, E.M. Pla d'atenció Sanitària a Les Persones Amb Deteriorament Cognitiu Lleu i Demència de Catalunya (PLADEMCAT). Available online: https://salutweb.gencat.cat/web/.content/_departament/ambits-estrategics/atencio-sociosanitaria/docs/plademcat/plademcat-model-asistencial.pdf (accessed on 26 December 2022).
45. Benejam, B.; Fortea, J.; Molina-López, R.; Videla, S. Patterns of Performance on the Modified Cued Recall Test in Spanish Adults with down Syndrome with and without Dementia. *Am. J. Intellect. Dev. Disabil.* **2015**, *120*, 481–489. [CrossRef] [PubMed]
46. Krinsky-McHale, S.J.; Devenny, D.A.; Silverman, W. Changes in Explicit Memory Associated with Early Dementia in Adults with Down's Syndrome. *J. Intellect. Disabil. Res.* **2002**, *46*, 198–208. [CrossRef]
47. Ball, S.L.; Holland, A.J.; Treppner, P.; Watson, P.C.; Huppert, F.A. Executive Dysfunction and Its Association with Personality and Behaviour Changes in the Development of Alzheimer's Disease in Adults with Down Syndrome and Mild to Moderate Learning Disabilities. *Br. J. Clin. Psychol.* **2008**, *47*, 1–29. [CrossRef]

48. Janicki, M.P.; McCallion, P.; Splaine, M.; Santos, F.H.; Keller, S.M.; Watchman, K. Consensus Statement of the International Summit on Intellectual Disability and Dementia Related to Nomenclature. *Intellect. Dev. Disabil.* **2017**, *55*, 338–346. [CrossRef]
49. Moss, S.; Ibbotson, B.; Prosser, H.; Goldberg, D.; Patel, P.; Simpson, N. Validity of the PAS-ADD for Detecting Psychiatric Symptoms in Adults with Learning Disability (Mental Retardation). *Soc. Psychiatry Psychiatr. Epidemiol.* **1997**, *32*, 344–354. [CrossRef]
50. Rubenstein, E.; Hartley, S.; Bishop, L. Epidemiology of Dementia and Alzheimer Disease in Individuals with Down Syndrome. *JAMA Neurol.* **2020**, *77*, 262–264. [CrossRef]
51. Association, A.P. *Diagnostic and Statistical Manual of Mental Disorders*, 5th ed.; American Psychiatric Publishing: Washington, DC, USA, 2013; ISBN 978-08-9042-555-8.
52. Kaufman, A.; Nadeen, L.; Kaufman, L. *Kaufman Brief Intelligence Test*, 2nd ed.; Pearson, Inc.: Minneapolis, MN, USA, 2004.
53. Sparrow, S.; Cicchetti, D.; Balla, D. *Vineland Adaptive Behavior Scales-2nd Edition Manual*, 2nd ed.; NCS, P., Ed.; Pearson, Inc.: Minneapolis, MN, USA, 2005.
54. Esteba-Castillo, S.; Peña-Casanova, J.; García-Alba, J.; Castellanos, M.A.; Torrents-Rodas, D.; Rodríguez, E.; Deus-Yela, J.; Caixàs, A.; Novell-Alsina, R. Test Barcelona Para Discapacidad Intelectual: Un Nuevo Instrumento Para La Valoración Neuropsicológica Clínica de Adultos Con Discapacidad Intelectual. *Rev. Neurol.* **2017**, *64*, 433–444. [CrossRef]
55. Organization(WHO), W.H. *The ICD-10 Classification of Mental and Behavioural Disorders*; World Health Organization: Genève, Switzerland, 1993; ISBN 9789241544559.
56. García-Alba, J.; Esteba-Castillo, S.; López, M.Á.C.; Hidalgo, E.R.; Vidal, N.R.; Díaz, F.M.; Novell-Alsina, R. Validation and Normalization of the Tower of London-Drexel University Test 2nd Edition in an Adult Population with Intellectual Disability. *Span. J. Psychol.* **2017**, *20*, E32. [CrossRef]
57. Krinsky-McHale, S.J.; Zigman, W.B.; Lee, J.H.; Schupf, N.; Pang, D.; Listwan, T.; Kovacs, C.; Silverman, W. Promising Outcome Measures of Early Alzheimer's Dementia in Adults with Down Syndrome. *Alzheimers Dement. Diagn. Assess. Dis. Monit.* **2020**, *12*, e12044. [CrossRef]
58. Fenoll, R.; Pujol, J.; Esteba-Castillo, S.; De Sola, S.; Ribas-Vidal, N.; García-Alba, J.; Sánchez-Benavides, G.; Martínez-Vilavella, M.G.; Deus, J.; Dierssen, M.; et al. Anomalous White Matter Structure and the Effect of Age in Down Syndrome Patients. *J. Alzheimers Dis.* **2017**, *57*, 61–70. [CrossRef] [PubMed]
59. Krinsky-McHale, S.J.; Silverman, W. Dementia and Mild Cognitive Impairment in Adults with Intellectual Disability: Issues of Diagnosis. *Dev. Disabil. Res. Rev.* **2013**, *18*, 31–42. [CrossRef]
60. Pujol, J.; Fenoll, R.; Ribas-Vidal, N.; Martínez-Vilavella, G.; Blanco-Hinojo, L.; García-Alba, J.; Deus, J.; Novell, R.; Esteba-Castillo, S. A Longitudinal Study of Brain Anatomy Changes Preceding Dementia in Down Syndrome. *NeuroImage Clin.* **2018**, *18*, 160–166. [CrossRef] [PubMed]
61. Sheehan, R.; Sinai, A.; Bass, N.; Blatchford, P.; Bohnen, I.; Courtenay, K.; Hassiotis, A.; Markar, T.; Mccarthy, J. Dementia Diagnostic Criteria in Down Syndrome. *Int. J. Geriatr. Psychiatry* **2015**, *30*, 857–863. [CrossRef] [PubMed]
62. Ramírez-Toraño, F.; García-Alba, J.; Bruña, R.; Esteba-Castillo, S.; Vaquero, L.; Pereda, E.; Maestú, F.; Fernández, A. Hypersynchronized Magnetoencephalography Brain Networks in Patients with Mild Cognitive Impairment and Alzheimer's Disease in down Syndrome. *Brain Connect.* **2021**, *11*, 725–733. [CrossRef]
63. Grissom, R.J. Probability of the Superior Outcome of One Treatment over Another. *J. Appl. Psychol.* **1994**, *79*, 314–316. [CrossRef]
64. Elliott-King, J.; Shaw, S.; Bandelow, S.; Devshi, R.; Kassam, S.; Hogervorst, E. A Critical Literature Review of the Effectiveness of Various Instruments in the Diagnosis of Dementia in Adults with Intellectual Disabilities. *Alzheimers Dement. Diagnosis, Assess. Dis. Monit.* **2016**, *4*, 126–148. [CrossRef]
65. Dekker, A.D.; Wissing, M.B.G.; Ulgiati, A.M.; Bijl, B.; van Gool, G.; Groen, M.R.; Grootendorst, E.S.; van der Wal, I.A.; Hobbelen, J.S.M.; De Deyn, P.P.; et al. Dementia in People with Severe or Profound Intellectual (and Multiple) Disabilities: Focus Group Research into Relevance, Symptoms and Training Needs. *J. Appl. Res. Intellect. Disabil.* **2021**, *34*, 1602–1617. [CrossRef]
66. Devinsky, O.; D'Esposito, M. Neurology of Cognitive and Behavioral Disorders: Sistema de Descoberta Para FCCN. Available online: https://vpn4.ulusofona.pt:10443/proxy/059de34c/https/eds.s.ebscohost.com/eds/detail/detail?vid=11&sid=33a120e4-04f2-4927-b84b-ad716e0b3a54%40redis&bdata=JkF1dGhUeXBlPWlwLHNoaWImbGFuZz1wdC1wdCZzaXRlPWVkcy1saXZlJnNjb3BlPXNpdGU%3D#AN=176888&db=e000bww (accessed on 12 October 2022).
67. Yew, B.; Alladi, S.; Shailaja, M.; Hodges, J.R.; Hornberger, M. Lost and Forgotten? Orientation Versus Memory in Alzheimer's Disease and Frontotemporal Dementia. *J. Alzheimers Dis.* **2012**, *33*, 473–481. [CrossRef]
68. Yamashita, K.; Uehara, T.; Prawiroharjo, P.; Yamashita, K.; Togao, O.; Hiwatashi, A.; Taniwaki, Y.; Utsunomiya, H.; Matsushita, T.; Yamasaki, R.; et al. Functional Connectivity Change between Posterior Cingulate Cortex and Ventral Attention Network Relates to the Impairment of Orientation for Time in Alzheimer's Disease Patients. *Brain Imaging Behav.* **2019**, *13*, 154–161. [CrossRef]
69. Bazydlo, A.; Zammit, M.; Wu, M.; Dean, D.; Johnson, S.; Tudorascu, D.; Cohen, A.; Cody, K.; Ances, B.; Laymon, C.; et al. White Matter Microstructure Associations with Episodic Memory in Adults with Down Syndrome: A Tract-Based Spatial Statistics Study. *J. Neurodev. Disord.* **2021**, *13*, 17. [CrossRef]
70. Fernández, A.; Ramírez-Toraño, F.; Bruña, R.; Zuluaga, P.; Esteba-Castillo, S.; Abásolo, D.; Moldenhauer, F.; Shumbayawonda, E.; Maestú, F.; García-Alba, J. Brain Signal Complexity in Adults with Down Syndrome: Potential Application in the Detection of Mild Cognitive Impairment. *Front. Aging Neurosci.* **2022**, *14*, 988540. [CrossRef]

71. Cole, J.H.; Annus, T.; Wilson, L.R.; Remtulla, R.; Hong, Y.T.; Fryer, T.D.; Acosta-Cabronero, J.; Cardenas-Blanco, A.; Smith, R.; Menon, D.K.; et al. Brain-Predicted Age in Down Syndrome Is Associated with Beta Amyloid Deposition and Cognitive Decline. *Neurobiol. Aging* **2017**, *56*, 41–49. [CrossRef]
72. Paiva, A.F.; Nolan, A.; Thumser, C.; Santos, F.H. Screening of Cognitive Changes in Adults with Intellectual Disabilities: A Systematic Review. *Brain Sci.* **2020**, *10*, 848. [CrossRef]
73. Lobo, A.; Ezquerra, J.; Gómez Burgada, F.; Sala, J.M.; Seva Díaz, A. Cognocitive Mini-Test (a Simple Practical Test to Detect Intellectual Changes in Medical Patients). *Actas Luso. Esp. Neurol. Psiquiatr. Cienc. Afines* **1979**, *7*, 189–202.
74. McGirr, A.; Nathan, S.; Ghahremani, M.; Gill, S.; Smith, E.E.; Ismail, Z. Progression to Dementia or Reversion to Normal Cognition in Mild Cognitive Impairment as a Function of Late-Onset Neuropsychiatric Symptoms. *Neurology* **2022**, *98*, e2132–e2139. [CrossRef]
75. Creese, B.; Arathimos, R.; Brooker, H.; Aarsland, D.; Corbett, A.; Lewis, C.; Ballard, C.; Ismail, Z. Genetic Risk for Alzheimer's Disease, Cognition, and Mild Behavioral Impairment in Healthy Older Adults. *Alzheimers Dement. Diagn. Assess. Dis. Monit.* **2021**, *13*, e12164. [CrossRef]

Disclaimer/Publisher's Note: The statements, opinions and data contained in all publications are solely those of the individual author(s) and contributor(s) and not of MDPI and/or the editor(s). MDPI and/or the editor(s) disclaim responsibility for any injury to people or property resulting from any ideas, methods, instructions or products referred to in the content.

Article

The Pictorial Screening Memory Test (P-MIS) for Adults with Moderate Intellectual Disability and Alzheimer's Disease

Emili Rodríguez-Hidalgo [1], Javier García-Alba [2], Maria Buxó [3], Ramon Novell [1,3] and Susana Esteba-Castillo [1,3,*]

[1] Specialized Service in Mental Health and Intellectual Disability, Institute of Health Assistance, Parc Hospitalari Martí i Julià, Catalonia, 17190 Girona, Spain
[2] Research and Psychology in Education Department, Complutense University of Madrid, 28040 Madrid, Spain
[3] Neurodevelopmental Group [Girona Biomedical Research Institute]-IDIBGI, Institute of Health Assistance (IAS), Parc Hospitalari Martí i Julià, Catalonia, 17190 Girona, Spain
* Correspondence: susanna.esteba@ias.cat; Tel.: +34-972-18-26-00

Abstract: In this study, we examined normative data and diagnostic accuracy of a pictorial screening test to detect memory impairment for mild cognitive impairment (MCI) and Alzheimer's disease (AD) in Spanish-speaking adults with intellectual disability (ID). A total of 94 volunteers with ID (60 controls, 17 MCI, and 17 AD), were evaluated by neuropsychological tests including the PMIS-ID in a cross-sectional validation study. Discriminative validity between the MCI, AD, and control group was analyzed by the area under the ROC curve. A cut-off score of 4.5 on the immediate recall trial had a sensitivity of 69% and a specificity of 80% to detect memory impairment (AUC = 0.685; 95% CI = 0.506–0.863) in the AD group. The PMIS-ID is a useful screening test to rule out a diagnosis of memory decline in people with moderate level of ID and AD, and it shows good psychometric properties.

Keywords: screening; memory; mild cognitive impairment; Alzheimer's disease; dementia intellectual disability

1. Introduction

Intellectual disability (ID) is a neurodevelopment disorder affecting intellectual functioning and adaptive behavior [1]. Globally, the prevalence of ID varies between 0.05 and 1.55% [2]. The underlying health conditions and the increased life expectancy of this population makes them more vulnerable to developing mild cognitive impairment (MCI) and dementia [3,4]. Although the epidemiological data of MCI and dementia in people with ID without Down's syndrome (DS) has not been accurately set, recently, in Japanese people, the prevalence data for MCI hovers around 3% from the age of 45 onwards, and from 0.8% to 13.9% in those aged between 45 and 74 years old for dementia [5].

There is increasing evidence of a link between neurodevelopment disorders as ID and dementia [6]. Specifically, Alzheimer disease (AD) is the most common syndrome of dementia in DS [7], with incidence rates from 75% to 100% in those aged 60 and older [8]. Beyond DS, people with autism spectrum disorder (ASD) with ID are also at high risk for developing early onset AD (EOAD) [9], and ASD behaviors may be present in geriatric people with MCI and AD without ID [10]. Cerebral palsy (CP) by itself increases the risk of EOAD and related dementias [11], having an accelerated aging that predisposes patients to MCI and AD [12]. Based on these facts, certain ID conditions increase the risk of suffering AD. Therefore, early detection of MCI and AD in people with ID is required to implement appropriate interventions on the optimal therapeutic window.

It is well-known that identifying MCI or AD in people with ID poses a challenge to clinicians. Strengths and weaknesses of the cognitive and behavioral phenotype of each etiology must be taken into account when considering changes that may herald MCI or dementia in aging [13]. Therefore, some studies try to cognitively characterize the stages of MCI and AD in ID population. In people with mild or moderate levels of ID and unspecified etiology, decline in orientation questions and depressive symptoms [14] or decline in memory measured by a paired-learning task [15] have been found. By the Dementia Questionnaire for Mentally Retarded People [16], memory and orientation were altered [17]. Furthermore, cognitive decline is similar between people with ID and the general population with AD [18], exhibiting difficulties in learning and visuoverbal memory, semantic verbal fluency, and attention/executive functions, measured with the Fuld Object-Memory Evaluation [19], the Controlled Oral Word Association Test [20], and the Color Trail Test [21], respectively. In people with moderate and severe levels of ID, significantly lower scores were found in autobiographical memory and orientation in people with AD compared to healthy people [22]. In this same work, performance on a modified Objective Memory Test was lower in the group with AD, but only in the immediate recognition trial and in both immediate and delayed memory subtests of a Picture Recognition Test, a visuoverbal learning and memory test developed for the purpose of their work, that has proven able to detect memory troubles in people with moderate and severe levels of ID and DS [23]. Despite the different etiologies studied, memory decline arises as a common factor associated with MCI or AD.

As AD is the most common form of dementia and it is especially linked with DS, the majority of studies focused on this population have used cognitive measures. In this sense, a recent study of functional brain connectivity in people with DS [24] showed that low scores on the Cambridge Cognitive Examination for Older Adults with Down's Syndrome (CAMCOG-DS) Spanish version [25] and decreased performance in verbal and visual memory appear to be key indicators of MCI and AD. Also, a slight impairment in delayed verbal and visual memory could be considered as a potential cognitive marker of MCI, with an increase in memory deficit in AD stage [26,27]. However, more important is the proposal model for MCI diagnosis in which decline or change in the Behaviour Regulaltion Index (BRI) from the Behaviour Rating Inventory of Executive Function-Informant's Report (BRIEF) [28], and in the delayed verbal and visual memory domains from the Barcelona Test for Intellectual Disability (TB-DI) [29] are good predictors for MCI diagnosis [30]. Upon collecting these data, it is evident that memory declines across the AD continuum. Hence, there is a need to develop sensitive and screening test for daily clinical practice to detect memory changes associated with MCI or AD in this population.

Memory tests including a delayed recall trial are useful to detect longitudinal changes [31], as are recognition trials that improve the sensibility to detect retrieval alterations [32]. The word-based Free and Cued Selective Reminding Test (FCSRT) [33] for the general population and the pictorial Cued Recall Test (CRT) [34] for people with DS are tests with controlled learning techniques to optimize the coding processes [35] that are specially altered in the early stage of AD. It is well-known that scores of word and pictorial versions are not equivalent [36,37], although it is suggested that poor results in the free recall essay are associated with a reduction of the hippocampal volume in both tests [38]. As of today, a few screening tests are available that yield robust data with high accuracy in detecting memory deficits in the general population. For instance, the Memory Impairment Screen (MIS) [39] is a brief tool of four items that controls learning and cued recall, providing excellent properties to detect individuals at higher risk to develop AD. Different MIS-based versions are currently available, such as the Picture-Based Memory Impairment Screen (PMIS) [40], with four pictorial stimuli for English people with low levels of education. A Spanish pictorial memory test is also available that reports preliminary results for the general population with amnesic MCI and AD [41], as well as for people with DS [42]. When compared to the general population, there is no picture memory screening test available for Spanish people with ID. Furthermore, the administration of the available tests is hard to acquire for people with ID and time is short for routine appointments. Clearly, there is a need to develop valid memory screening tests suitable for primary care and specialized services in this population.

In light of these facts, the main aims of the current study were (a) to adapt the PMIS [40] for people with ID, (b) to provide normative data, and (c) to assess its feasibility as a screening tool for memory decline to discriminate healthy ID subjects from those with amnestic impairment typical of MCI or AD.

2. Materials and Methods

2.1. Participants

We undertook a prospective single-center cross-validation study with a convenience sample from December 2017 to December 2018. A total of 116 subjects recruited from the Specialized Service in Mental Health Unit for Adults with ID (SESM-DI, Parc Hospitalari Martí i Julià, Girona, Spain) were identified. All the participants were 18 years old or older, with a mild or moderate level of ID according to DSM-5 criteria (5th ed.; DSM-5) and with no drug treatment that could had significant effects on cognition. Those showing psychiatric or neurological conditions that could cause a dementia-like presentation or cognitive decline (depression, clinical hypo/hyperthyroidism, uncontrolled B9/B12 vitamin deficiency, seizures, delirium) and uncorrected auditory or visual sensory impairment that would make a neuropsychological assessment impossible were excluded. Of the subjects selected, 12 did not agree to participate in the study, 4 were excluded due to an absence of expressive language, and 6 more were excluded due to non-stable medical conditions at the moment of the assessment. The final sample consisted of 94 adults with ID (mean age = 47.33 ± 5.18 years; males = 57.4%, females = 42.6%) due to different etiology (54 Down's syndrome, 4 tuberous sclerosis, 4 fragile X syndrome, 2 cerebral palsy, and 30 unknown). The baseline level of at least one year of all participants was available through annual follow-up in our service, in which most of the cognitive and functional tests that are part of the present study are routinely administered. The sample was divided into three groups: CN group (subjects without symptoms of MCI or AD), MCI group (subjects fulfilling criteria for MCI diagnosis), and AD group (subjects with AD diagnosis). The diagnosis of MCI or AD was based on expert multidisciplinary clinical judgment according to recent publications [27,30,43–46]. The diagnosis of MCI was made when participants presented a single or multiple cognitive decline(s) without significant functional loss. On the other hand, the diagnosis of AD was made in participants with memory decline and another cognitive impairment as aphasia, apraxia, agnosia, or disexecutive syndrome, and loss of functionality. In both conditions, changes from previous level of performance had to be supported by information obtained from a close caregiver [27,43,45].

The CN group included 60 subjects (47.47 ± 5.78 years; males = 65%, females = 25%) and was used to obtain normative data of the PMIS-ID. Both the MCI group, composed of 17 subjects (45.76 ± 4.22 years; male = 47.05%, females = 52.95%), and the AD group, composed of 17 subjects (48.41 ± 3.34 years; males = 41.18%, females = 58.52%), were used to gain the diagnostic accuracy properties of the PMIS-ID.

2.2. Instruments

Each participant underwent a comprehensive clinical and neuropsychological assessment. A neuropsychologist administered a large cognitive evaluation and informed-based measures during three different sessions.

2.2.1. To Detect ID Level

- Kaufman Brief Intelligence Test manual, second edition (K-BIT-2) [47];
- Vineland Adaptive Behaviour Scales-Second Edition (Vineland II) [48];

2.2.2. Neuropsychological Assessment with Cognitive Tools Adapted and Validated for ID Spanish-Speaking Population

- Barcelona Test for people with Intellectual Disability (TB-DI) [29]. This neuropsychological test battery consists of different subtests related to eight cognitive domains (language, working memory, orientation, praxis, attention, executive function, visuoconstruction, and memory). For this study, orientation and verbal learning were used (internal consistency of $\alpha = 0.87$ and $\alpha = 0.73$, respectively);
- CAMCOG-DS Spanish version [25]. This is the cognitive assessment module of the CAMDEX-DS Spanish version. It covers different cognitive domains mainly memory. For this study, memory subtests were used (new learning, remote, recent and memory total score).
- Picture Memory Impairment Screen for people with Intellectual Disability (PMIS-ID). It was applied at the beginning of the cognitive exam to mitigate the possible interferences with the rest of the tests.

2.2.3. Parents Interview

- Cambridge Examination for Mental Disorders of Older People with Down's syndrome and Others with Intellectual Disabilities (CAMDEX-DS) Spanish version [25]. It consists of a structured informant-based interview, cognitive evaluation, diagnostic criteria guide, and recommendations for the interventions. The Spanish version presents an internal consistency of $\alpha = 0.93$, considering performance on the memory subtest of the cognitive form and the memory section of the informant interview.

2.2.4. Picture Memory Impairment Screen for People with Intellectual Disability (PMIS-ID)

The PMIS-ID consists of four-color photographs semantically unrelated in each quadrant of a DIN-A4 sheet. It includes four distinct parts: Identification (I), Learning (L), Immediate Recall (IR), and Delayed Recall (DR).

In the I and L parts, a sheet with four different categories of photographs (*horse, ludo, sofa, cherry*) is presented to the subject who has to name each one. Afterwards the subject has to identify them according to a cue (category) provided by the examiner (*animal, board game, fruit, furniture*). If the subject does not recognize or identify a photograph, the administration is ruled out. If items are correctly identified, the sheet is removed and the subject is told that they will be asked to repeat the words in a short time. Exploration must go on with another non visuoverbal task.

After three minutes, in the IR part, the participant is asked to recall the name of the four photographs (Immediate Free Recall, IFR). If any of the four items is missed, the examiner provides a category cue [Immediate Cued Recall (ICR)]. In case of failure, the target stimulus and two more distracters of an equal semantic category are orally provided (*cherry, pear, kiwi; goose game, cards, ludo; table, sofa, chair; horse, cow, tiger*) and the subject has to detect the right stimulus [Immediate Recognition (IRC)]. Correct stimulus has to be provided again if failure persisted. Finally, after twenty minutes, the DR part is administered, with the same tasks as in the IR part: Delayed Free Recall (DFR), Delayed Cued Recall (DCR) and a Delayed Recognition Recall (DRC).

The scores are calculated as two points for each correct response in FR, one point for each one in CR task, and 0.5 point in the RC. Immediate Total Recall (ITR) and Delayed Total Recall (DTR) are calculated separately (FR scores + CR scores + RC scores) of the FR, the CR and the RC parts. Total PMIS-ID (TPMIS-ID) score (0–16) is the sum of ITR and DTR, both ranging from 0 to 8.

- PMIS-ID adaptation

The PMIS test [40] was adapted by: (1) introducing different items and categories suitable for people with mild and moderate ID; (2) translating the instructions with easiest vocabulary; (3) introducing Delayed Recall (DR) and Recognition (RC) tasks both for the Immediate Recall (IR) and Delayed Recall (DR) trials; and (4) by implementing a new scoring system. The numbers of items were consistent with the original version. An iterative procedure in line with practices recommended by Muñiz, Elosua, and Hambleton (2013) was followed, considering the particularity of this memory visuoverbal test. A pool of 12 color photographs belonging to four different semantic categories according to Spanish typicality norms were extracted [49,50]. To provide the sufficient complexity and avoid the ceiling effect, six stimuli corresponded to the first third while the other six to the second third of the total responses by category. The photographs were shown to 30 volunteers with mild and moderate ID (men age 43.8 ± 3.55; males = 55%; females = 45%) who were not enrolled in the validation study. Then, stimuli were reduced to the four most recognized and the remaining ones were introduced as distracters for the recognition task. Two native-English specialized psychologists in ID translated the test instructions. The two versions were discussed by the research team. An independent English linguist completed the back-translation of the document. Finally, a neurologist and a speech therapist reviewed the process and agreed to a pre-final version. The pre-final version was rounded off to implement further modifications during a pilot test in the same sample for the stimuli selection phase. During test administration, the examiner controlled the execution time and also checked the comprehension of the instructions, asking the volunteer to repeat and to explain them with their own words. The PMIS-ID was applied again in a convenience subsample of 20 participants within four weeks to assess test–retest reliability and in another 20 participants by two different examiners (SEC, ERH) to assess inter-rater reliability.

2.3. Data Analysis

The working database includes entries from February to December 2018. A descriptive analysis was applied to the entire group sample to describe the demographic variables (age and sex), the ID level, and performance on the cognitive protocol (TB-DI memory and orientation, CAMCOG-DS memory subtest). Due to the small sample size in some subgroups, a nonparametric statistical analysis was conducted. Means comparisons were made by independent samples t-test or ANOVA for qualitative data, and χ^2-test for category data. These data were presented as median and interquartile range (IQR) and were compared by Kruskal–Wallis test with Bonferroni adjustment. Multiple linear regression analysis was used to verify the possible influence of sociodemographic variables (age, sex) and the level of ID (mild, moderate) on the PMIS-ID immediate total score, delayed total score, and total score. Reliability was estimated by the test–retest and inter-rater methods and by calculating Pearson and intraclass correlation coefficients, respectively. For the MCI and AD groups, a descriptive analysis was applied for the sociodemographic variables (age, sex, and ID level). Construct validity of the PMIS-ID was verified using the coefficient corrected kappa statistic between the PMIS-ID total score and MCI and AD groups. Spearman's rho was run to evaluate convergent validity between the PMIS-ID total score and the memory subtest performance of the TB-DI and the CAMCOG-DS. Normative data was presented in line of the assumption of the MCI or AD prevalence (%) for the different PMIS-ID cut-scores (PPV and NPV). Receiver operating characteristic curve (ROC) and the Youden index were used to determine the optimal cut-off point of the PMIS-ID (immediate, delayed, and total scores) as a screening memory test for MCI or AD. The areas under the curve (AUC) were compared between the different trials [51].

All statistical analyses were conducted using the software program G-Stat (version 2.0) and the statistical software program SPSS (version 27.0; SPSS Inc., Chicago, IL, USA). Bilateral significance levels were set at a p-value of less than 0.05.

3. Results

3.1. Demographics

Results in Table 1 shows that the CN group was similar to the MCI and AD groups in mean age ($p = 0.315$), level of ID ($p = 0.159$), and sex distribution ($p = 0.136$).

Table 1. Demographic characteristics and cognitive performance by group.

	Control	MCI	AD
n	60	17	17
Age	47.47 ± 5.78 (40–60)	45.76 ± 4.22 (42–55)	48.41 ± 3.34 (43–54)
SEX			
Male	39 (65%)	8 (47.06%)	7 (41.18%)
Female	21 (35%)	9 (52.94%)	10 (58.82%)
ID LEVEL			
Mild	32 (46.67%)	10 (58.82%)	5 (29.41%)
Moderate	28 (53.33%)	7 (41.18%)	12 (70.59%)
TB-DI			
Verbal learning	26.7 (20–33.5)	24.4 (16–31)	17.6 (9–24) ***
Delayed free recall	4.7 (2.5–7)	3.6 (0–6)	1.6 (0–3) ***
False positives	3.5 (0–6.5)	6.1 (1–12) *	8.5 (4–12) ***
Delayed word recognition	10.2 (10–12)	11.4 (12–12)	10.6 (10–12)
CAMCOG-DS			
New learning	13.5 (11–16)	11.5 (8–15)	8.8 (7–11) ***
Remote	2.7 (2–4)	2.6 (2–4)	1.5 (0–2) ***
Recent	2.6 (2–4)	1.9 (1–3)	0.9 (0–2) ***
Memory total	18.8 (15–23)	16.1 (11–21)	11.2 (9–15) ***

Values are given by means and range; sex in percentages for each group. ID, intellectual disability; TB-DI, Barcelona Test for People with Intellectual Disability; CAMCOG-DS, Cambridge Examination for Mental Disorders of Older People with Down's Syndrome and Others with Intellectual Disability (brief neuropsychological battery); MCI, mild cognitive impairment; AD, Alzheimer's disease. * $p < 0.05$, *** $p < 0.001$, using Kruskal–Wallis with Bonferroni correction or χ^2-test for category data between MCI and AD groups compared with the control group.

3.2. Between-Group Comparison of Cognitive Performance

Compared to the CN group, the scores were significantly lower for the AD group on verbal learning, delayed free recall subtest, and false positive scores of the TB-DI and on new learning, remote, recent, and memory total score subtest of the CAMCOG-DS. Performance on the subscales of both tests was similar between the MCI and CN groups (Table 1).

In people with mild ID, the performance of the CN and MCI groups was similar on the entire subtest. Between the CN group and AD group, significant differences were shown in performance on verbal leaning, delayed free recall, and false positives of the TB-DI. No significant differences were observed on the subtests of the CAMCOG-DS (Table 2).

Table 2. Cognitive scores by group for mild intellectual disability sample.

	CN	MCI	AD
n	32	10	5
TB-DI			
Verbal learning	31.2 (26–36)	26 (17–33)	20 (17–24) **
Delayed free recall	5.9 (4–8)	3.8 (0–7)	1.8 (1–3) **
False positives	2.2 (0–3)	4.2 (1–9)	6.8 (3–12) *
Delayed word recognition	10.5 (10–12)	10.9 (9–12)	11.2 (10–12)
CAMCOG-DS			
New learning	14.2 (12–16)	12.6 (9–15)	11.8 (10–11)
Remote	2.9 (2–4)	2.9 (2–4)	2.2 (2–3)
Recent	2.9 (2–4)	2.2 (1–4)	1.4 (0–2)
Memory total	19.9 (17–23)	17.7 (13–21)	15.4 (11–19)

Values are given by means and range. TB-DI, Barcelona Test for People with Intellectual Disability; CAMCOG-DS, Cambridge Examination for Mental Disorders of Older People with Down's Syndrome and Others with Intellectual Disability (brief neuropsychological battery); CN, control group; MCI, mild cognitive impairment; AD, Alzheimer's disease. * $p < 0.05$, ** $p < 0.01$, using Kruskal–Wallis with Bonferroni correction between MCI and AD groups compared with the control group.

In people with moderate ID, no significant differences were observed between the CN group and the MCI group on all the subtests. Significant differences were observed on the false positives score, and no significant differences but moderate decline were observed on verbal learning and delayed free recall subtests of the TB-DI. Significant differences were observed on new learning, remote, recent, and memory total score of the CAMCOG-DS (Table 3).

Table 3. Cognitive scores by group for moderate intellectual disability sample.

	CN	MCI	AD
n	28	7	12
TB-DI			
Verbal learning	21.5 (17–26)	22.1 (15–24)	16.6 (4.5–24)
Delayed free recall	3.3 (1–4)	3.4 (0–6)	1.6 (0–2)
False positives	4.9 (0–10)	9.3 (6–12)	8.9 (3–12) **
Delayed word recognition	9.9 (7.5–12)	12 (12–12)	10.4 (10–12)
CAMCOG-DS			
New learning	12.8 (11–15)	10 (5–13)	7.6 (4.5–11) ***
Remote	2.6 (2–4)	2.3 (2–3)	1.3 (0–2) **
Recent	2.3 (0.5–4)	1.6 (0–2)	0.7 (0–2) **
Memory total	17.5 (15–21)	13.9 (9–18)	9.5 (5.5–13) ***

Values are given by means and range. TB-DI, Barcelona Test for People with Intellectual Disability; CAMCOG-DS, Cambridge Examination for Mental Disorders of Older People with Down's Syndrome and Others with Intellectual Disability (brief neuropsychological battery); CN, control group; MCI, mild cognitive impairment; AD, Alzheimer's disease. ** $p < 0.01$, *** $p < 0.001$, using Kruskal–Wallis with Bonferroni correction between MCI and AD groups compared with the control group.

3.3. Between-Group Comparison of PMIS-ID Performance

The AD group performance differs from the CN group on free recall and total scores from both immediate and delayed part, as well as on the total PMIS-ID score, whereas the performance of the MCI and CN groups was similar on all the trials (Table 4). Analyses according the ID level show that these differences were valid for adults with a moderate level of ID, but not for those with mild ID (Table 5).

Table 4. PMIS-ID descriptive scores by group.

	CN	MCI	AD
n	60	17	17
Immediate			
Free recall	4 (3–4)	3 (2–4)	2 (0–4) **a
Cued recall	0 (0–1)	0 (0–1)	0 (0–1)
Recognition	0 (0–0)	0 (0–0)	0 (0–1)
Total	8 (7–8)	7 (6–8)	6 (2.5–8) **a
Delayed			
Free recall	4 (3–4)	3 (0–4) *b	0 (0–3) ***a
Cued recall	0 (0–1)	0 (0–1)	1 (0–2)
Recognition	0 (0–0)	0 (0–1)	0 (0–1)
Total	7.5 (6.5–8)	7 (2.5–8)	3.5 (1–6.5) ***a
Total PMIS-ID	15 (11.8–16)	13 (9.5–16)	10.5 (4–13) **a

Median (first quartile–third quartile) for each variable is summarized. PMIS-ID, Picture Memory Impairment Screen for People with Intellectual Disability; CN, control group; MCI, mild cognitive impairment; AD, Alzheimer's disease; a Between CN and AD group. b Between MCI and AD group. * $p < 0.05$, ** $p < 0.01$, *** $p < 0.001$ using Kruskal–Wallis with Bonferroni correction between MCI and AD groups compared with the control group.

Table 5. PMIS-ID descriptive scores by group and level of intellectual disability.

	Mild ID			Moderate ID		
	CN	MCI	AD	CN	MCI	AD
n	32	10	5	28	7	12
Immediate						
Free recall	4 (3–4)	4 (2–4)	2 (1–4)	4 (3–4)	3 (0–4)	1.8 (0–3.5)
Cued recall	0 (0–1)	0 (0–1)	1 (0–2)	0 (0–1)	0 (0–1)	0 (0–1)
Recognition	0 (0–0)	0 (0–0)	0 (0–0)	0 (0–0)	0 (0–1)	0 (0–1)
Total	8 (7–8)	8 (6–8)	6 (3.5–8)	8 (7–8)	6.5 (0.5–8)	5.2 (1.3–7.5) *ab
Delayed						
Free recall	4 (3–4)	4 (2–4)	2 (1–4)	3 (2–4)	0 (0–3)	0 (0–2.5) **a
Cued recall	0 (0–1)	0 (0–1)	1 (0–1)	0 (0–1)	1 (0–2)	0.5 (0–2)
Recognition	0 (0–0)	0 (0–0)	0 (0–0)	0 (0–0)	0 (0–1.5)	0.3 (0–1)
Total	8 (7–8)	8 (6–8)	5 (3–8)	7 (3.5–8)	2.5 (1–7)	0.3 (0–6.3) **a
Total PMIS-ID	16 (14–16)	15.5 (12–16)	11 (6.5–16)	14 (11–16)	10 (1–13.5)	10.5 (1.3–12.3) **a

Median (first quartile–third quartile) for each variable is summarized. PMIS-ID, Picture Memory Impairment Screen for People with Intellectual Disability; ID, intellectual disability; CN, control group; MCI, mild cognitive impairment; AD, Alzheimer's disease. [a] Between CN and AD group. [b] Between MCI and AD group. * $p < 0.05$, ** $p < 0.01$, using Kruskal–Wallis with Bonferroni correction between MCI and AD groups compared with the control group.

3.4. Analysis of Control Group

To study the demographics and level of ID impact on the PMIS-ID scores, a multiple linear regression analysis for the PMIS-ID immediate total score ($r2adj = 0.032$; $F = 1.006$; $p = 0.397$), delayed total score ($r2adj = 0.515$; $F = 1.102$; $p = 0.356$), and total score ($r2adj = 1.357$, $F = 1.271$; $p = 0.293$) was performed for the CN group. Neither the level of ID (immediate: $t = -1.523$, $p = 0.133$, $B = -0.615$; delayed: $t = -1.419$, $p = 0.161$, $B = -0.895$; total: $t = -1.509$, $p = 0.069$, $B = -1.509$) nor the age (immediate: $t = -1.078$, $p = 0.286$, $B = 0.0.38$; delayed: $t = -0.689$, $p = 0.494$, $B = -0.037$; total: $t = -0.001$, $p = 0.999$, $B = -0.001$) nor sex (immediate: $t = -0.602$, $p = 0.549$, $B = -0.615$; delayed: $t = -0.350$, $p = 0.7274$, $B = -0.222$; total: $t = -0.568$, $p = 0.572$, $B = -0.466$) were significantly related to the PMIS-ID total scores. Hence, no adjustment of the PMIS-ID total scores was required.

3.5. Reliability

The Pearson's correlation coefficient for the total PMIS-ID score was 0.90 ($p < 0.0001$), a very strong test–retest association. The inter-examiner agreement was found to be good, with a mean intra-class correlation coefficient (ICC) of 0.96 ($p < 0.0001$).

3.6. Validity

3.6.1. Convergent Validity

The correlations patterns between the PMIS-ID total score for the whole sample and by level of ID and the TB-DI and CAMCOG-DS subtest are displayed in Table 6.

Considering the total sample, the overall correlations were significant. For the mild ID sample, the total score of the PMIS-ID was low but positive in correlation with the verbal learning and delayed free recall subtest of the TB-DI and with the new learning ant total memory score of the CAMCOG-DS. In the moderate sample, satisfactory positive correlations were found between verbal learning and delayed free recall subtest of the TB-DI, and new learning, recent, and total memory score subtest of the CAMCOG-DS. Low negative correlation was found between false positives score of the TB-DI and total PMIS-ID total score. Weak positive and negative correlations were found for the other subtest of both sample and the PMIS-ID total score.

Table 6. Convergent validity values by groups.

	PMIS-ID Total Score		
	Total	Mild ID	Moderate ID
TB-DI			
Verbal learning	0.622 **	0.409 **	0.665 **
Delayed free recall	0.549 **	0.381 **	0.558 **
False positives	−0.459 **	−0.216	−0.522 **
Delayed word recognition	−0.215 *	−0.138	−0.289 *
CAMCOG-DS			
New learning	0.688 **	0.519 **	0.763 **
Remote	0.395 **	0.182	0.398 *
Recent	0.454 **	0.186	0.560 **
Total memory	0.679 **	0.481 **	0.743 **

TB-DI, Barcelona Test for People with Intellectual Disability; CAMCOG-DS, Cambridge Cognitive Examination Adapted for Individuals with Down Syndrome; PMIS-ID, Picture Memory Impairment Screen for People with Intellectual Disability; ID, intellectual disability. * $p < 0.05$, ** $p < 0.01$ (two-tailed test), using Spearman's correlation coefficient.

3.6.2. Discriminative Validity

Three ROC curves for each total PMIS-ID trial with enough discriminatory power between CN and AD groups with moderate ID were plotted (Figure 1) and comparisons between AUCs were calculated (Table S1 of the Online Supplement). The AUCs to discriminate between CN and AD groups had good diagnostic utility. For immediate total recall (ITR), the AUCs were 0.685 (CI 95%: 0.506–0.863) and 0.757 (CI 95%: 0.612–0.903) for the total delayed recall (TDR) and 0.749 (CI 95%: 0.597–0.901) for the TPMIS-ID. Paired comparison of the AUCs of the three totals scores were not statistically significant ($z = -0.842$, $z = -1.021$, $z = 0.229$). Hence, immediate total recall (ITR) was the best and most time-efficient trial for our purpose.

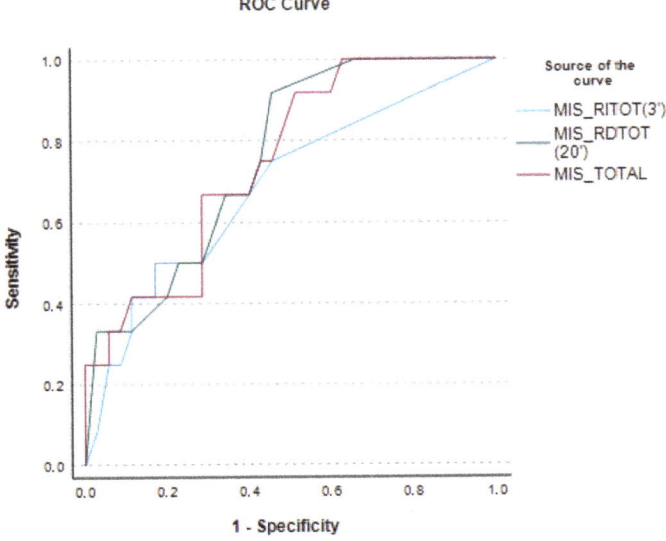

Figure 1. Receiver operating characteristics (ROC) of the PMIS-ID as a screening memory tool for AD in people with a moderate level of ID.

3.7. Normative Data

The values of sensitivity, specificity, positive likelihood ratio (+ LR), negative likelihood ratio (−LR), and the Youden indexes for various cuts-off scores of the PMIS-ID for the AD group with mild and moderate level of ID were calculated. For the group with moderate level of ID, the delayed and total recall trials normative data are presented in Tables S2 and S3 of the Online Supplement, and for the immediate recall (IR) in Table 7. Data for the sample with mild ID and AD is presented in Tables S4–S6 of the Online Supplement. Considering that the base rate in the moderate ID sample was 25.5%, for the immediate total recall (ITR), a cut-off score of ≤4.5 provided a moderate sensitivity (69%) and a high level of specificity (80%).

Table 7. Normative data of the PMIS-ID immediate total score for different cut-off points for AD in moderate level of ID sample.

Cut-Off Points	S	Sp	J	PPV [a]	NPV [a]
0	0.00	1.00	0.00	0.64	1.00
0.5	0.31	1.00	0.31	0.67	1.00
1	0.50	1.00	0.50	0.71	1.00
1.5	0.50	1.00	0.50	0.72	1.00
2	0.50	0.86	0.36	0.72	0.94
2.5	0.50	0.96	0.46	0.74	0.94
3	0.56	0.96	0.52	0.76	0.94
3.5	0.56	0.90	0.46	0.74	0.84
4	0.62	0.90	0.52	0.76	0.84
4.5	0.69	0.86	0.55	0.76	0.80
5.5	0.69	0.83	0.52	0.75	0.76
6.5	0.75	0.79	0.54	0.74	0.73
7.5	0.87	0.62	0.49	0.78	0.59
8	1	0.00	0.00	1.00	0.36

MIS-ID, Picture Memory Impairment Screen for People with Intellectual Disability; S, sensitivity; Sp, specificity; J, Youden's J statistic; PPV, positive predictive values; NPV, negative predictive values. [a] 25.5% is the prevalence of AD in the sample.

4. Discussion

This is the first validation study of a pictorial screening memory test for people with ID, providing normative data and assessing its diagnostic utility to detect memory decline. The PMIS-ID demonstrates good discriminant validity for distinguishing between people with moderate ID and AD from healthy population with ID, and exhibits good convergence validity and reliability.

Our results show that it is possible to detect memory impairment with the PMIS-ID in people with moderate ID in a quick and simple way. It is easy to administer, brief (no more than five minutes), and cost-effective. Also, it shows good convergent validity with memory subtest of the TB-DI and CAMCOG-DS. Considering that the verbal memory subtest of the TB-DI presents good internal consistency [29] and the CAMCOG-DS is recommended for follow-up studies [52], this proves that the PMIS-ID measures memory processes. Furthermore, AUC is acceptable (above 0.7) and the discriminant validity for the proposed cut-off score of the PMIS-ID (4.5) shows good specificity (86%) and appropriate sensitivity (69%). Values of specificity are in line with the majority of the MIS-based screening tests in the general population that yield specificities values higher than 80%: the MIS [39], MIS-S [53], MIS-E [54], MIS-D [55], and PMIS [40]. The PMIS-ID also identifies healthy subjects correctly as the aforementioned screening tests. Consequently, the PMIS-ID is an excellent screening memory test for use in daily clinical specialized services for people with moderate ID.

Data gained from the immediate total recall (ITR) part of the PMIS-ID in isolation well enable detection of memory impairment in adults with moderate ID and AD. The inclusion of a delayed recall is tautological, opposite to the improvement described in the general population with MCI [53], but closer to the use of pictorial memory test based in learning trials without delayed recall in people with low educational level [41] and in people with ID [42]. Our results reveal that when performance is scarce in the immediate recall, it is also in the delayed recall. Moreover, in our sample, people with lower performance in free recall do not gain with the inclusion of a cued recall in the immediate or in the delayed recall. These results are aligned with those described for the MIS-S [54] and cued recall test [42]. Also, learning of relational material depends on the functionality of the hippocampus [55] and free recall trials of the FCSRT picture versions could be considered as an indicator of hippocampus structural integrity [38]. Furthermore, longitudinal memory score variation is specifically associated with volume change in the hippocampus [45,56]. For these reasons, it can be concluded that the PMIS-ID is a noninvasive tool to detect memory impairment due to hippocampus dysfunction in people with moderate ID and AD.

In our study, significant memory decline is the predominant symptom in people with moderate level of ID and AD. Memory decline has been described in MCI and AD in the general population and those with ID [57]. Especially, in people with DS, a slight memory impairment is usually found in MCI, with a significant decline in AD [24,26,27,30,58]. Possibly, memory processes in people with moderate level of ID are not semantic-dependent, and other strategies should be considered because deep processing is beyond their capability [59]. Other promising alternatives could involve developing a test under the associative learning paradigm (binding) that depends on the integrity of the medial temporal lobe structures, as in the general population with hopeful results for AD [60], MCI [41], and in adults with mild and moderate ID [61].

Although stimuli selection in our work was accurate, the scores on the PMIS-ID have a low ceiling effect. Despite the apparent easiness of the four proposed pictorial stimuli, the PMIS-ID measures the same function as a standard memory test. High concordance was obtained between the PMIS-ID total score and memory subtests of the CAMCOG-DS [25] and the TB-DI [29], especially for people with a moderate level of ID. For instance, the satisfactory concordance in our study for the verbal learning subtest of the TB-DI ($r = 0.62$, $p < 0.001$) has also been described between the MIS-E [62] and the analogue subtest of the original version of the TB-DI, the Barcelona Test [63] ($r = 0.78$; $p < 0.001$) in the general population. In this sense, it is important to consider that assessing memory in people with ID is a complex task for clinicians. In clinical practice, pictorial tests seem to be better accepted due to an increased feeling ability to solve the task. In return, the ceiling effect in pictorial tests has already been considered in the general population because the selected drawings are excessively simple and with little ecological validity [64]. This is consistent with the enhancement of performance with pictorial memory test in older adults [37] and in a Spanish population with amnesic MCI [41] and with AD [36] compared with word memory test. Our results confirm the classical dual-coding information theory [65] that postulates superiority in picture processing against words. In this context, increasing the number of stimuli could reduce the ceiling effect, improving its diagnostic capacity for adults with mild ID.

Our results show a slight decrease of the performance on the PMIS-ID for MCI compared with the CN group, both for mild and moderate level of ID groups. Medians are similar in both groups for each trial, but values of the first and third quartile are wider again in each trial, especially for the moderate ID group. This fits with the discrete accuracy to detect MCI compared with the satisfactory data for AD in people with ID. Until recently, few studies had shed light on how to detect preclinical or prodromal stages of AD. Thus, in the recent proposed diagnostic criteria for MCI in DS [30], three variables from a comprehensive neuropsychological examination have proven sensitive enough for this fact: the BRI of the BRIEF and the abstraction and delay memory subtest from the TB-DI. Also, the PAL first-trial memory is one of the most sensitive variables to detecting changes between the preclinical and prodromal phases of AD in people with DS [7]. Furthermore, it is feasible to diagnose AD with neuropsychological tools such as the CAMCOG-DS or the modified Cued Recall Test (mCRT) [34]. In this sense, a decline of performance on both tests was evident in the continuum of AD, but performance on the mCRT was not discriminative for people with DS in the prodromal stage of AD. Analyzing these results, one can deduce that the most tangible changes occur when AD is established, but not in the prodromal phases. Possibly, the course of AD is different in comparison to the general population, in which MCI can be considered a slowly progressive transitional phase in cases of conversion to AD; sensitive neuropsychological instruments are available to detect these changes. Based on results in subjects with ID, changes between the preclinical and prodromal phase would be minimal and undetectable with current neuropsychological instruments, and are only sensitive when performance declines abruptly. From this data, it can be hypothesized that memory deficits with more or less intensity are part of the phenotype of almost all people with ID, and this implies that falls in memory are more difficult to detect than in the general population, in which the margins of scores are greater. This also might suggest that the course of the disease may not be slowly progressive and early detection is essential to initiate proper intervention. Therefore, neuropsychological tools with normative data for all ID ranges are needed to reduce misdiagnosis and to interpret cognitive profiles better in normal and pathological ageing.

Overall, our clinical experience reveals that in the general population, the diagnostic of MCI or DA poses a challenge in those with high educational level, just as learning disorders can be masked in exceptional children. In this sense, intelligence, education, and occupational level influence the onset and course of deterioration due to the reserve cognitive assumption [66]. This is also evident in people with ID in which the presentation and natural history of AD varies according to the level of ID [46]. Furthermore, declines in CAMCOG-DS scores are more evident in people with moderate ID [56], and adults with Klinefelter syndrome with higher values in intelligence tests performed better in working memory and executive functions [67]. Thus, the impact of the level of intelligence on neuropsychological tool performance seems contrasted. That is why sufficiently reliable neuropsychological tools should be available for different ranges of intellectual capacity and the level of cognitive reserve must be regarded.

There are some limitations that need to be considered when interpreting our findings; some caution is required.

First, even if the sample is acceptable for a preliminary study, participants were classified by level of ID, decreasing the size of the MCI and AD groups and limiting statistical and discriminatory power. Therefore, future research should be carried out with a representative sample, calculating power estimation before the onset of the study.

Second, alternatives forms are desirable to use in clinical practice and research in neuropsychology. In our study, the PMIS-ID stimuli were chosen according to the data in the general population, which could contribute to the ceiling effect of the scores. To avoid this bias and to expand its use for people with mild ID, we recommend carrying out studies to provide norms for word prototipicity and picture familiarity, according to appropriate cultural context, for people with ID.

Third, the predictive capacity of the PMIS-ID cannot be evaluated reliably because it is a cross-sectional study. Also, we have not considered the stage or severity degree of AD. Our objective was to develop a rapid measure of memory decline associated with MCI or AD to be applied in daily primary care, but it is well-known that follow-up of cognitive decline is required in people with ID to confirm a diagnosis of MCI or AD. Therefore, we recommend carrying out longitudinal studies with various time points and adapting current staging scales in the general population for people with ID.

5. Conclusions

Limitations notwithstanding, the PMIS-ID is a valid memory screening test for people with a moderate level of ID for use in primary health care centers and in clinical specialized services. The findings in the current pilot study suggest that the PMIS-ID does not provide a comprehensive memory assessment but may be useful as a first step in the diagnostic process to help clinicians in healthcare settings to determine the need to carry out a broader diagnostic evaluation.

Supplementary Materials: The following supporting information can be downloaded at: https://www.mdpi.com/article/10.3390/ijerph191710780/s1, Table S1: Paired comparisons of the areas under the curve of the PMIS-ID trials diagnostic accuracy; Table S2: Normative data of the PMIS-ID delayed total score for different cut-off points for AD in moderate level of ID sample; Table S3: Normative data of the PMIS-ID total score for different cut-off points for AD in moderate level of ID sample; Table S4: Normative data of the PMIS-ID immediate total score for different cut-off points for AD in mild level of ID sample; Table S5: Normative data of the PMIS-ID delayed total score for different cut-off points for AD in mild level of ID sample; Table S6: Normative data of the PMIS-ID total score for different cut-off points for AD in mild level of ID sample.

Author Contributions: Conceptualization, E.R.-H. and S.E.-C.; methodology, E.R.-H. and S.E.-C.; software, E.R.-H. and M.B.; validation, S.E.-C. and J.G.-A.; formal analysis, M.B.; investigation, E.R.-H. and S.E.-C.; data curation, M.B.; writing—original draft preparation, E.R.-H.; writing—review and editing, S.E.-C. and J.G.-A.; supervision, S.E.-C.; project administration, S.E.-C., J.G.-A. and E.R.-H.; funding acquisition, S.E.-C., J.G.-A. and R.N. All authors have read and agreed to the published version of the manuscript.

Funding: This research was funded by the Spanish Government, grant number PI12/02019, PSI-2014-53524-P. The APC was funded by R.N.'s SESMDI research start-up funds.

Institutional Review Board Statement: The study was conducted in accordance with the Declaration of Helsinki and approved by the Institutional Review Board (or Ethics Committee) of Research Ethics Committee of the Parc Hospitalari Martí i Julià (Approval Code: S041-775; Approval Date: 4 July 2012).

Informed Consent Statement: Informed consent was obtained from all subjects involved in the study.

Data Availability Statement: The data presented in this study are available on request from the corresponding author.

Acknowledgments: The authors would like to thank the Down Syndrome Foundation of Girona (ASTRID-21), Els Garrofers Foundation, and participants and their families enrolled in this study.

Conflicts of Interest: The authors declare no conflict of interest. The funders had no role in the design of the study; in the collection, analyses, or interpretation of data; in the writing of the manuscript; or in the decision to publish the results.

References

1. American Psychiatric Association. *Diagnostic and Statistical Manual of Mental Disorders*, 5th ed.; American Psychiatric Publishing: Washington, DC, USA, 2013; ISBN 978-08-9042-555-8.
2. McKenzie, K.; Milton, M.; Smith, G.; Ouellette-Kuntz, H. Systematic Review of the Prevalence and Incidence of Intellectual Disabilities: Current Trends and Issues. *Curr. Dev. Disord. Rep.* **2016**, *3*, 104–115. [CrossRef]
3. Coppus, A.M. People with intellectual disability: What do we know about adulthood and life expectancy? *Dev. Disabil. Res. Rev.* **2013**, *18*, 6–16. [CrossRef] [PubMed]
4. Arvio, M.; Bjelogrlic-Laakso, N. Screening of dementia indicating signs in adults with intellectual disabilities. *J. Appl. Res. Intellect. Disabil.* **2021**, *34*, 1463–1467. [CrossRef] [PubMed]
5. Takenoshita, S.; Terada, S.; Kuwano, R.; Inoue, T.; Cyoju, A.; Suemitsu, S.; Yamada, N. Prevalence of dementia in people with intellectual disabilities, Cross-sectional study. *Int. J. Geriatr. Psychiatry* **2020**, *35*, 414–422. [CrossRef]
6. Magnin, E. Neurodevelopmental and Neurodegenerative Similarities and Interactions: A Point of View about Lifelong Neurocognitive Trajectories. *J. Alzheimer's Dis.* **2021**, *79*, 1397–1407. [CrossRef] [PubMed]
7. Startin, C.M.; Hamburg, S.; Hithersay, R.; Al-Janabi, T.; Mok, K.Y.; Hardy, J.; LonDownS Consortium; Strydom, A. Cognitive markers of preclinical and prodromal Alzheimer's disease in Down syndrome. *Alzheimer's Dement.* **2019**, *15*, 245–257. [CrossRef] [PubMed]
8. McCarron, M.; McCallion, P.; Reilly, E.; Dunne, P.; Carroll, R.; Mulryan, N. A prospective 20-year longitudinal follow-up of dementia in persons with Down syndrome. *J. Intellect. Disabil. Res.* **2017**, *61*, 843–852. [CrossRef]
9. Vivanti, G.; Tao, S.; Lyall, K.; Robins, D.L.; Shea, L.L. The prevalence and incidence of early-onset dementia among adults with autism spectrum disorder. *Autism. Res.* **2021**, *14*, 2189–2199. [CrossRef]

10. Rhodus, E.K.; Barber, J.M.; Bardach, S.H.; Nelson, P.T.; Jicha, G.A. Autistic spectrum behaviors in late-life dementia are associated with an increased burden of neurofibrillary tangles in the frontal lobe. *Alzheimer's Dement.* **2020**, *16*, e043927. [CrossRef]
11. Mahmoudi, E.; Lin, P.; Kamdar, N.; Gonzales, G.; Norcott, A.; Peterson, M.D. Risk of early- and late-onset Alzheimer disease and related dementia in adults with cerebral palsy. *Dev. Med. Child. Neurol.* **2021**, *64*, 372–378. [CrossRef]
12. Ng, T.K.S.; Tagawa, A.; Ho, R.C.-M.; Larbi, A.; Kua, E.H.; Mahendran, R.; Carollo, J.J.; Heyn, P.C. Commonalities in Biomarkers and Phenotypes Between Mild Cognitive Impairment and Cerebral Palsy: A Pilot Exploratory Study. *Aging* **2021**, *13*, 1773–1816. [CrossRef] [PubMed]
13. McKenzie, K.; Metcalfe, D.; Murray, G. A review of measures used in the screening, assessment and diagnosis of dementia in people with an intellectual disability. *J. Appl. Res. Intellect. Disabil.* **2018**, *3*, 725–1342. [CrossRef] [PubMed]
14. Harper, D.C.; Wadsworth, J.S. Dementia and depression in elders with mental retardation: A pilot study. *Res. Dev. Disabil.* **1990**, *11*, 177–198. [CrossRef]
15. Shultz, J.; Aman, M.; Kelbley, T.; Wallace, C.L.; Burt, D.B.; Primeaux-Hart, S.; Loveland, K.; Thorpe, L.; Bogos, E.S.; Timon, J.; et al. Evaluation of Screening Tools for Dementia in Older Adults with Mental Retardation. *Am. J. Ment. Retard.* **2004**, *109*, 98–110. [CrossRef]
16. Evenhuis, H.M. Further evaluation of the Dementia Questionnaire for Persons with Mental Retardation (DMR). *J. Intellect. Disabil. Res.* **1996**, *40*, 369–373. [CrossRef]
17. Kirk, L.; Hick, R.; Laraway, A. Assessing dementia in people with learning disabilities. *J. Intellect. Disabil.* **2006**, *10*, 357–364. [CrossRef]
18. Palmer, G.A. Neuropsychological profiles of persons with mental retardation and dementia. *Res. Dev. Disabil.* **2006**, *27*, 299–308. [CrossRef]
19. Fuld, P.A. Guaranteed stimulus-processing in the evaluation of the memory and learning. *Cortex* **1980**, *16*, 255–271. [CrossRef]
20. Spreen, O.; Strauss, E. *A Compendium of Neuropsychological Tests*, 2nd ed.; Oxford University Press: New York, NY, USA, 1998.
21. D'Elia, L.F.; Satz, P.; Uchiyama, C.L.; White, T. *Color Trails Test Professional Manual*; Psychological Assessment Resources: Odessa, FL, USA, 1996.
22. Pyo, G.; Kripakaran, K.; Curtis, K.; Curtis, R.; Markwell, S. A preliminary study of the validity of memory tests recommended by the Working Group for individuals with moderate to severe intellectual disability. *J. Intellect. Disabil. Res.* **2007**, *51*, 377–386. [CrossRef]
23. Pyo, G.; Ala, T.; Kyrouac, G.A.; Verhulst, S.J. A pilot study of a test for visual recognition memory in adults with moderate to severe intellectual disability. *Res. Dev. Disabil.* **2010**, *31*, 1475–1480. [CrossRef]
24. Ramírez-Toraño, F.; García-Alba, J.; Bruña, R.; Esteba-Castillo, S.; Vaquero, L.; Pereda, E.; Maestú, F. Hypersynchronized Magnetoencephalography Brain Networks in Patients with Mild Cognitive Impairment and Alzheimer's Disease in down Syndrome. *Brain Connect.* **2021**, *11*, 725–733. [CrossRef] [PubMed]
25. Esteba-Castillo, S.; Dalmau-Bueno, A.; Ribas-Vidal, N.; Vilà-Alsina, M.; Novell-Alsina, R.; García-Alba, J. Adaptación y validación del Cambridge Examination for Mental Disorders of Older People with Down's Syndrome and Others with Intellectual Disabilities (CAMDEX-DS) en población española con discapacidad intelectual. *Rev. Neurol.* **2013**, *57*, 337–346. [CrossRef] [PubMed]
26. Firth, N.C.; Startin, C.M.; Hithersay, R.; Hamburg, S.; Wijeratne, P.A.; Mok, K.Y.; Hardy, J.; Alexander, D.C.; LonDowns Consortium; Strydom, A. Aging related cognitive changes associated with Alzheimer's disease in Down syndrome. *Ann. Clin. Transl. Neurol.* **2018**, *5*, 741–751. [CrossRef]
27. García-Alba, J.; Ramírez-Toraño, F.; Esteba-Castillo, S.; Bruña, R.; Moldenhauer, F.; Novell, R.; Romero-Medina, V.; Maestú, F.; Fernández, A. Neuropsychological and neurophysiological characterization of mild cognitive impairment and Alzheimer's disease in Down syndrome. *Neurobiol. Aging* **2019**, *84*, 70–79. [CrossRef] [PubMed]
28. Gioia, G.A.; Isquith, P.K.; Guy, S.C.; Kenworthy, L.; Baron, I.S. Behavior rating inventory of executive function. *Child. Neuropsychol.* **2000**, *6*, 235–238. [CrossRef]
29. Esteba-Castillo, S.; Peña-Casanova, J.; García-Alba, J.; Castellanos, M.A.; Torrents-Rodas, D.; Rodríguez-Hidalgo, E.; Deus-Yela, J.; Caixas, A.; Novell-Alsina, R. Test Barcelona para discapacidad intelectual: Un nuevo instrumento para la valoración neuropsicológica clínica de adultos con discapacidad intelectual. *Rev. Neurol.* **2017**, *64*, 433–444. [CrossRef] [PubMed]
30. Esteba-Castillo, S.; García-Alba, J.; Rodríguez-Hildago, E.; Vaquero, L.; Novell-Alsina, R.; Moldenhauer, F.; Castellanos, M.A. Proposed diagnostic criteria for mild cognitive impairment in Down syndrome population. *J. Appl. Res. Intellect. Disabil.* **2022**, *35*, 495–505. [CrossRef]
31. Sano, M.; Raman, R.; Emond, J.; Thomas, R.G.; Petersen, R.; Schneider, L.S.; Aisen, P.S. Adding Delayed Recall to the Alzheimer Disease Assessment Scale is Useful in Studies of Mild Cognitive Impairment But Not Alzheimer Disease. *Alzheimer Dis. Assoc. Disord.* **2011**, *25*, 122–127. [CrossRef]
32. Lezak, M.; Howieson, D.; Bigler, E.; Tranel, D. *Neuropsychological Assesment*, 5th ed.; Oxford University Press: New York, NY, USA, 2012.
33. Buschke, H. Cued Recall in Amnesia. *J. Clin. Neuropsychol.* **1984**, *6*, 433–440. [CrossRef]
34. Benejam, B.; Videla, L.; Vilaplana, E.; Barroeta, I.; Carmona-Iragui, M.; Altuna, M.; Valldeneu, S.; Fernandez, S.; Giménez, S.; Iulita, F.; et al. Diagnosis of prodromal and Alzheimer's disease dementia in adults with Down syndrome using neuropsychological tests. *Alzheimer's Dement. Diagn. Assess. Dis. Monit.* **2020**, *12*, 11. [CrossRef] [PubMed]

35. Tulving, E.; Thomson, D.M. Encoding specificity and retrieval processes in episodic memory. *Psychol. Rev.* **1973**, *80*, 352–373. [CrossRef]
36. Delgado, C.; Muñoz-Neira, C.; Soto, A.; Martínez, M.; Henríquez, F.; Flores, P.; Slachevsky, A. Comparison of the Psychometric Properties of the "word" and "picture" Versions of the Free and Cued Selective Reminding Test in a Spanish-Speaking Cohort of Patients with Mild Alzheimer's Disease and Cognitively Healthy Controls. *Arch. Clin. Neuropsychol.* **2015**, *31*, 165–1753. [CrossRef] [PubMed]
37. Zimmerman, M.E.; Katz, M.J.; Wang, C.; Burns, L.C.; Berman, R.M.; Derby, C.A.; L'Italien, G.; Budd, D.; Lipton, R.B. Comparison of "Word" vs. "Picture" version of the Free and Cued Selective Reminding Test (FCSRT) in older adults. *Alzheimer's Dement. Diagn. Assess. Dis. Monit.* **2015**, *1*, 94–100. [CrossRef] [PubMed]
38. Slachevsky, A.; Barraza, P.; Hornberger, M.; Muñoz-Neira, C.; Flanagan, E.; Henríquez, F.; Bravo, E.; Farías, M.; Delgado, C. Neuroanatomical Comparison of the "word" and "picture" Versions of the Free and Cued Selective Reminding Test in Alzheimer's Disease. *J. Alzheimer's Dis.* **2017**, *61*, 589–600. [CrossRef]
39. Buschke, H.; Kuslansky, G.; Katz, M.; Stewart, W.F.; Sliwinski, M.J.; Eckholdt, H.M.; Lipton, R.B. Screening for dementia with the Memory Impairment Screen. *Neurology* **1999**, *52*, 231–238. [CrossRef]
40. Verghese, J.; Noone, M.; Johnson, B.; Ambrose, A.; Wang, C.; Buschke, H.; Pradeep, V.G.; Salam, K.A.; Shaji, K.S.; Mathuranath, P.S. Picture-Based Memory Impairment Screnn for Dementia. *J. Am. Geriatr. Soc.* **2012**, *60*, 2116–2120. [CrossRef]
41. Rodrigo-Herrero, S.; Mendez-Barrio, C.; Sánchez-Arjona, M.B.; De Miguel Tristancho, M.; Graciani-Cantisán, E.; Carnero-Pardo, C.; Franco-Macías, E. Evaluación preliminar de una versión pictórica y abreviada del Free and Cued Selective Reminding Test. *Neurología* **2019**, *27*, 192–198. [CrossRef]
42. Benejam, B.; Fortea, J.; Molina-López, R.; Videla, S. Patterns of performance on the modified Cued Recall Test in Spanish adults with down syndrome with and without dementia. *Am. J. Intellect. Dev. Disabil.* **2015**, *120*, 481–489. [CrossRef]
43. Fenoll, R.; Pujol, J.; Esteba-Castillo, S.; De Sola, S.; Ribas-Vidal, N.; García-Alba, J.; Sánchez-Benavides, G.; Martínez Vilavella, G.; Deus, J.; Dierssen, M.; et al. Anomalous White Matter Structure and the Effect of Age in Down Syndrome Patients. *J Alzheimer's Dis* **2017**, *57*, 61–70. [CrossRef]
44. Krinsky-McHale, S.J.; Silverman, W. Dementia and mild cognitive impairment in adults with intellectual disability: Issues of diagnosis. *Dev. Disabil. Res. Rev.* **2013**, *18*, 31–42. [CrossRef]
45. Pujol, J.; Fenoll, R.; Ribas-Vidal, N.; Martínez-Vilavella, G.; Blanco-Hinojo, L.; García-Alba, J.; Deus, J.; Novell-Alsina, R.; Esteba-Castillo, S. A longitudinal study of brain anatomy changes preceding dementia in Down syndrome. *NeuroImage Clin.* **2018**, *18*, 160–166. [CrossRef]
46. Sheehan, R.; Afia, A.; Hassiotis, A. Dementia in intellectual disabilities. *Curr. Opin. Psychiatry* **2014**, *27*, 852–856. [CrossRef] [PubMed]
47. Kaufman, A.; Nadeen, L.; Kaufman, L. *Kaufman Brief Intelligence Test*, 2nd ed.; American Guidance Service: Circle Pines, MN, USA, 2004.
48. Sparrow, S.; Cicchetti, D.; Balla, D. *Vineland Adaptive Behavior Scales: Second Edition (Vineland II), Survey Interview Form/Caregiver Rating Form*, 2nd ed.; Pearson Assessments: Livonia, MN, USA, 2005.
49. Moreno-Martínez, F.J.; Montoro, P.R. An ecological alternative to Snodgrass & Vanderwart: 360 high quality colour images with norms for seven psycholinguistic variables. *PLoS ONE* **2012**, *7*, e0037527. [CrossRef]
50. Soto, P.; Sebastián, M.V.; García-Bajos, E.; del Amo, T. *Categorización y datos Normativos en España*; Visor: Madrid, ES, USA, 1994; ISBN 84777410260.
51. Hanley, J.A.; McNeil, B.J. A method of comparing the areas under receiver operating characteristic curves derived from the same cases. *Radiology* **1983**, *148*, 839–843. [CrossRef]
52. Paiva, A.F.; Nolan, A.; Thumser, C.; Santos, F.H. Screening of cognitive changes in adults with intellectual disabilities: A systematic review. *Brain Sci.* **2020**, *10*, 848. [CrossRef]
53. Labos, E.; Trojanowski, S.; Schapira, M.; Seinhart, D.; Renato, A. Nuevos predictores en Alzheimer prodrómico: Fase diferida en el test MIS de recuerdo de palabras. *Vertex* **2016**, *4*, 45–61.
54. Böhm, P.; Peña-Casanova, J.; Gramunt, N.; Manero, R.M.; Terrón, C.; Quiñones Úbeda, S. Versión española del Memory Impairment Screen (MIS): Datos normativos y de validez discriminativa. *Neurología* **2005**, *20*, 402–411.
55. Davachi, L.; Wagner, A.D. Hippocampal contributions to episodic encoding; Insights from relational and item-based learning. *J. Neurophysiol.* **2002**, *88*, 982–990. [CrossRef]
56. Fortea, J.; Vilaplana, E.; Carmona-Iragui, M.; Benejam, B.; Videla, L.; Barroeta, I.; Fernández, S.; Altuna, M.; Pegueroles, J.; Montal, V.; et al. Clinical and biomarker changes of Alzheimer's disease in adults with Down syndrome, a cross-sectional study. *Lancet* **2020**, *395*, 1988–1997. [CrossRef]
57. Krinsky-McHale, S.J.; Devenny, D.A.; Silverman, W. Changes in explicit memory associated with early dementia in adults with Down's syndrome. *J. Intellect. Disabil. Res.* **2002**, *46*, 198–208. [CrossRef]
58. Fonseca, L.M.; Padilla, C.; Jones, E.; Neale, N.; Haddad, G.G.; Mattar, G.P.; Barros, E.; Clare, I.C.; Busatto, G.F.; Bottino, C.M.; et al. Amnestic and non-amnestic symptoms of dementia, An international study of Alzheimer's disease in people with Down's syndrome. *Int. J. Geriatr. Psychiatry* **2020**, *35*, 650–661. [CrossRef]

59. Dulaney, C.L.; Ellis, N.R. Long-term recognition memory for items and attributes by retarded and nonretarded persons. *Intelligence* **1991**, *15*, 105–115. [CrossRef]
60. Gramunt, N.; Sánchez-Benavides, G.; Buschke, H.; Diéguez-Vide, F.; Peña-Casanova, J.; Masramon, X.; Fauria, K.; Gispert, J.D.; Molinuevo, J.L. The Memory Binding Test, Development of Two Alternate Forms into Spanish and Catalan. *J. Alzheimer's Dis.* **2016**, *52*, 283–293. [CrossRef] [PubMed]
61. McPaul, A.; Walker, B.; Law, J.; McKenzie, K. An Exploratory Study Investigating How Adults with Intellectual Disabilities Perform on the Visual Association Test (VAT). *J. Appl. Res. Intellect. Disabil.* **2017**, *30*, 824–829. [CrossRef] [PubMed]
62. Pérez-Martinez, D.A.; Baztán, J.J.; González-Becerra, M.; Socorro, A. Evaluacion de la utilidad diagnostica de una adaptacion espanola del Memory Impairment Screen de Buschke para detectar demencia y deterioro cognitivo. *Rev. Neurol.* **2005**, *40*, 644–648. [CrossRef]
63. Peña-Casanova, J. *Normalidad, Semiología y Patología Neuropsicológicas*; Masson: Barcelona, ES, USA, 1991; ISBN 84-458-1472-9.
64. Laws, K.R.; Gale, T.M.; Leeson, V.C.; Crawford, J.R. When is category specific in Alzheimer's disease? *Cortex* **2005**, *41*, 452–463. [CrossRef]
65. Paivio, A. *Imagery and Verbal Processes*; Holt, Rinehart, and Winston: New York, NY, USA, 1971.
66. Barulli, D.; Stern, Y. Efficiency, capacity, compensation, maintenance, plasticity: Emerging concepts in cognitive reserve. *Trends Cogn. Sci.* **2013**, *17*, 502–509. [CrossRef]
67. Skakkebæk, A.; Moore, P.J.; Pedersen, A.D.; Bojesen, A.; Kristensen, M.K.; Fedder, J.; Laurberg, P.; Hertz, J.M.; Østergaard, J.R.; Wallentin, M.; et al. The role of genes, intelligence, personality, and social engagement in cognitive performance in Klinefelter syndrome. *Brain Behav.* **2017**, *7*, 61–70. [CrossRef]

MDPI
St. Alban-Anlage 66
4052 Basel
Switzerland
Tel. +41 61 683 77 34
Fax +41 61 302 89 18
www.mdpi.com

International Journal of Environmental Research and Public Health Editorial Office
E-mail: ijerph@mdpi.com
www.mdpi.com/journal/ijerph

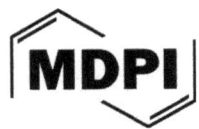